Professional Praise

"*Taking Charge of Your Fertility* is a fantastic book, loaded with practical and beautifully presented information that will transform and empower every woman's relationship with her fertility. I recommend it to women of all ages."
> —Christiane Northrup, M.D., author of *Women's Bodies,*
> *Women's Wisdom* and *The Wisdom of Menopause*

"This beautifully written guide to a woman's fertility signs is packed with knowledge, wisdom, and humor—a must for the bookshelf."
> —Co-authors of *The New Our Bodies, Ourselves*

"With fascinating, reliable, and up-to-date explanations, Toni Weschler reveals all that we should know about our fertility and sexuality while demystifying the wondrous nature of reproduction. Her practical approach to Fertility Awareness is presented in a compassionate and empowering way. Whether you want to be pregnant or to avoid pregnancy, or simply understand female fertility better, this is the book for you."
> —Penny Simkin, PT, author of
> *Pregnancy, Childbirth, and the Newborn:*
> *The Complete Guide* and *The Birth Partner:*
> *Everything You Need to Know to Help a Woman Through*
> *Childbirth*

"This well-established book by Toni Weschler is a 'must read' for all infertile couples who wish to gain a basic understanding of their ovulatory cycle, how to evaluate their infertility, avoid unnecessary and expensive testing, and get right to the heart of their problem with minimal delay. This book clears up a great deal of confusion that couples may have about the optimal methods of achieving pregnancy with a conventional, non-technological approach. The illustrations are superb, and the explanations easy to follow. I highly recommend reading this book as a beginning point in treating infertility."
> —Sherman J. Silber, M.D., Director,
> Infertility Center of St. Louis at St. Luke's Hospital
> and author of *How to Get Pregnant with the New*
> *Technology*

"*Taking Charge of Your Fertility* is an invaluable resource for women seeking to better understand their reproductive cycles and take an active role in their own healthcare. It serves as a significant diagnostic tool to both evaluate fertility-related concerns and monitor ovulation treatment, and thus I highly recommend it for both clinicians and patients alike."
> —Mark Perloe, M.D.,
> Medical Director, Georgia Reproductive Specialists,
> Atlanta, Georgia

"Toni Weschler's book, *Taking Charge of Your Fertility,* provides couples with the tools to do just that, empowering them with knowledge and hope at a time when they may feel out-of-control. Infertility often robs couples of a lifetime of expectations, replacing them with an increasing sense of loss. Toni helps couples reclaim control of their lives with a simple and compassionate approach to understanding their fertility. There is no other book like it on the market, and I strongly recommend that it be read by physicians and patients alike."
> —Lee R. Hickok, M.D.,
> Pacific Gynecology Specialists,
> Seattle, Washington

Excerpts from Letters to the Author

"Yesterday I received your book, *Taking Charge of Your Fertility*. I finished it today. What an incredible book. It is so full of information that I could read it 10,000 times and pull something different out each time. Thank you for writing such an informative book."
—Cindi Aschenbrenner
Enterprise, Oregon

"Your book is absolutely fabulous; I refer to it as my bible. As I began reading it little light bulbs started going on; everything finally made sense. It's very informative and detailed. I only wish I had found it sooner. It really has changed my perception of fertility, and someday soon I know it will have changed my life. Thanks for writing such a great book."
—Debi Avocato
Kingsland, Georgia

"I love your book, *Taking Charge of Your Fertility*! It has opened my eyes to the wonders of my body. Your work is vital to a world that is becoming less and less in tune with their bodies."
—Denise Evarts
New York, New York

"I am 33 years old and have been married for over ten years and finally have discovered that my body doesn't have to be a guessing game anymore! Thanks to your book!"
—Diane Carswell
Ohio

"I am writing to you out of a page of my Fertility Awareness notebook, which accompanied your book—I love it! Your book is the first one I have read that is straightforward—no bones about it! Cheers to your hard work that is reflected in these pages."
—Heather LoVecchio
Mendham, New Jersey

"Your book is part of why I am where I am right now, a place where I trust my body, mind, and spirit. I thank you for that. . . . I recently read 'society honors live conformers and dead trouble makers.' I hope, for once, society will listen to an important message while the 'prophet' is still living!"
—Jackie Schmidt
Seattle, Washington

"Your book has made a wonderful and dramatic impact on me. I feel as if I've awoken from a long, deep sleep into a world of clarity and beauty! I finally understand what is happening in my own body. It is exciting and fascinating. I am now pregnant. Most importantly I am empowered! Thank you for such a wonderful gift. If I have a daughter you can be sure your book will be presented as a most treasured gift at the appropriate time. Meanwhile, any woman close to me will be hearing about your book."
—Janet Villani-Garratt
Woodstock, New York

"The book was a godsend. I devoured it voraciously, absolutely barraging my husband with the information that I acquired about both my own body and his. I can't thank you enough for educating me about my own reproductive system. For fourteen years I have participated in the fertility cycle and have known next to nothing about the mechanisms responsible for it. I was unappreciative to the wonder of my own body. . . . What was especially valuable about your book is that it went beyond the baseline experience of FAM. You explored the various patterns that women will practically encounter in their charting. The recognition of these variables is important so that every woman will appreciate her uniqueness and not feel she is abnormal if she does not conform to the standard. . . . I cannot contain my enthusiasm about FAM. I am in command of my own body now and I am elated. You should be incredibly proud for the service that you have done all women in the sharing of your knowledge. Thank you again for your wonderful book."
—Jennifer Chellis Olivieri
New York, New York

"Marvelous book. . . . It is the most complete and empowering book on this subject matter I have read. Your format and coverage of this topic is exceptional. Every woman should know and understand their bodies, and you have certainly succeeded in relaying this important information. Thanks for helping us to achieve this miracle. We feel very fortunate to experience pregnancy again and credit your book with giving us the knowledge to maximize our chances."
—Jennifer Dunn
Clearwater, Florida

"I can't tell you how pleased I am with this book. I think that I have read it all the way through twice. . . . I would like to thank you for providing me with a renewed sense of self-esteem because I now have control over my body and don't have to rely on anyone."
—Kim Taylor
Platte City, Missouri

"I came across your book, *Taking Charge of Your Fertility,* several years ago and was immediately impressed by how you made the information on fertility cycles accessible through humor, anecdotes, and plain language, while still making the information current and useful. Not a physiology textbook rehash! I've widely recommended your book because it is one of the few women's health books that actually gives information, not just simplified commentary."
—Louise Smith
Fort Langley, British Columbia, Canada

"We were absolutely blown away by your book arriving in the mail. What a thoughtful, generous, and special gift. It is a masterpiece—a book I wish I had fourteen years ago."
—Ming Lu
Santa Monica, California

"Quite simply, your book has changed my life. I can't thank you enough for taking the time, and making the effort required, to create such an informative work. From the moment I opened *Taking Charge of Your Fertility*, I was mesmerized. I sat in the bookstore for an hour, reading the appendixes. So many of my questions were right there on the page! So many of my concerns were addressed. I brought the book home and read it, cover to cover, in one sitting. Your gift to me through *Taking Charge of Your Fertility,* has value beyond measure! Thank you again from the bottom of my heart!"

—Pamela M.
Seattle, Washington

"Your book was a GODSEND! . . . My doctors both expressed how much my charts are helping them to help me. It really surprised me that not every woman with fertility problems is doing her charts and checking her cervical fluid. I also learned a tremendous amount about fertility, the woman's body, and also about ourselves. We are deeply grateful and appreciative for your wonderfully comprehensive and excellently written book."

—Sacha Willsey
Bloomington, Indiana

"I wanted to write to thank you for writing your book, *Taking Charge of Your Fertility.* My friend had been trying to get pregnant for two years. After charting for only two months, she became pregnant. . . . You have helped me in more than one way, and I don't know how to thank you enough. . . . My husband and I were trying for three years to get pregnant. I am now four-months pregnant, and also I finally can feel at ease with my female reproductive organs. I wish that every woman could get a hold of your book. You have done such a great service for women by presenting this information in such a clear and compassionate manner."

—Sharon Maitino
Chicago, Illinois

"I am so thankful that you wrote such an informative book. Your words empowered me to tell everyone I know about this book and method. I wish this book had been available when I was in college. I have gained invaluable knowledge about myself, and I am so thankful that it is available now. THANK YOU!!!"

—Wendy Baughman
Warner Robins, Georgia

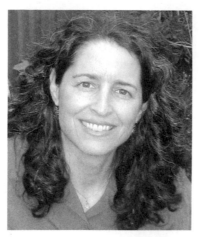

Roger Sandwick

About the Author

TONI WESCHLER is a nationally respected women's health educator and speaker with a master's degree in Public Health. She founded Fertility Awareness Counseling and Training Seminars (FACTS) in 1986, and has lectured at hospitals, clinics, and universities since 1982. She recently helped develop cycle-tracking software as an adjunct to her book, *Taking Charge of Your Fertility*. The TCOYF Fertility Software is available at www.TCOYF.com. She is a frequent guest on television, radio, and Internet Web sites, where she continues to advocate the dissemination of Fertility Awareness education as an empowering body of knowledge for all women of reproductive age. She lives in Seattle, Washington, USA.

Taking Charge of Your Fertility

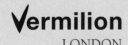 The Definitive Guide to
Natural Birth Control,
Pregnancy Achievement,
and Reproductive Health

Revised Edition

TONI WESCHLER, MPH

Vermilion
LONDON

Ms. Weschler is available for public speaking engagements, as well as professional seminars for medical schools, hospitals, and clinics. In addition, any comments or suggestions for future editions of this book would be greatly appreciated. She can be reached at:

Toni Weschler, MPH
P.O. Box 31094
Seattle, WA 98103
USA

For those interested in combining the benefits of FAM with the power of computerized charting, the affiliated Web site, www.TCOYF.com, has been designed to supplement this book.

Grateful acknowledgment is made for permission to reprint the following:

Cartoons: page 17, printed with special permission from John Callahan/Levin Represents; page 45, copyright © Los Angeles Times Syndicate; page 84, copyright © Viv Quillin, "The Opposite Sex"; page 89, "Between Friends" reprinted with special permission of King Features Syndicate; page 124, OFF THE LEASH reprinted by permission of UFS, Inc.; page 156, copyright © 1982, 1991 by Lynn Johnston Productions Inc. and Lynn Johnston, reprinted from *David, We're Pregnant!* with permission of its publisher, Meadowbrook Press; pages 167 and 168, "Greeting Card Pregnancy Test" reprinted with special permission of Skip Morrow; page 208, copyright © David Horsey, *Seattle Post-Intelligencer;* page 239, copyright © 1988, Los Angeles Times Syndicate, reprinted by permission; page 259, "The Brink of Madness," PMS Attacks, by Steve Phillips, copyright © 1986 by Steve Phillips, used by permission of Ten Speed Press, P.O. Box 7123, Berkeley, CA; page 264, "Maxine's Crabby Road," 2001, reprinted with special permission from Hallmark Licensing, Inc.

Adaptation of the graph on efficacy rates from *Contraceptive Technology* on page 355; *Contraceptive Technology,* Hatcher, R. A.; Trussell, J.; Stewart, F.; Stewart, G. K.; Kowal, P.; Guest, F.; Cates, W.; Policar, M. S., Irvington Publishers, 1998.

Color insert: pages 1-2 of insert, photographs by Frankie Collins; page 3, photographs by Lennart Nilsson, *A Child Is Born,* Dell Publishing Company; page 4, ovulation photographs by Erlandsen/Magney: *Color Atlas of Histology,* 1992; page 5, hormone graph by Kate Sweeney; page 6, photograph of egg in fallopian tube by Lennart Nilsson, *A Child Is Born,* Dell Publishing Company, and photographs of cervical fluid and baby by Bruce Bobman.

10

Published in 2003 by Vermilion, an imprint of Ebury Publishing
First published in the United States by HarperCollins in 2002

Ebury Publishing is a Random House Group company

Copyright © Toni Weschler 1995, 2003

Toni Weschler has asserted her right to be identified as the author of this Work in accordance with the Copyright, Designs and Patents Act 1988.

The Random House Group Limited Reg. No. 954009

Addresses for companies within the Random House Group can be found at www.randomhouse.co.uk

A CIP catalogue record for this book is available from the British Library

The Random House Group Limited supports The Forest Stewardship Council® (FSC®), the leading international forest certification organisation. Our books carrying the FSC label are printed on FSC® certified paper. FSC is the only forest certification scheme endorsed by the leading environmental organisations, including Greenpeace. Our paper procurement policy can be found at www.randomhouse.co.uk/environment.

Printed and bound in China by C&C Offset Printing Co.,Ltd.

ISBN 9780091887582

Copies are available at special rates for bulk orders. Contact the sales development team on 020 7840 8487 or visit www.booksforpromotions.co.uk for more information.

To buy books by your favourite authors and register for offers, visit www.randomhouse.co.uk

In loving memory of my mother,
Franzi Toch Weschler,
whose strength always amazed me

Contents

Acknowledgements

They say women are blessed with the ability to forget the pain of childbirth so they will be able to have more children later on. I often wonder whether the same principle applies to the pain of writing a book. Had another author warned me about what a monumental task it would be, I'm not sure I would have been so insane as to pursue the dream. And even now, revising the book years later, I am struck once again with the age-old question: "What were you thinking?"

But I suppose writers are a deluded bunch, or perhaps their memories are simply fried from their own projects! Either way, I've come away from having written the original and revised book having experienced the gamut of human emotion, from total frustration and misery to incredible joy and pride. Along the way, as the following list will attest, I've had the privilege of being supported by numerous people to whom I owe a debt of gratitude.

To the many health practitioners and professionals who supported me when the first edition was but a concept in my head: Andrea Brass, Suzannah Cooper Doyle, Michael Greer, M.D., Vivien Webb Hanson, M.D., Joan Helmich, Patricia Kato, M.D., Nancy Kenney, Ph.D., Chris Leininger, M.D., Zora Pesio, M.S.N., Molly Pessl, B.S.N., Suzanne Poppema, M.D., Deb Van Derhei, and especially Rebecca Wynsome, N.D., whom I would like to single out for being especially helpful in this project and providing invaluable professional expertise. And for the revision, to Dr. Lee Hickok and Dr. Mark Perloe for their endless patience and willingness to review various tables in the book.

To the individuals who were kind enough to wade through the initial drafts of the first manuscript, including Diana Brement, Emilie Coulter, Barbara Feldman, Stephanie Irving, Miriam Labbok, M.D., Susan Specht, and Janet Yoder.

To the research assistants I had over the years from the University of Washington, three of whom stood out: Melanie Warren (my first assistant, and the standard by which I judged all others), Wendy Blair, and Robin Cutler. In fact, I am eternally grateful to Melanie for freeing me to focus on the first edition of the book. Her sense of humor and positive attitude contributed to this project in ways she'll never know.

To my literary agent, Joy Harris, and her assistants, Leslie, Paul, and Stephanie, for guiding me through the ominous publishing maze. And to the editors of the first edition, Jenna Hull, for her sweet encouragement and direction, and Janet Goldstein, as well as her team at HarperCollins, including Betsy Thorpe, Pam LaBarbiera, and Linda Dingler, for their wizardry in pulling it all together at the eleventh hour. And for this equally challenging revision, to the wonderful new group of professionals under the guidance of Susan Weinberg, including Elliott Beard, Aimee Boyer, Heather Burke, Dori Carlson, Erin Clermont, Jennifer Hart, Lizz Pawlson, and most especially, Kate Travers, my endlessly patient and supportive editor during times that I'm sure cost her as many nights sleep as I lost. How lucky I was to be paired with her!

To my medical illustrator, Kate Sweeney, and her assistant, Christine Shafner, for their gorgeous visuals. And to my graphics illustrator, Rosy Aronson, for her beautiful artwork, but more important, for her incredibly sweet and wonderful attitude. It was a pleasure to work with her, especially under such intense deadlines. And to my photographer, Frankie Collins, who had the perfect disposition to be on call every time a cervix model phoned to inform her that her cervix or cervical fluid were at just the right phase to be photographed.

To the model whom I ultimately chose for her incredibly photogenic cervix, Deanna Hope, who was so proud of her contribution to the enlightenment of women that she wanted to be mentioned by name.

To my coterie of other sundry supports and life-savers, including Lana Newman, Michal Schonbrun, and Shelley Watson. In addition, I want to especially thank Jay Weinland, whose amazing knowledge and patience saved me from myself over and over whenever my computer travails reduced me to a driveling puddle of tears, and Tamela Graling Goeden, whose willingness to help me with anything and everything made her a pleasure to work with. To my dear friend Susan Jacoby Stern, who sacrificed precious sleep and time for the cause.

To my TCOYF software developers and cofounders of Ovusoft, Gene Grant and Phil Boyer, for their unbelievably hard work and dedication to the development of Fertility Awareness software to match the book, and for their tolerance when I would disappear amid piles of research for the revision.

To my brother Lawrence Weschler, whose remarkable literary achievements gave me the inspiration to write this book. And to my brother Robert Weschler, for his numerous insightful contributions.

To my cherished friends who tried to help me maintain a sense of perspective when I kept wondering whether I would ever have a life again. Especially Audrey, Cathy, Barbara, and Linda. And of course, to Roger, who willingly contributed hours of his time on seemingly endless tasks, and whose presence over the years helped give me the sanity and stability to get through it all.

To the scores of clients and readers who continue to swell my "Thank You" file with their poignant letters of gratitude for the ways I have apparently enriched and changed their lives. It is this type of appreciation which buoys me when I occasionally feel disheartened by a medical community which has yet to fully grasp the scientific validity and endless benefits of the Fertility Awareness Method.

To my incredible assistant for the revised edition, Cricky Kavanaugh, my total Godsend, whose intelligence, ingenuity, and attention to detail were surpassed only by her warmth and wonderful sense of humor. I feel privileged that she has come into my life, and almost tempted to write another book just for the joy of working with her again.

Finally, and most important, to my younger brother Raymond, without whom this book could never have been written. He was an indispensable editor, researcher, and organizer, as well as an endless source of wit and moral support throughout this project. The fact is that we talked about sharing authorship credit, but he insisted that the book came from my passion and experiences, not his, and ultimately it was written with my voice. Perhaps, but truth be told, Raymond was my cowriter. I am eternally grateful to him for all he's done, although more than any of that, I thank him for simply being the best brother that any sister could have.

Preface to the Revised Edition

When I first began to think about revising *Taking Charge of Your Fertility,* I found myself asking if the subject matter really justified a revision. After all, the basic biological principles of the Fertility Awareness Method (FAM) have not changed, and like women's cycles themselves, they are unlikely to do so in the future. Still, people over the years have given me excellent suggestions to improve on the original, and just as important, I soon concluded that as timeless as Fertility Awareness education is, it does not exist in a vacuum.

In some cases, advances in medicine may influence how you interpret your primary fertility signs and, of course, the progress in reproductive technologies continues unabated. Given that a large majority of my readers have been those couples seeking to conceive, this edition significantly updates and expands discussion of these topics. I have done this knowing full well that while FAM will be the only thing many couples need to become parents, others may have to treat fertility charting as just the first step on the path to a successful pregnancy— invaluable but perhaps not sufficient.

Regardless, I have also had exciting new ideas on how to make this a better book; more specifically, on how to more efficiently promote FAM as part of a woman's basic health education. Thus there is the usual updating and revising that one would expect, but in addition there are new features that I hope will serve to popularize this timeless information, which can be empowering to so many women for so many reasons. Among the new features for this revised edition are the following:

- A dramatically improved charting system that will make Fertility Awareness even easier and more intuitive.
- A series of new master charts, including those specifically for birth control, pregnancy achievement, and menopause, as well as a version in Celsius for those outside the United States.
- A greatly expanded and updated exploration of the most recently discovered impediments to conception and the latest high-tech fertility treatments.

- Easy-to-read boxes that summarize the various fertility drugs that are now most commonly prescribed.
- A tear-out appendix written exclusively for physicians and other health care practitioners that quickly introduces them to FAM's basic principles and also explains its importance in helping to diagnose and treat many of their patients' gynecological problems.
- New TCOYF software specifically designed to match this book, now available on the Internet (www.TCOYF.com).
- A specially written epilogue that puts the Fertility Awareness Method in historical context, emphasizing its relationship to the many women's health movements of the past and the inevitable expansion of high-technology in the reproductive health care of the future.

Ultimately, it is my simple hope that the new information in this revised edition will further assure FAM's place in the history of the movements I refer to in the epilogue. Of course, no matter how many times this or any other book is revised, its basic scientific principles will indeed remain the same, and thus with a little societal wisdom, FAM will become the common knowledge of each new generation of maturing young women—curious, confident, and biologically self-aware.

Introduction

I still cringe when I recall my college years and what ironically led me to pursue the field of fertility education. I cannot count the number of times I ran off to the gynecologist with what I thought was a vaginal infection. Most women will agree that no matter how many times they've had a pelvic exam, the experience is still unpleasant and sometimes even traumatic. Yet I remember returning, seemingly every month, with the same apparent problem. As usual, I'd be sent home with an unsatisfying assurance that "there's really nothing there." So I would leave, feeling like a hypochondriac, only to meekly return when I had what appeared to be the signs of yet another infection.

Along with my frustration at this recurring problem were the inevitable side effects of the various methods of birth control I tried. If I wasn't dealing with weight gain and headaches caused by the Pill, I was enduring urinary tract infections from the diaphragm or irritation from the sponge. Yet, every time I asked the gynecologist for a natural, *effective* alternative to the dismal selection of birth control methods available, I was informed that the only "natural" method was Rhythm, and everyone knew that the Rhythm Method simply didn't work. So back to square one I would go, seeming to have infections all the time and without an acceptable method of birth control.

It wasn't until years later when I took a class in Fertility Awareness that I realized I was absolutely healthy all that time. What I had been perceiving as infections was in fact normal cervical fluid, one of the healthy signs of fertility that all women experience as they approach ovulation. But since discussing one's vaginal secretions is hardly your typical topic of social chitchat, I had no idea that my experiences were normal, universal, and perhaps most important, cyclical.

Because of misleading and inadequate health education, women are rarely taught how to distinguish between normal signs of fertile cervical fluid produced every cycle and the signs of a vaginal infection. Other than the unnecessary expense, inconvenience, and anxiety that women experience, what are the consequences of such a basic omission in upbringing and education? I think that such ignorance can lead to lowered self-esteem and confusion about sexuality.

My negative gynecological experiences gradually led to an interest in women's health that evolved into a real passion. It was that passion which led me to interview for a position as a health educator at a women's clinic—a disastrous experience, which in hindsight provided the final catalyst in my decision to pursue fertility education as a career.

While sitting in the waiting room anticipating my interview with the clinic director, my eyes wandered, glancing over the all-too-familiar paraphernalia of all women's clinics: the posters warning against spreading sexually transmitted diseases, the charts comparing methods of birth control (with their inherent side effects and risks in tiny print), and the plastic models of the female reproductive system.

I remember being suddenly struck with the futility of my situation. Here I was, applying to be a health educator in a women's clinic, with absolutely no training in the field. While fidgeting, I noticed a brochure about classes on the Fertility Awareness Method that were available at the clinic.

I could not believe that this supposedly reputable clinic seemed to be teaching the discredited Rhythm Method. I was in a dilemma. The cover of the brochure mentioned natural birth control, but I knew of no natural contraceptive methods that weren't synonymous with Rhythm. Should I risk losing this coveted position by expressing my dismay, or should I keep my mouth shut and get the job?

In the end, I would have felt dishonest if I said nothing. My heart skipped a beat when the clinic director called my name. The pressure was on. The director was cordial, but I barely gave her a moment to introduce herself before I blurted out: "I don't understand why you teach Rhythm here. Everybody knows it doesn't work!"

"Oh really? We teach *what?*" she inquired with obvious surprise. "Don't you teach the Rhythm Method?" I muttered shyly. "I noticed your brochure here about the Fertility Awareness Method. Isn't that the same thing?" She looked a bit irritated and responded, "Actually, Toni, no. It's not the Rhythm Method, and frankly, your lack of knowledge about such an important facet of women's health wouldn't bode well at our clinic."

Needless to say, I didn't get the job. But that embarrassing experience years ago helped transform my perspective about women's health care. After swallowing my pride, I took the clinic's class on Fertility Awareness—and was amazed. What I learned is that not only was it possible for me to take control of my cycles, but I no longer needed to feel uncertain about various secretions, pains, and symptoms. I could finally understand the subtle changes I experienced every month. I could place my menstrual cycle in the context of my overall health—both physiological and psychological. And no more unnecessary trips to the gynecologist.

By taking just a couple of minutes a day, I am able to utilize a highly effective method of natural birth control in which I can accurately determine those days of my cycle when I am potentially fertile. In addition, if I want to get pregnant, I can avoid the guessing game so many couples play by learning precisely when to time intercourse. I can also identify for myself problems that could potentially impede pregnancy achievement. And the fact is, so can you.

Probably the best thing to come out of my years using the Fertility Awareness Method is the privilege I feel in being so knowledgeable about such a fundamental part of being a woman. I no longer question when I will get my period. I always know. I know what to expect physically and emotionally at different times in my cycle. I've also gained confidence in a way that is reflected in other areas of my life.

Your menstrual cycle is not something that should be shrouded in mystery. By the end of this book, I hope that you will also experience the liberation of feeling in control of your body. Beyond its practical value in giving you the tools to avoid or achieve pregnancy naturally, this information about your cycle and body will empower you with numerous facets of self-knowledge that you rightly deserve.

PART ONE

BREAKING FERTILE GROUND: TOWARDS A NEW WAY OF THINKING

CHAPTER 1

Fertility Awareness: What You Should Know and Why You Probably Don't

How often have you heard that a menstrual cycle should be 28 days and that ovulation usually occurs on Day 14? This is a myth, pure and simple. And yet it is so accepted that it's sadly responsible for countless unplanned pregnancies. Furthermore, it has prevented many couples who have desired a pregnancy from attaining one. Much of this fallacy is a legacy of the dangerously inaccurate Rhythm Method, which falsely assumes that individual women have cycle lengths that, if not precisely 28 days, are reliably consistent over time. The result is that Rhythm is nothing more than a flawed statistical prediction using a mathematical formula based on the average of *past* cycles to predict *future* fertility.

In reality, cycles vary tremendously among women and often within each woman herself, though most cycle lengths are 24 to 36 days. The myth of Day 14 can affect individuals in the most astounding ways:

Ilene and Mick were virgins when they got married on May 21. They wanted to start a family soon after their wedding, so they had their joint medical insurance start on May 15. When they discovered that Ilene had gotten pregnant on their honeymoon, they were pleasantly surprised that it happened so fast. Imagine their shock when the insurance company refused to cover the pregnancy and delivery, claiming that since her last period started on April 19, she must have gotten pregnant about three weeks before the wedding.

"That's impossible, she insisted, "we were both virgins until our wedding day." She tried to explain to them that her cycles had become quite long and irregular since she started jogging and dieting in order to be a "picturesque bride."

The insurance company wouldn't hear of it. They adhered to the frequently used pregnancy wheel, the calculating device that doctors rely on to determine a woman's due date. It is based on the assumption that ovulation always occurs on Day 14. As Ilene lamented, "We were sunk. How does one prove virginity in a courtroom? And why should it be anyone else's business?"

Needless to say, the Day 14 myth had very expensive consequences for Ilene and Mick. The only consolation they took from their experience was the fact that their son was born just when they expected, three weeks after the insurance company's due date! He was, in the words of Ilene, "worth all the trouble anyway."

Luckily, with advances in our understanding of human reproduction, we now have a highly accurate and effective method of identifying the woman's fertile phase: The Fertility Awareness Method (FAM). Fertility Awareness is simply a means of understanding human reproduction. It is based on the observation and charting of scientifically proven fertility signs that determine whether or not a woman is fertile on any given day. The three primary fertility signs are waking temperature, cervical fluid, and cervical position (the last one being an optional sign that simply corroborates the first two). FAM is an empowering method of natural birth control or pregnancy achievement, and it is an excellent tool for assessing gynecological problems and understanding your body.

ℂ WHY THE FERTILITY AWARENESS METHOD IS NOT BETTER KNOWN

As you read in the introduction, probably the greatest resistance to the acceptance of FAM has been its dubious misassociation with the Rhythm Method. Unfortunately, just the phrases "Natural Birth Control" or "Fertility Awareness" inevitably conjure up jokes along the lines of "What do you call Rhythm Method users?"—"Parents." Given the prevalence of this type of joke and the confusion of Rhythm with Fertility Awareness, is it any wonder that FAM is so misunderstood?

Furthermore, because the Rhythm Method is still practiced by people morally opposed to artificial methods of birth control, FAM tends to be falsely perceived as used *only* by such individuals. But in fact women from all over the world have been drawn to FAM simply because it is free of the chemicals associated with hormonal methods such as the Pill. Just as important, it allows them to minimize the time they need to use the devices that make other methods unpleasant, impractical, or unspontaneous. Many of these people tend to be oriented toward leading a natural and health-conscious life in other ways besides taking control of their fertility and reproduction.

It is true that many religious people have discovered the benefits of Fertility Awareness, though they may technically practice "Natural Family Planning" (NFP). The primary distinction between FAM and NFP is that those who use NFP choose to abstain rather than use barrier methods of contraception during the woman's fertile phase. But regardless of the differing values that often divide users of FAM and NFP, all are drawn by the desire for a natural method of effective contraception.*

FAM's Conspicuous Absence from Medical School

If FAM has so many benefits as a method of birth control (and as an aid to pregnancy achievement, as you will later read), why, then, is it not better known? One of the most critical and mystifying reasons that people have rarely heard of it is that doctors are still seldom taught a comprehensive version of this scientific method in medical school. It is amazing to think that women who practice the Fertility Awareness Method are often more knowledgeable about their own fertility than gynecologists who are trained to be experts in female physiology! †

> *Years ago when I taught at a women's clinic, the entire staff except one doctor took my seminar to use FAM as a method of contraception. One day, the one who had never attended pulled me aside and whispered, "Toni, I'll be honest with you. I don't refer my patients to your classes." "Oh really, why is that?" I casually asked, trying not to act surprised. "I got pregnant using your method and haven't trusted it since," she replied. "You're kidding! What rules did you use?" I inquired. "What do you mean, what rules?" she asked. "You know, did you observe the rules for both waking temperature and cervical fluid or just one of them?" She looked at me totally confused, as if she had no clue about what I had just asked. It was then that I realized just how widespread ignorance of Fertility Awareness was in the medical community. Even among many doctors, I thought, Fertility Awareness still meant Rhythm, or perhaps a flower child's intuition.*

---

* Appendix D extensively discusses contraceptive efficacy rates.
† For this reason, I have created Appendix O, a succinct six-page tear-out on FAM specifically written for medical professionals. I strongly encourage you to share it with your doctor.

What is especially remarkable about the glaring omission of Fertility Awareness education from medical school curricula is the fact that the method's effectiveness is based on purely biological principles, all discussed in greater detail in Chapter 4. They include the functions of oestrogen, progesterone, luteinizing hormone, and the corpus luteum, all of which have been scientifically proven.

Because Fertility Awareness is useful not only for birth control and pregnancy achievement but for promoting gynecological health in general, it is even more surprising that this information is not part of a complete medical education. Indeed, FAM can be a vital aid to doctors and their patients in diagnosing a number of conditions, including:

1. anovulation (lack of ovulation)
2. late ovulation
3. short luteal phases (the second phase of the cycle)
4. infertile cervical fluid
5. hormonal imbalances (such as polycystic ovary syndrome [PCOS])
6. insufficient progesterone levels
7. occurrence of miscarriages

Another advantage of charting the three fertility signs is that it facilitates diagnosis of gynecological problems. Women who chart are so aware of what is normal for themselves that they can help their clinician determine irregularities based on their own cycles. Examples of potential gynecological problems that can be more easily diagnosed through daily charting include:

1. irregular or abnormal bleeding
2. vaginal infections
3. urinary tract infections
4. cervical anomalies
5. breast lumps
6. premenstrual syndrome
7. miscalculated date of conception

By not being taught FAM, doctors are denied an excellent tool with which to better diagnose and counsel their female patients. Moreover, this lack of knowledge on the part of doctors often results in patients being unnecessarily subjected to invasive, painful, and frequently expensive tests to diagnose an apparent menstrual problem. Of course, if women were taught how to chart for their fertility-related health, they would not need to visit their doctor nearly as often and substantial numbers of useless medical procedures could be avoided.

As the list on page 6 should make clear, charting would reveal a myriad of potential impediments to pregnancy, ranging from the woman not ovulating to her simply not producing the cervical fluid necessary for conception. It may even show that this woman is consistently getting pregnant, but having repeated miscarriages of which neither she nor her doctor had been aware. And for those seeking to *prevent* pregnancy, charting would eliminate the anxiety so many feel as they run off to the store or their gynecologist for expensive and inconvenient pregnancy tests. Women who chart know if they are pregnant just by observing their waking temperatures, and thus they can eliminate that recurrent doubt while awaiting the arrival of a "late period."

Politics, Profit, and Natural Contraception

Another reason this method is not better known or promoted for birth control is that it is not profitable for either physicians or the major pharmaceutical companies such as those that produce the Pill or IUDs. In other words, beyond the initial investment in a book or class, and a thermometer, there is little further cost to the woman or couple using FAM. Compare this to the cost of the Pill, which can range from $2,000 to $4,000 for a ten-year supply in the USA, but is free in the UK under prescription from the NHS.*

Given the profitability of other contraceptives, is it any wonder that FAM is not promoted more enthusiastically by the medical community? It's no secret that great sums of money are spent to present the Pill as a contraceptive panacea, but what is often overlooked is the bias with which various pharmaceutical companies distort the effectiveness and validity of other birth control methods, particularly Fertility Awareness.

Corporate literature that summarizes the various contraceptives for public consumption is consistently filled with blatant inaccuracies, such as one pamphlet entitled "Contraception: The Choice Is Yours," which claims that "Natural Family Planning is based on the fact that fertilization is most likely to occur just before, during, and just after ovulation." This would almost make sense, except for the tiny detail that fertilization cannot take place without an egg present, so it would be no small feat for fertilization to take place before the egg is released!

Of course, more important than any individual misrepresentation is the overall way FAM and NFP are portrayed. This particular pamphlet was typical in that its "Natural Family Planning" heading was followed by a clarification in parentheses, which as you could guess, simply said "the Rhythm Method."

---

* Of course, you will still incur the cost of barriers for the fertile phase if you choose not to abstain while using Fertility Awareness.

Aside from birth control, it's fairly apparent that for those doctors and companies involved in providing the high-tech reproductive treatments that have given hope to so many, there is little incentive in promoting a virtually free system of knowledge that could obviate the need for their services. While these reproductive technologies are often a clear necessity, you will learn throughout this book why they are not required for many couples for whom education alone would help them achieve their dreams.

The Language of "Palatability"

Finally, the last reason FAM is not better known is that it suffers from the misfortune of being a method that many, especially in the media, refer to as "unpalatable." Why is this?

> *We have a doctor on the Seattle news who does medical stories every week. I had approached him about the possibility of doing a feature about the Fertility Awareness Method a number of times over the years, but he was always noncommittal while still acknowledging that he sincerely believed the method was effective. I could never grasp why he felt it wouldn't be suitable for the news until he finally admitted that he felt the subject was simply unpalatable for the general public.*
>
> *Perhaps his concern was about the term used for one of the three fertility signs: "cervical mucus." Maybe if it were referred to as "cervical fluid" he would find it suitable for the evening news. No sooner had I written him with that suggestion when he called to tell me he thought the change in vocabulary was just the modification necessary to make FAM acceptable for the news. Within a few weeks, he did a story about Fertility Awareness.*

It took that experience to make me realize how powerful language can be in the acceptance of FAM. Since that news feature years ago, I have found that people are infinitely more attentive to and interested in FAM when cervical *mucus* is referred to by the more neutral term cervical *fluid*. Perhaps the increased acceptability of that terminology is less puzzling when you consider that the woman's *cervical* fluid is analogous to the man's *seminal* fluid. One would never refer to seminal fluid as seminal *mucus*, and yet the purpose of the fluid in both the man and woman is comparable: to nourish and provide a medium in which the sperm can travel.

Of course, the media is an extension of our culture, which tends to promote a sanitized, unrealistic view of human physical processes. The purpose of FAM, however, is to enlighten people with a clear and empowering knowledge of their bodies' functioning. Thus, if coining a term such as "cervical fluid" makes that task easier, so much the better.

৫ৎ WHY SOME DOCTORS FAMILIAR WITH THE FERTILITY AWARENESS METHOD DO NOT INFORM THEIR PATIENTS

Many doctors know that FAM is a scientifically validated, natural method of effective birth control, pregnancy achievement, and health awareness, but they may still cite various reasons why they don't recommend it to their patients. Some say that women cannot be bothered to learn it because it's complicated and difficult to use, requires high intelligence in order to apply, and takes too much time to learn and practice. But for the vast majority of women, I believe that these assertions are simply not valid.

It is unfortunate that some physicians believe and help disseminate the erroneous assumption that FAM is complicated and difficult to use. Actually, it is generally simple and easy, once you learn its basic principles. (Many will be able to learn those principles in this book. Others will need to take a class, where a certified instructor can typically teach a comprehensive course in a couple of evening sessions.) The method is no different from many skills in life, such as learning to drive a car. It may seem intimidating at first, until a little practice gives you the confidence you need.

Some doctors may genuinely believe that women are not smart enough to understand and assimilate the information taught in FAM classes. While I find this perspective discouraging, I understand why they believe this. It is true that the type of people attracted to FAM tend to be quite educated. However, I think this is more a function of the way in which people have initially learned about it, and not the inherent intelligence required to use it. It often takes a very motivated individual to seek out information about a subject which, until now, has typically been reserved for the few who are resourceful enough to research the topic.

I personally have taught FAM to over 1,500 clients and can assure you that virtually all women can internalize the method and its biological foundation within a few hours. I also suspect few of them are particularly burdened by the couple of minutes a day it takes to apply.

In Defense of Doctors

The above is not meant to be a diatribe against the medical community. In an industry that is becoming increasingly high-tech, many doctors may be truly skeptical, precisely because FAM is so *non*-tech. Indeed, they may believe that they are not active enough in their patients' care if they do not prescribe drugs or perform procedures.

GPs do have charts and booklets available on FAM but are more likely to suggest alternative contraceptive methods such as the Pill, or the coil, simply because they don't realistically have the time to thoroughly explain the method in a typical office visit, and thus few women ever learn it. Ultimately, there is a perpetual circle of ignorance, for even those physicians who are especially supportive of women taking control of their own reproductive health cannot be as effective as they would like to be. Indeed, the benefits of FAM cannot become commonplace in the doctor-patient relationship until more women do *their* part by charting their cycles.

Taking Control of Your Reproductive Health

During every cycle, a woman's body prepares for a potential pregnancy, much to the frustration of those who prefer not to become pregnant. But a woman is actually fertile only a few days per cycle, around ovulation (when the egg is released). The only practical, non-invasive way to reliably identify that fertile time is through observing the woman's waking temperature and cervical fluid, as well as the optional sign of cervical position. By charting these primary fertility signs, a woman can tell on a day-to-day basis whether or not she is capable of getting pregnant on any given day. Because the actual day of ovulation can vary from cycle to cycle, the determination of those few days around ovulation becomes critical, and therein lies the value of the Fertility Awareness Method.

THE POLITICS OF NATURAL BIRTH CONTROL

> *We want far better reasons for having children than not knowing how to prevent them.*
>
> —Dora Russell

Why are so many women frustrated with the state of contraception today? Why is the vast majority of birth control designed for women to use even though it is men who are fertile every single day? Wouldn't it make more sense for birth control to be developed for the gender that is the most fertile? Consider the following table:

METHODS OF BIRTH CONTROL AVAILABLE TODAY
(listed from most to least invasive)

For Women	For Men
Tubal Ligation	Vasectomy
Norplant (being phased out in the UK)	Condom
Depo-Provera	Withdrawal
Pill	
IUD (intrauterine device)	
Diaphragm	
Cervical Cap	
Sponge	
Female Condom	
Suppositories	
Spermicides	
Natural Methods	

Given that women are fertile only a few days per cycle, it's ironic that they're the ones who risk the vast array of side effects and physical ramifications of birth control. These include increased risk of blood clots, strokes, breast cancer, irregular spotting, severe pelvic inflammatory disease or uterine perforation, heavy and crampy periods, urinary tract infections, cervical inflammation, and allergic reactions to spermicides and latex, to name a few. And for what? To protect themselves from a man, who produces millions of sperm per hour!

Imagine the reaction of most males to the following announcement:

A NEW INTRAPENAL CONTRACEPTIVE

The newest development in male contraception was unveiled recently at the American Women's Surgical Symposium. Dr. Sophia Merkin announced the preliminary findings of a study conducted on 763 unsuspecting male graduate students at a large midwestern university. In her report, Dr. Merkin stated that the new contraceptive—the IPD—was a breakthrough in male contraception. It will be marketed under the trade name "Umbrelly."

The IPD (intrapenal device) resembles a tiny folded umbrella which is inserted through the head of the penis into the scrotum with a plungerlike instrument. Occasionally there is perforation of the scrotum, but this is disregarded since it is known that the male has few nerve endings in this area of his body. The underside of the umbrella contains a spermicidal jelly, hence the name "Umbrelly."

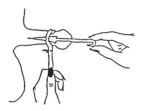

Experiments on a thousand white whales from the continental shelf (whose sexual apparatus is said to be closest to man's) proved the Umbrelly 100% effective in preventing production of sperm, and eminently satisfactory to the female whale since it doesn't interfere with her rutting pleasure.

Dr. Merkin declared the Umbrelly to be statistically safe for the human male. She reported that of the 763 grad students tested with the device, only two died of scrotal infection, three developed cancer of the testicles, and 13 were too depressed to have an erection. She stated that the common complaints ranged from cramping and bleeding to acute abdominal pain. She emphasized that these symptoms were merely indications that the man's body had not yet adjusted to the device. Hopefully, the symptoms would disappear within a year.

One complication caused by the IPD was the incidence of massive scrotal infection necessitating the surgical removal of the testicles. "But this is a rare occurrence," said Merkin, "too rare to be statistically important." She and the other distinguished members of the Women's College of Surgeons agreed that the benefits far outweighed the risk to any individual man.

—©1974 Written by Belita H. Cowan. Reprinted with permission.

Illustration by Frankie Collins.

Although the above is only a parody, in reality the notorious Dalkon Shield IUD rendered many women infertile by causing severe pelvic inflammatory disease. It is but one example of the type of medical nightmares to which many women have been subjected; history reveals countless ways in which women's bodies and those of their potential offspring have been exposed to dangerous drugs and procedures.

From the tragedies caused by thalidomide and DES in the 1950s to the more recent controversies over the side effects of Norplant and Depo-Provera, we've seen an endless stream of revelations that call into question the level of safety that female patients are assured. Beyond the often dubious nature of the drugs we've been prescribed, both contraceptive and otherwise, we've witnessed the anguish surrounding the use of breast implants. In addition, we're now aware of the wide overuse of such medical procedures as C-sections and hysterectomies, adding even more confusion to the average woman's relationship with her medical practitioners.

Whether men would submit to all the "inconveniences" is not really the issue. Given all that women have been through, it's only natural that they would desire to take control of their own medical and reproductive needs with the most effective, least intrusive means possible.

Why Unplanned Pregnancies Occur

> *I remember . . . a friend described her first experience with a contraceptive device, which shot out a bathroom window into the college quadrangle. She never retrieved it. I wouldn't have, either.*
> —ANNA QUINDLEN

To understand the politics of natural birth control, we must examine the concept of unplanned pregnancies. Why do unplanned pregnancies occur? * There are four primary reasons:

1. People do not use birth control because they are "swept away with the moment."
2. People do not use birth control because of ignorance.
3. People do not use birth control because they feel no method is acceptable.
4. People use birth control, but the method fails.

How does the Fertility Awareness Method fit into the above scheme? Let us examine each situation individually:

People Do Not Use Birth Control Because They Are Swept Away with the Moment

All barrier methods leave people vulnerable to the type of passion that reduces them to a momentary lapse in judgment. Who among us has not thought at one time or another, "Oh, I'm sure we're fine." However, if a woman knows when she is fertile, it eliminates guessing. Being unlucky is no longer an excuse.

---

* By unplanned pregnancies, I am not referring here to the unfortunate practice of many unmarried teenage girls who engage in an intentional pattern of unprotected sex, either out of indifference to the consequences or because they actually want to have babies. This issue, the subject of intensive sociological analysis and public policy debate, is beyond the scope of this book.

People Do Not Use Birth Control Because of Ignorance

Many people would be more inclined to use birth control if they understood the likelihood of pregnancy occurring at specific times in the cycle. There are so many myths perpetuated about human fertility that it's no wonder there are so many unplanned pregnancies. The classic one responsible for probably the most unplanned pregnancies is that ovulation occurs on Day 14. In actuality, ovulation *may* occur on Day 14; it may also occur on Day 10, Day 18, or Day 37. In other words, ovulation is not the consistent event it is presumed to be. But the fallacy of Day 14 is so prevalent that even clinicians perpetuate it.

If a couple thinks a woman can only get pregnant on Day 14, they may feel safe having unprotected intercourse up to Day 13 and again from Day 15 on. Some couples may even feel that they are being conservative if they put a buffer zone of several days on either side of Day 14. But if the woman ovulates on Day 20, for example, no amount of abstinence between Days 11 and 17 will prevent an unplanned pregnancy! The dangerous fiction of Day 14 is but one example in which people simply do not understand human reproduction.

What about the faulty assumption that women cannot get pregnant from intercourse during their periods? (See page 372.) Another common belief is that sperm can only live up to three days. (In reality, sperm can survive up to five days *if* fertile-quality cervical fluid is present.) Combine this belief with that of ovulation always occurring on Day 14, and undesired results are almost inevitable.

These are just some of the more common misperceptions that people have about basic human biology. Suffice it to say, many unplanned pregnancies occur because people believe such fallacies. Obviously, education is key in dealing with this problem.

People Do Not Use Birth Control Because They Feel No Method Is Acceptable

It is hardly surprising that most people find today's contraceptive choices far from ideal. Aside from sterilization, our options include such alternatives as a method that infuses the woman's body with hormones (the Pill), may increase a woman's risk of breast cancer or osteoporosis (Depo-Provera), involves inserting six matchstick-size silicone tubes under the skin of the arm (Norplant), maintains the uterus in a constant state of inflammation, causing painful periods (the IUD), fills the woman's vagina with a latex dome that leaks gooey spermicide for at least 24 hours after intercourse (the diaphragm), can be uncomfortable and cause cervical anomalies (the cervical cap), is notorious for causing vaginal infections (the sponge), completely covers the woman's clitoris (the female condom), and places a rubber sheath between the two individuals (the male condom).

Is it any wonder that unplanned pregnancies occur, given the choice of methods people perceive as their only options? With FAM, couples can experience the freedom of effective contraception without devices, chemicals, or side effects for most of the cycle.

People Use Birth Control, but the Method Fails

One of the most inflammatory opinions certain people hold is that if a couple has an unplanned pregnancy, it is their fault because they were being careless by not using birth control. Often this is simply not true. According to the Alan Guttmacher Institute, a leading think tank for population research, of the nation's three million annual unplanned pregnancies, at least 50% result from the failure of various birth control methods. Many of those failures could have been avoided if couples understood the woman's menstrual cycle better. The Family Planning Association in the UK state that 'how effective any contraceptive is depends on how old you are, how often you have sex and whether you follow the instructions. If too sexually active women don't use any contraception 80 to 90% of them will become pregnant in a year.'

This fact is particularly interesting given that so many of the barrier methods advertise such impressive "effectiveness rates," often around 95% or higher. These statistics are inherently misleading primarily because they are based on the faulty assumption that women can get pregnant throughout their cycles, when in fact a woman can only get pregnant for about one-fourth of a typical cycle. If a method is going to fail, it is only going to fail during the short fertile phase when her body is even capable of getting pregnant.

Given this information, people should know *when* in the cycle a contraceptive has the potential to fail. They can then make an educated decision as to whether they want to abstain or double up on methods of birth control during that very risky phase to reinforce effectiveness of the methods. For example, if a couple normally used the diaphragm and knew that the woman was especially fertile on a particular day, they would be able to increase its effectiveness by using extra spermicide.

Women, Men, and Contraceptive Responsibility

A common theme in women's conversations is the frustration they often feel when saddled with the full burden of birth control. Once people understand that women are only fertile for a fraction of the time men are, they are especially struck with the inequity of it all. So it is particularly interesting to examine the

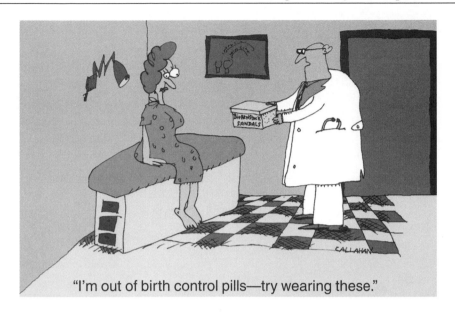

"I'm out of birth control pills—try wearing these."

ways in which women have been disproportionately exposed to side effects throughout their cycle. For example, there are many who will concede that while the Pill was originally designed to sexually emancipate women, what also transpired was burdening the woman with the sole responsibility of birth control.

Susan and Joe were a very loving couple who grappled with the issue of inequality. Susan had been on the Pill for years even though she often suffered nausea and migraine headaches. So when she suggested they take a class in the Fertility Awareness Method, Joe was more than willing. Three years later, they joke about the fact that, even today, every time the alarm rings, he gets up, puts the thermometer in her mouth, brushes his teeth, comes back and removes the thermometer, records it on her chart, and shakes it down. Susan, for her part, remains half asleep, snuggled in bed. No more nausea. No more headaches.

Unlike most other methods, FAM affords men the opportunity to lovingly and actively share in the responsibility of contraception. In fact, the method is so conducive to male involvement that many couples claim that FAM has strengthened their relationship.

❦ THE POLITICS OF PREGNANCY ACHIEVEMENT

I'll never forget that day my client Terry called. She had been trying to get pregnant for over a year before taking my seminar. It was two weeks follow-ing the class, and there was a slight hint of panic in her voice as she asked me whether she and her husband should make love that night. They were worried because she thought she had a serious vaginal infection that might affect their chances of conceiving. Just as she began describing what was "coming out of her," I heard someone pick up the other extension. It was her husband, James, on the other end. "You cannot believe what is leaking out of Terry right now."

"Wait a second, you guys. Let me ask you several questions. Is it clear?"
"Yes."
"Is it slippery?"
"Definitely."
"Is it stretchy?"
"Toni, it's ten inches!"
"Well then, what the hell are you doing talking to me? I joked, "Get off the phone and take advantage of it!"

Before making love that night, Terry and James took a dozen photos of her fertile cervical fluid. Nine months later, their little son was born.

It is unclear whether the incidence of infertility is actually increasing or peo-ple are simply seeking treatment in higher numbers today. Most likely it's a com-bination of both, in large part because more women now delay having children until at least their mid-30s. Of course, as you have no doubt heard many times before, the unfortunate reality is that a woman's fertility diminishes as she grows older. Regardless of what the reason is, infertility touches about 1 in 6 couples; however, what is often *referred* to as infertility may not necessarily *be* infertility.

The standard definition of infertility is not becoming pregnant after one year of unprotected intercourse. Nevertheless, there are many couples whose infertil-ity problem is so minor that Fertility Awareness alone would facilitate pregnancy. This is not to imply that all infertility can be treated through education. Nor is it to imply that those who are having a fertility problem are uneducated or igno-rant. But the medical community itself often inadvertently perpetuates myths that prevent couples from attaining pregnancy.

The classic myth, already discussed in Chapter 1, is that ovulation occurs on Day 14. To use this as an example: A couple may spend one year trying to time intercourse around Day 14, only to discover that in their particular case, the woman doesn't usually ovulate until about Day 20. If the couple gets pregnant after learning this information about her particular cycle, would one say that they were infertile up until that point? Clearly they were not. But the emotional and financial consequences are often so great that it's as if they really were.

Why People Are Often Misled to Believe They Are Infertile

Before discussing the impact on a couple of being inappropriately labeled "infertile," let us examine why people are often misled in the first place.

1. Infertility is assumed if pregnancy has not occurred after a year.

If a couple has been unable to get pregnant after a year of unprotected intercourse, the standard wisdom is to assume there is probably a fertility problem, when in reality there may be no medical problem whatsoever.

2. Irregular cycles are assumed to be potentially problematic.

The concept that normal cycles are 28 days and ovulation occurs on Day 14 is so entrenched in the medical profession that when a woman's cycles vary from that standard, the variation is often presumed to be a potential concern. "Irregular" cycles are seen as problematic in part because gynecologists need to time fertility procedures around when the egg is released. But if a couple is taught how to identify approaching ovulation to time intercourse appropriately, then it is irrelevant whether it occurs on Day 14, 19, or 25. (Of course, if your cycle lengths vary *dramatically*, you might want to see a clinician to rule out hormonal or other possible conditions, as discussed on page 113.)

> One of my clients was a woman who first called me in a very depressed state because it had been over a year since she and her husband had started trying to get pregnant. She mentioned that she thought the reason she may not be getting pregnant was because her cycles were not a "normal" length. I learned that they were about 35 days, an absolutely normal period of time, but certainly longer than the prototype 28 days. She went on to say that her husband got so frustrated with their apparent infertility that they would have intercourse only up to Day 14, then stop until the next cycle. No wonder they weren't getting pregnant! If a woman has long cycles, by definition she ovulates later than Day 14. Within a month of taking my fertility seminar, the couple got pregnant.

3. Doctors often overlook the most obvious solutions.

Doctors are trained to identify disease and illness, often by diagnosing and treating with the use of high-tech procedures. The result is that the most obvious solutions are often overlooked. A good example of this is the relationship between frequency of intercourse and pregnancy. A couple may have sex twice a week for a year and wonder why they have not gotten pregnant. A doctor may proceed with a fertility workup (including invasive and painful tests) on the assumption that the couple may have a fertility problem, without considering the most rudimentary question, namely, whether the couple is having intercourse *at the right time* in the woman's cycle. It is quite possible to have intercourse twice a week for a year and still be missing the fertile phase each cycle, especially if the woman has only a day or so of fertile cervical fluid, or the man's sperm count is marginal. This is not a fertility problem but an education problem.

This overlooking of fundamental principles is exemplified by Abraham Kaplan's theory, The Law of the Instrument:

> Give a small boy a hammer,
> and he will find that everything
> he encounters needs pounding.

Doctors have a vested interest in using the tools that they have perfected through years of study. It should come as no surprise, then, that infertility specialists initially apply the high-tech tools of the trade. This is very helpful for scores of couples dealing with actual infertility. However, there are many couples for whom the use of these tests and procedures is simply unnecessary. *Before any high-tech tests or treatments are employed, the man should have a semen analysis. In addition, the couple should chart the woman's fertility signs to both identify when she is the most fertile and to determine any possible impediments to pregnancy achievement.*

4. Doctors tend to focus on basal temperatures rather than cervical fluid.

Doctors will usually focus on basal body temperatures to the exclusion of the most important fertility sign for timing intercourse effectively: cervical fluid. In fact, physicians may unintentionally create a fertility problem by advising their patients to time intercourse for either the drop or rise in temperature. This advice is not only misleading, it can actually impede pregnancy achievement! Cervical fluid is the key to timing intercourse for becoming pregnant, yet many infertility doctors simply assume that women wouldn't want to take the few seconds a day necessary to chart. Informed women should decide that for themselves.

One of the most glaring examples of a doctor reinforcing the notion of depending on past temperatures to indicate future fertility took place at, of all places, a conference of the infertility organization RESOLVE. The doctor's keynote address was about all the myths surrounding fertility. She was making the correct point that basal body temperatures only indicate fertility after it is too late, after ovulation has already occurred. While sitting in the audience, I remember thinking how gratifying it was to finally hear a physician stress the point that temperatures are invalid for predicting fertility. Imagine my surprise, then, when she continued: "Therefore, to predict impending fertility, you must look back at your previous temperature shifts to predict your upcoming fertile time."

I was stunned. Here she was, reinforcing the idea of looking at past cycles to predict future fertility, without so much as mentioning the most important fertility sign for pregnancy achievement: the cervical fluid. The irony of the moment would have been amusing if it wasn't such blatantly bad advice, and addressed to such a vulnerable group of people.

The reason that temperatures don't help determine the best time to achieve pregnancy is *because by the time the temperature shifts up, the egg is typically already dead and gone.* However, the temperature is still very useful in terms of determining several facts about the woman's cycle, including: (1) whether she is ovulating at all, (2) whether the second phase of the cycle (from ovulation until her period) is long enough for the egg to implant in the uterus, and (3) whether she has achieved a pregnancy that particular cycle. (See Chapter 11.)

5. Many fertility tests are often timed inappropriately (or simply needlessly performed).

If infertility is suspected, doctors will often perform a postcoital test to determine if the man's sperm are swimming freely in the woman's cervical fluid. With this test, the couple has intercourse, then the woman goes to the doctor's office within several hours. A few drops of the semen are removed from her vagina and examined under a microscope to determine if sperm are alive and moving in the fluid. The purpose is basically to determine two facts: whether the woman's cervical fluid is conducive to sperm viability, and whether her partner's own sperm will survive in it.

One of the most common mistakes made is the procedure's timing. Many doctors continue to perform it around Day 14 of the woman's cycle, regardless of when she actually ovulates. Unless the woman does ovulate close to that day, the test is usually invalid, and leads many couples to believe they have a fertility problem when they do not.

I will never forget a lecture I gave to a group of nurse practitioners experienced in infertility treatment. As I explained that tests are useless if performed at the wrong time in a woman's cycle (for numerous women, Day 14 is simply too early) I could feel the anger build. Finally, one nurse blurted out sarcastically: "And just who do you expect us to refer our patients to for postcoitals where they will be willing to test them based on the woman's cycle rather than the availability of the staff?" All I could think of at that point was that I was not there to tell them what they wanted to hear, but rather what works.

There are certain medical events over which we simply have no control. Childbirth does not occur merely between the hours of 9 to 5, Monday through Friday. Certainly trauma is treated when it occurs, not just when the clinic is open. To the extent possible, a woman's ovulation should be no different.

A test is only useful if it is both reliable and valid. In the case of the post-coital test, the only information to be obtained from performing it on Day 14 on a woman who ovulates on Day 20, for example, is to prove that Fertility Awareness can also be effectively used as a method of birth control! Sperm die within a few hours of intercourse when a woman is not in her fertile phase, and that phase is only the few days surrounding ovulation. If performed at any other time, the test is useless.

Another frequently mistimed test is the endometrial biopsy, which involves removing a small segment of the uterine lining close to the estimated time of menstruation. This is done in order to determine if the woman is ovulating and producing a suitable lining for implantation. But again, practitioners will often simply assume a Day 14 ovulation, whether this really occurred or not, and thus the procedure's accuracy and relevance are questionable. (Had ovulation actually taken place on Day 21, one should expect both endometrial development and the next period to be a week behind.) Clearly, women undergoing these procedures deserve useful information, which is only possible if they are appropriately timed.

It should also be mentioned here that some tests are performed well before it is appropriate to do so, especially given how painful and intrusive they can be. For example, the hysterosalpingogram (HSG) is a dye test used to determine if the woman's fallopian tubes are open. It is actually quite revealing, but given its potential discomfort and cost, it should only be performed after it has been determined that possible ovulatory and cervical fluid problems have been ruled out. And needless to say, it is completely useless if in fact the fertility problem is determined to be due to miscarriages. Charting would have revealed all of these problems.

6. Women are often needlessly prescribed the ovulatory drug Clomid (clomiphene citrate).

If a couple is presumed to be infertile the woman is often put on an ovulatory drug called Clomid, whether or not she is actually ovulating. This is especially unfortunate since recent studies continue to suggest that Clomid may increase the risk of ovarian cancer or tumors, particularly for women exposed to the drug for at least a year or more. The purpose of the drug is to stimulate egg development in the ovaries. What the couple is usually not told is that it has two paradoxical side effects. One is that it can dry up the cervical fluid that is vital for sperm transport through the cervix. The other is that it can cause the second phase of the cycle to be abnormally short, preventing an egg from being able to implant in the uterus. So while this potent medication is given to increase a woman's fertility, it can, ironically, act to prevent a pregnancy. (Sometimes, the only way to remedy this former problem is through intrauterine insemination, where the sperm is deposited directly in the uterus, bypassing the cervix altogether.) I have had many clients achieve a pregnancy specifically after discontinuing Clomid.

This is not to suggest that Clomid does not have a role in infertility treatment. Certainly many women do get pregnant by using it, and indeed, it may be possible to alleviate some of the side effects. However, the use of Clomid should be an informed decision, rather than a routine first step. Women should ask their doctors why they think a prescription would be beneficial in their particular case, especially if they already know from charting that they are ovulating normally.

7. The commonly used ovulation predictor kits can be misleading.

With the advent of ovulation predictor kits, which are so readily available in drugstores now, many women are led to believe they have a fertility problem if the kits do not show the expected color surge indicating ovulation is about to occur. But even if the kits do show a color surge, it does not necessarily mean the woman is fertile. The reasons they can be misleading are all discussed in Chapter 11.

8. Women are often led to believe they are not getting pregnant, when they are actually having miscarriages.

There is a huge difference in terms of the fertility of a woman who has never achieved a pregnancy and one who gets pregnant, but then miscarries.

I do not mean to imply that women who continually miscarry do not have a fertility problem. However, the diagnostic steps taken for the two women should be drastically different.

The problem with miscarriages is that they can be difficult to diagnose since they often happen so early in the woman's cycle. They may be mistaken for nothing more than a menstrual period. But a woman trained in Fertility Awareness knows that she needs a history of at least 10 days from ovulation to menstruation for implantation to later occur, and that 18 consecutive high temperatures after ovulation almost always indicates a pregnancy. She would therefore be able to determine with a high degree of accuracy whether or not she was indeed pregnant before she bled. But since most women are not taught how to take control of their cycles, they are unable to interpret what is occurring in their bodies. Thus, they may needlessly subject themselves to painful and invasive diagnostic procedures to rule out an infertility problem that may not exist.

My client Julie thought she might finally be pregnant because she had taken my class and knew that 18 high temperatures most likely indicated a pregnancy. Upon hearing from her, I suggested she come in to the clinic to get a blood test to confirm her pregnancy. Sure enough, she was pregnant. In fact, she had conceived so early in her cycle (about Day 11) that by the time 18 high temps had been recorded, she was only on Day 29, not a day that most women typically associate with pregnancy! But she knew she was pregnant earlier than most women would typically know because she had educated herself through Fertility Awareness. Unfortunately, within a few days of her positive pregnancy test, she had a miscarriage. Although it was sad she had the miscarriage, the fact that she conceived was nevertheless very helpful in terms of what it told her about her fertility at that time:

> *a. She was ovulating.*
> *b. Her fallopian tubes were open.*
> *c. Her cervical fluid was suitable for sperm penetration.*
> *d. Her partner's sperm count was fine.*

What Julie learned from this experience is that she had undoubtedly been having other miscarriages while trying to get pregnant, but would never have known had she not learned how to identify pregnancy through charting. FAM taught her that her problem seemed to be related to a shortened phase of progesterone in the second part of her cycle (the luteal phase). Rather than start the infertility workup from square one, with all of the inherently intrusive tests, she was able to show her charts to her doctor and immediately address the problem. Several months later, after being treated for a short luteal phase, she got pregnant and carried her baby daughter to term.

The Infertility Diagnosis: Staying in Control

As you can see, there are a number of reasons people are led to believe they are infertile when they actually may not be. The physical and emotional ramifications of this misdiagnosis are far-reaching and hard to overstate. The cost of infertility diagnosis and treatment is also a major contributing factor. In the UK we have the National Health Service to which we pay a contribution of our salaries and everybody is entitled to receive free treatment. The case for IVF treatment differs from one health authority to another; you can find details of individual clinics on the HFEA website www.hfea.gov.uk. In reality it depends on postcode and age. If it is not available on the NHS then the couple have to fund it themselves. Fertility treatment can run into tens of thousands of pounds and although some private health insurance plans will cover the cost of the initial consultation and tests, treatment is not usually covered. For a list of the main UK health insurers and their policy on funding for tests see the fertility confidential website (www.fertility confidential.com).

While men are impacted to a certain extent, the woman is usually the partner most affected by the whole process. Because a woman's fertility is so integrally related to her menstrual cycle, she must visit the doctor several times a cycle to determine potential fertility problems. Since doctors' offices are rarely open at night or on weekends, many must make arrangements to miss work numerous times, or in some cases quit their jobs to pursue fertility diagnosis and treatment.

As you've read, many of the diagnostic tests are quite uncomfortable or even painful. Even worse, they are often mistimed and simply not needed. But by charting their three primary fertility signs, women can inform their doctors of numerous facts about their fertility, which can quickly narrow the range of possible diagnoses. In so doing, they can help exclude those procedures that would serve no purpose, and help to most appropriately time those tests which could reveal valuable information.

Indeed, imagine how much more confident a woman would feel if she could say to her physician:

Hi, Dr. Smith. Yes, I am basically fine, thank you. But I do have a couple of concerns I wanted to discuss with you. I practice Fertility Awareness and have noticed that my luteal phase is a little short. We plan to get pregnant this spring and would like to try to lengthen it to avoid risking a miscarriage. What would you suggest?

In other words, women and couples can become *active* participants in their health care. By charting, couples facing fertility issues will reduce their feelings of vulnerability, and most important, increase their chances of pregnancy, whether medical intervention is required or not.

Knowing When: Identifying the Date If Conception Occurs

Interestingly enough, some clinicians may inadvertently lead couples who have *gotten* pregnant to believe there is a problem when there is not. Once again, it all reverts back to the erroneous assumption that women usually have 28-day cycles and ovulate on Day 14.

Dana was a 25-year-old woman who had recently come off the Pill, so her cycles had not yet returned to normal. Because she and her husband wanted to get pregnant, they practiced Fertility Awareness to determine her fertile phase. After she became pregnant, her doctor asked her the date of her last menstrual period to apply the standard pregnancy wheel. Dana mentioned that the pregnancy wheel would be inaccurate in her particular case since it assumes ovulation on Day 14. She explained that she practiced FAM and knew that she didn't ovulate until about Day 37, so it would inaccurately predict her due date a full three weeks earlier than it really should be.

You can imagine Dana's surprise when the doctor not only did not give credence to her charts, but actually expressed great concern when his pelvic exam revealed that the fetus was "extremely small for dates." Had this women not been practicing Fertility Awareness, she would have been distressed to be told by the doctor that there was something wrong with her fetus, all because he was basing her cycles on the average woman's day of ovulation, rather than her own. As if that wasn't enough, he actually red-flagged her chart with a "medical alert" tag, indicating that her pregnancy was high risk and needed to be followed carefully.

Although the use of ultrasound would eliminate this confusion, there are a great many women who would prefer to avoid such high-tech pregnancies, and thus pregnancy wheel estimations should be approached with caution. Indeed, such miscalculations can and have led to the induced labor of many a premature baby.

⅋ FERTILITY AWARENESS FOR DETECTING GYNECOLOGICAL PROBLEMS AND UNDERSTANDING THE HEALTHY BODY

How often have you felt a sudden sharp pain in your side, noticed spotting at odd times, or even felt a breast lump that caused you to panic? While all of these experiences may seem confusing, they can be normal occurrences *if they take place at the appropriate time in your cycle.*

The benefits of charting extend far beyond knowing when a woman can and cannot get pregnant. There are many gynecological conditions that can be identified through observing your fertility signs. Women who chart can determine whether they are experiencing normal occurrences or true gynecological problems such as vaginal or urinary tract infections and cervical anomalies. Those who chart are so aware of what is normal for themselves that they can help their clinician determine irregularities based on their *individual* symptoms rather than the average woman's symptoms.

This has tremendous advantages, as seen in the classic example of a woman who may have occasional midcycle spotting, which is usually harmless and often referred to as ovulatory bleeding. But because spotting can be an indication of other potentially serious problems (such as cervical cancer), doctors often feel obligated to pursue unnecessary testing and examinations, needlessly worrying and inconveniencing their patients. A woman who charts would know when this type of bleeding is normal, and thus not seek medical attention unless she really needed it.

Of course, certain unpleasant medical procedures will always be necessary. Most women would say that a pelvic exam is hardly one of their favorite activities. The average woman would probably rather be scrubbing a toilet than lying on the exam table, her legs in stirrups, trying to maintain a semblance of dignity. Especially when the doctor walks in, smiling and acting as if there's nothing the least bit awkward about her lying there stark naked under a 2-by-2-inch hospital gown.

And what is the first thing that physicians say when they sit down at the foot of the exam table? "Scoot down, please." It's hardly a coincidence that doctors must always request that of their patients. After all, how many women of their own volition would choose to have their derriere hanging off the table if they didn't have to?!

Now granted, no amount of fertility consciousness will free you from this unpleasant experience. But taking responsibility for your own health care will at least give you some integrity and a sense of control often lost in a typical office visit. Charting the menstrual cycle allows a woman and her health care practitioner to work together as a team, with the patient contributing to her own well-being.

In addition, FAM will put you so in tune with the normal occurrences of your cycle that it will greatly reduce the number of times you feel a need to consult with your doctor in the first place. For example, how many times have you gone to your gynecologist complaining of an infection only to be assured you were fine? Unfortunately, information about women's fertility signs is not typically taught in school; therefore, many girls and young women grow up thinking they are unhealthy or even dirty. What they really are is simply uninformed.

So That's What It Is!

There is nothing more confusing than sitting in the library studying for physics one night when you feel a sudden, slippery, wet sensation (you know that physics has never excited you *that* much). What's going on? You run to the bathroom, thinking you may be bleeding, but you find no discoloration on your underwear. In reality, you are no doubt experiencing what is commonly referred to as "eggwhite" cervical fluid, an extremely slippery and fertile secretion that is released as you approach ovulation. As you will learn, such secretions are healthy and normal.

> *The first time Barbara ever noticed fertile cervical fluid as a young teenager, she was horrified. She couldn't imagine what was hanging from her vagina when she went to urinate. The only thing she could think to do in order to remove it was wad up balls of toilet paper and hurl them at this seemingly foreign blob. Barbara is now a FAM instructor!*

Many women today refuse to remain ignorant. They are beginning to actively participate in all facets of their health care, enhancing their understanding of their fertility in the process. FAM gives women these opportunities. Most women are thrilled with the sense of control they feel after spending just a couple of minutes a day charting their cycle, cherishing the privilege of finally under-standing their bodies.

Fertility Awareness as Basic Education

I fully admit that Fertility Awareness is not the best choice of birth control for all women. Indeed, given the realities of AIDS and other sexually transmitted dis-eases (STDs), FAM as contraception is only recommended for monogamous cou-ples with the maturity and discipline to follow the method correctly. However, even if a woman never uses it for contraceptive purposes, this book will clearly show that the biological principles that form the foundation for FAM should be seen as part of every woman's basic education. If this came to pass, women would be far less dependent on doctors for fundamental answers that should be a part of their own knowledge and understanding.

> *Audrey, one of my clients, had been charting her cycles for several years when she volunteered to be a control for an ultrasound study in abnormal ovula-tion. Over five months, her ovaries were monitored to determine if she was re-leasing an egg. Every time she went in, she would announce confidently that she was about to ovulate, and as usual the technician would raise her eye-brows in surprise. "Oh, really?" she would say. She would then check the mon-itor and say, "Oh, it looks like you're about to ovulate." "I know, that's what I just told you." And sure enough, the following day, Audrey would indeed ovu-late.*
>
> *When she returned the next day, she would say, "By the way, I think you'll find that I've already ovulated." "Oh, really?" the technician would say, scratching her head. She would then check the monitor and say, "Oh, it looks like you already ovulated." "I know, that's what I just told you," Audrey would reply, feeling a real sense of confidence about her ability to interpret her fer-tility signs.*

It is worth noting that the renowned scientist Dr. Carl Djerassi, often hon-ored as the father of the Pill, acknowledges that women should be privy to such basic biological occurrences. "Eventually," he has written, "many a woman in our affluent society may conclude that the determination of when and whether she is ovulating should be a routine item of personal health information to which she is entitled as a matter of course."

PART TWO

REDISCOVERING YOUR CYCLE AND YOUR BODY

There's More to Your Reproductive Anatomy Than Your Vagina

What woman doesn't remember awkwardly gathering with other sixth-grade girls to learn about the mysteries of their bodies and the fascinating world of sanitary napkins they were soon to embark upon? The funny thing is, when all was said and done, most of us came away from the uninspired instruction with hardly a clue as to what was really about to happen to us. We proceeded to grow up with the menstrual cycle still cloaked in mystery, the subject of numerous myths.

We were all led to believe that the main event of every cycle was menstruation, and the primary lesson was proper tampon and sanitary pad etiquette. I can still remember giggling in the corner with my friends as we whispered the joke that was pathetically transformed from one of Stevie Wonder's most popular songs: "What's all right, uptight, and outta sight?" Tampons, of course. We were *so* adult now. We sixth-graders could joke about these sorts of things—things the fifth-graders surely would just not get. We were so cool.

So it should come as no surprise that after spending hours in the "feminine hygiene" aisle of the drugstore, most of us find that we still know basically nothing about our bodies, but can tell you pretty much anything you ever wanted to know about mini- versus maxipads, napkins with wings versus those with superduper adhesive strips, extra-wide versus extra-long panty shields, and superabsorbent versus regular tampons.

This is where Fertility Awareness comes in. It is about so much more than merely understanding female hygiene and menstruation. At its core is a philosophy of taking control of, understanding, and demystifying the menstrual cycle and all its effects on you. This is because sexuality, fertility, childbirth, and menopause are all facets of being female, and charting is the edifying window into these aspects of a woman's life. The self-knowledge available from Fertility Awareness is a valuable resource for all kinds of personal decision-making. Perhaps most important, it encourages women to value and trust knowledge provided by their own bodies.

Gynecologists are experts in women's physiology so it only makes sense that women tend to turn to doctors rather than themselves to interpret their bodies. Reliance on physicians would be understandable if the knowledge doctors possessed about women's cycles was incomprehensible to the general public. But this is basic fertility, not brain surgery. In reality this information is quite simple, and not the mystery so many people believe it is.

To understand your cycle, though, you should first have a general knowledge of human reproductive biology. The following pages should familiarize you with both female and male anatomy.

❧ INTERNAL FEMALE REPRODUCTIVE ANATOMY

Do you realize that a part of every single one of us resided inside our maternal *grandmother's* uterus, even before our own mothers were born? Unlike male fetuses which contain no sperm, female fetuses already contain all the eggs that the newborn child will ever have. What that means, practically speaking, is that when your mother was just a fetus inside her mother, she already had developed one of the eggs that eventually became you.

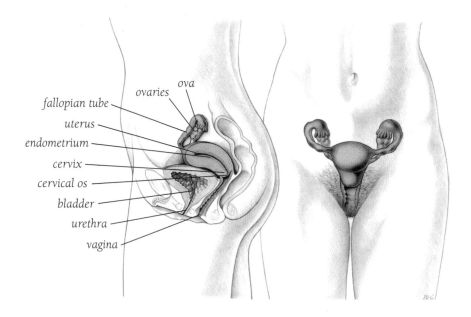

fallopian tube
uterus
endometrium
cervix
cervical os
bladder
urethra
vagina

ovaries
ova

CROSS-SECTION OF THE UTERUS

Uterus: The womb. A hollow, muscular, pear-shaped organ (about the size of a small lemon) that builds up and releases a blood-rich lining every cycle and acts as an "incubator" for the developing fetus if conception occurs. In most women, the uterus curves forward.

Fallopian tubes: The 4- to 5-inch-long narrow tubes that transport the egg from the ovary to the uterus.

Ova (ovum): Granule-sized eggs stored in the ovaries, only one of which is usually released each cycle. The ovulated ova may unite with sperm during fertilization to form the eventual fetus.

Ovaries: Two almond-sized primary sex glands that contain up to a million immature eggs at birth. Each egg (or ovum) is surrounded by a group of cells called a follicle. The ovaries produce estrogen and progesterone during the reproductive years.

Endometrium: Lining of the uterus that builds up in preparation for a potential pregnancy and is shed every cycle in the form of menstruation.

Cervix: The lower opening of the uterus. The only part of the uterus that can be felt protruding into the upper vagina. Lined with channels that cyclically develop cervical fluid in which sperm thrive.

Vagina: The elastic 4- to 6-inch-long muscular passage between the vulva and cervix. During sexual arousal, the vagina expands to receive the penis during intercourse and stretches to become the birth canal during childbirth.

Cervical os: The small opening of the cervix that becomes larger around ovulation (referred to as "cervical tip" in this book).

One of the major differences between male and female anatomy has to do with when the sex cells (or gametes) are developed. As mentioned above, girls are born with all the eggs they will ever have. The eggs start to mature and be released at puberty, continuing to usually expel one egg per cycle until menopause. Boys, on the other hand, don't develop sperm until adolescence, but then continually produce sperm every day until they die. The box below reflects the three major differences between male and female fertility.

DIFFERENCES BETWEEN MALE AND FEMALE FERTILITY	
Males	**Females**
Fertile all the time, since sperm are produced on a daily basis.	Fertile only a few days per cycle, since ovulation occurs only once a cycle.
Fertile from puberty until death.	Fertile from puberty until menopause (about 50 years old).
Do not develop any sperm until puberty.	Born with all the eggs they will ever have.

🙢 EXTERNAL FEMALE REPRODUCTIVE ANATOMY

It is amazing how few women really know what their external anatomy looks like. Sadly, most girls are led to believe that they are "dirty down there," and are therefore reluctant to even examine themselves. Boys, however, are usually socialized to believe they possess a treasure in which to take pride.

Although the illustration on the next page should be self-explanatory, there are several points I would like to make regarding external anatomy. One thing women should understand is that there are probably as many variations of sizes and shapes of vaginal lips as there are women. The enormous variation between women's vaginas and vaginal lips merely adds spice and uniqueness. Aside from the obvious external differences between men and women, they also differ both sexually and in terms of certain potential physical problems.

EXTERNAL FEMALE REPRODUCTIVE ANATOMY

Vulva: The external female genitalia.

Mons pubis: The soft fleshy tissue beneath the pubic hair that protects the internal reproductive organs.

Hood of clitoris: The protective covering of the clitoris, formed by the joining of the two inner vaginal lips.

Clitoris: The pea-sized organ that becomes filled with blood during sexual arousal, causing it to become firm and erect. As the primary site of orgasm for the majority of women, it is filled with more sexual nerve endings than any other part of the body. The female analog to the tip of the male penis.

Vaginal lips (outer): Soft padding, which contains oil-producing glands and a small amount of pubic hair.

Vaginal lips (inner): Folds of very soft, sleek skin. Typically covers the vagina unless the woman becomes sexually aroused, at which point the inner lips tend to fill with blood and blossom out to allow for insertion of the penis. They may also become full and separate around ovulation.

Urethra: The narrow tube that carries urine from the bladder out of the body.

Introitus (Vaginal opening): The outer entrance to the vagina. The opening for the release of menstrual blood, as well as cervical fluid. The site through which a baby's head comes out during childbirth.

Vagina: The elastic 4- to 6-inch-long muscular passage between the vulva and cervix, acting as the receptor of the penis during intercourse and the birth canal during childbirth.

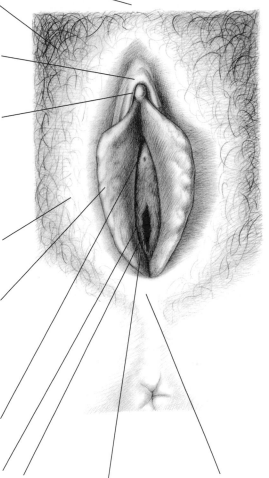

Bartholin's glands: Two tiny glands on each side of the vaginal opening that produce a thin lubricant when a woman becomes sexually aroused.

Perineum: The membrane between the vaginal opening and the anus that remarkably stretches during childbirth to allow a baby's head to emerge through the vaginal opening.

Women, for example, tend to be more prone to urinary tract infections (UTIs). This is because a woman's urethra is shorter, so bacteria have less distance to travel from its opening to the bladder. In addition, its location so close to the vaginal opening makes it more vulnerable to external bacteria, as well as occasional irritation during intercourse. Finally, the contraceptive diaphragm can obstruct the flow of urine by pressing against the urethra, creating a perfect medium for bacterial growth.

In addition to UTIs, women may develop occasional vaginal infections due to the delicate pH balance in the vagina. As you know, discharge from infections should not to be confused with healthy cervical fluid which women usually produce every cycle around ovulation. (True vaginal infections are discussed in Chapter 15.)

Differences in anatomy affect the way men and women experience sexuality. This seems obvious on the surface, but there are so many subtle distinctions in this area that I have devoted much of Chapter 16 to discussing it. Still, one difference is certainly worth mentioning in this context: orgasms.

Women do not achieve orgasms the way men do. They're simply not built the same. A man's most sensitive nerves are just below the tip of the penis, which is the part most stimulated during sexual intercourse. It should come as no surprise that men achieve orgasm fairly easily due to the physical nature of intercourse.

Why do women not achieve orgasms during intercourse the same way men do? The answer is straightforward. The most sensitive sexual nerves in women are in the clitoris, which is outside and above the vagina. So during traditional intercourse (with the couple face-to-face in the missionary position), while the man is having a grand ol' time, the woman may be compiling a grocery list for dinner that night. It's not that the sensation of intercourse isn't wonderful for most women. And for the lucky 30% or so who achieve orgasms from intercourse, the experience can be fantastic. But the point is that women are built differently than men, plain and simple.

The most graphic way to explain this is by illustrating how a human being develops while in the uterus. Before a fetus evolves into a boy or girl, the exact same cells that would become the tip of the penis in the boy become the clitoris in the girl. And the same cells that would become the scrotum in the boy become the vulva in the girl. Perhaps the best way to help men understand women's sexuality would be to ask them whether they would be able to achieve an orgasm from merely being stroked on the scrotum. Who knows? Maybe, maybe not. Or maybe after, say, two hours! Yet high expectations cause men and women alike to get frustrated when women don't have orgasms as readily as men do.

EMBRYONIC DEVELOPMENT OF FEMALE AND MALE GENITALIA

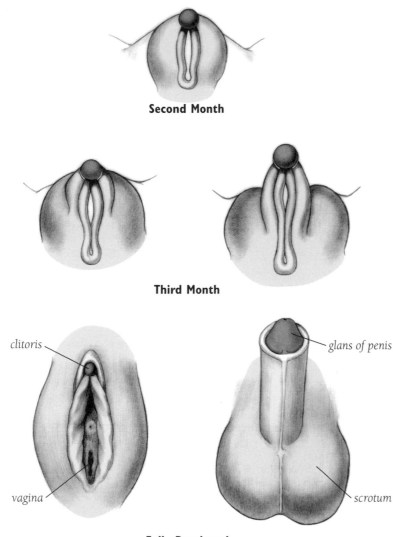

Second Month

Third Month

clitoris

vagina

glans of penis

scrotum

Fully Developed

How embryonic development determines pleasure during intercourse. The clitoris and the tip of the penis evolve from the same sensitive cells. The vulva and the scrotum evolve from less-sensitive cells. The vagina, however, is comprised of cells of very low sensitivity, and has no analog in the male. Thus, during sexual intercourse, a man's most sensitive area is directly stimulated, while a woman's is not.

If you could be a fly on the wall of bedrooms throughout the world, I think you'd be amused to discover how often women blame their partners for "lousy technique," which prevents them from having orgasms during intercourse. Meanwhile, men blame their partners for not being "womanly enough" to automatically have orgasms. Alas, this often leads to conflict between the sexes.

Sex between men and women can be extremely sensual and gratifying if both partners learn about each other's bodies and needs. Satisfying your partner means taking the time to ask questions and being willing to be vulnerable. Chapter 16 further discusses how to enrich your sex life by charting.

MALE REPRODUCTIVE ANATOMY

Mary is one of those rare individuals who leads a charmed life out in the country with her husband and three-year-old. The adorable little boy loves to run around naked in the warm sun. One beautiful spring day, as my friend Linda was sitting out on Mary's patio sipping iced tea and chatting with her, little Josh ran over, pointed down and innocently asked, "Mom, this little guy at the end of my penis—is it my brain?" As Linda tells it, the reaction on his mother's face seemed to say "No, honey, but when you get older, it might as well be."

Have you ever noticed that bald men almost always have hairy chests? Long before I became a fertility educator, I knew there must be some association between the two. It has to do with testosterone, the hormone responsible for the development of male sex traits. Although the exact mechanism is not fully understood, there is a correlation between a higher amount of testosterone and the two characteristics.

Of course, testosterone is also related to fertility, since it is responsible for sperm production. But so often when we think of fertility, the tendency is to think only of women. After all, they are the ones who have menstrual cycles and ultimately bear children. Yet, if it weren't for the minor detail of men's sperm, women would obviously never get pregnant. In addition, whenever there is a fertility problem with a couple, it is attributable as often to the man as to the woman.

As you have seen from the last few pages, there are significant differences between men and women's fertility and sexuality. Interestingly enough, there are also distinct similarities between male and female reproductive anatomy. Just as women develop eggs in their ovaries, men produce the male counterpart, sperm, in their testes. And just as the woman's egg is picked up and drawn into the fallopian tube, a man's sperm travels through a tube called the vas deferens. Finally, the woman's uterus and the man's prostate, both in approximately the same location, produce nutrients for the egg and sperm, respectively.

MALE REPRODUCTIVE ANATOMY

Bladder: The muscular reservoir that stores urine before being released during urination.

Prostate gland: A walnut-sized gland that produces a thin, milky fluid which acts to nourish sperm and provide part of the substance that forms semen. Surrounds the junction of the vas deferens and the urethra.

Cowper's gland: Two pea-sized glands that produce a clear, lubricating fluid designed to provide nutrients for sperm survival. It also helps to neutralize the acidity of any urine remaining in the urethra.

Vas deferens: A pair of approximately 15-inch-long tubes that carry sperm to the seminal vesicles. The inner channel is as thin as a hair.

Penis: The male organ through which urine and semen are emitted. Becomes erect for intercourse.

Urethra: The narrow 8-inch tube that can carry either urine or semen through the penis and out of the body.

Testes (testicles): The pair of oval-shaped sex glands that produce testosterone and an average of 200 million sperm daily. The left testes usually hangs lower than the right.

Seminiferous tubules: Microscopic tubes in the testes in which sperm are produced.

Scrotum: The loose, thin skin pouch surrounding the testicles, which thins out and contracts in response to external temperatures.

Seminal vesicles: Saclike structures that produce a nourishing substance for sperm and form about 65% of the seminal fluid in which sperm travel.

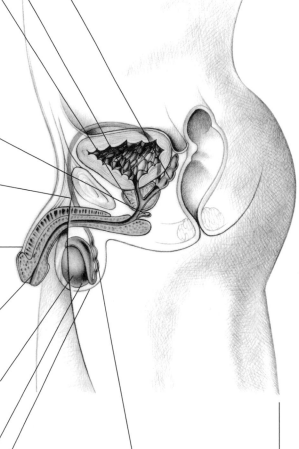

Epididymis: A 20-foot-long series of ultra-thin, tightly coiled tubes that mature and store young sperm cells. Takes about 2 to 12 days for sperm to pass through, during which time they develop swimming ability and attain fertilization capability. Together the epididymis and vas deferens store about 700 million sperm at a time.

It is no coincidence that men's testes are situated outside their bodies, since the sperm require 3 to 4 degrees below normal body temperature to develop. Apparently, that design works quite well, because most men produce 100 to 300 million sperm a *day!* To assure that the testicles remain cool, the scrotum that surrounds the testes thickens and thins in response to the external temperature. For example, if a man jumps into a cold lake, the scrotum contracts, becoming very thick and pulling the testes against his body. But if he takes a hot shower, the scrotum thins out, allowing the testes to drop down. In this way, the body maintains a steady testicular temperature in various thermal conditions.

Even though sperm are produced on a daily basis, the production of individual sperm can take about 72 days to complete. They begin their reproductive journey inside the long, thin seminiferous tubules in the testes before going into "cold storage" in the epididymis, a series of 20-foot-long tightly coiled tubes that act as a school for sperm to perfect their swimming technique. It takes them anywhere from about 2 to 12 days to pass through the epididymis.

Before ejaculation, the cowper's gland releases a slippery, clear fluid designed to facilitate sperm survival and neutralize the acidity of the urethra. People often confuse these few drops of "leaking" with a man's inability to control his ejaculation. In reality, it is an absolutely healthy and necessary sexual function. But the pre-ejaculate may contain live sperm, which is why "withdrawal" is not recommended for birth control (though, in fact, it is more effective than having completely unprotected intercourse). At ejaculation itself, the prostate and seminal vesicles supply the nutrient-rich fluid in which sperm travel. One of the reasons it takes a while for men to be able to ejaculate again is that the seminal vesicle and prostate need time to manufacture more seminal fluid.

While we are on the subject of what men emit during ejaculation, you can rest assured that one of the things they do not emit is urine! One of the reasons it's difficult for a man to urinate when he is sexually aroused is that a muscular sphincter closes the opening of the bladder, preventing him from urinating and ejaculating simultaneously. Women can breathe a collective sigh of relief.

What does happen at ejaculation is that the sperm travel from the epididymis through the vas deferens and out the urethra. On the way, the fluid from the seminal vesicles also enters the vas deferens and mixes with the sperm. The seminal vesicles are two saclike structures that produce part of the seminal fluid in which the sperm travels. The other source of fluid for semen comes from the prostate gland.*

---

* Question: What did the epididymis say to the seminal vesicle? Answer: There's a vas deferens between us. (Thanks to Robert Mecklosky, New York City's most beloved science teacher.)

If a man ejaculates inside a woman, the length of time the sperm can survive is directly related to where the woman is in her cycle. If a woman is nowhere near ovulation, and is therefore infertile, the sperm won't survive more than a couple of hours or so. However, if she is approaching ovulation, and has wet quality cervical fluid, sperm can live up to five days. This is discussed in greater detail later.

The initial gelatinlike consistency of the semen acts to prevent early leakage out of the vagina, while sugar within the gel provides instant energy for sperm motility. But once it has served this purpose, the gel tends to melt and leak out in the ensuing hours, much to the chagrin of many women.

Sperm comprise a surprisingly small fraction of the semen itself. The composition of semen is approximately as follows:

Fluid from the seminal vesicles:	65%
Fluid from the prostate gland:	30%
Sperm and testicular fluid:	5%

Portions of the following list should shed light on why it is that many women who are trying to avoid pregnancy have good reason to be cautious:

Number of sperm produced per day:	100–300 million
Typical number of sperm per ejaculate (2–6 ml):	100–400 million
Typical number of sperm per milliliter:	20–200 million
Number of days sperm can live in fertile cervical fluid:	5 days

The good news is that with a method like FAM, women need not concern themselves with whether men produce one or ten million sperm per hour. The point is that once women determine when they are not fertile themselves, it doesn't matter how many sperm the man produces. If there is no egg to be released, there is no physiological way a pregnancy can occur.

CHAPTER 4

Finally Making Sense of Your Menstrual Cycle

*K*eri and Brent are the classic example of educated people being misinformed about normal cycle lengths. They weren't clients of mine, but Brent told me his theory about the effect of stress on women's cycles when he heard that I was writing a book on Fertility Awareness. He said his wife was so paranoid about getting pregnant that she would consistently worry herself into having delayed periods. Keri's anxiety would lead her to continually buy pregnancy tests that would always be negative, followed by menstruation within a day or two of the test. Based on this pattern, Brent deduced that anxiety itself was causing the delay, and that the reassuring news allowed her to finally relax enough for her period to start. Seems logical, right?

Wrong. As you will learn, starting to worry abut a pregnancy just a few days before your period is due will not delay it, since the time from ovulation to menstruation (the luteal phase) is a finite length that is not affected by external factors such as stress. In reality, what was undoubtedly happening was that Keri had longer than average cycles, perhaps 32 days or so. But since she was under the commonly held illusion that cycles were 28 days, she would start to panic when Day 30 or 31 arrived. Finally, by Day 32, she would take a pregnancy test, it would come out negative, and lo and behold she would get her period the next day. But it wasn't the negative test results that were allowing her menstruation to begin. It was that her cycles were almost certainly about 32 days anyway.

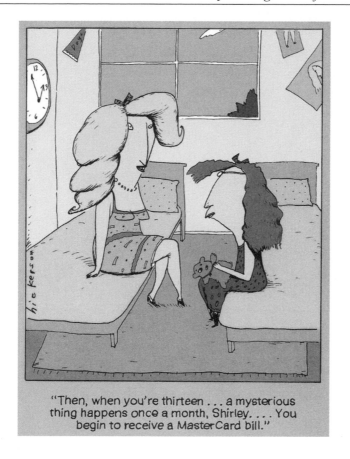

"Then, when you're thirteen . . . a mysterious thing happens once a month, Shirley. . . . You begin to receive a MasterCard bill."

🙢 THE GREAT RACE

There's a time when you have to explain to your children why they were born, and it's a marvelous thing if you know the reason by then.
—HAZEL SCOTT

Oh, yawn, here we go again . . . the menstrual cycle. Now, before you start whining about how boring this section is going to be, trust me. It's really one of the most remarkable things that happens within your body. The menstrual cycle is like a fine-tuned symphony, a fascinating interplay of hormones and physiological responses. By the end of this chapter, I think you, too, will agree.

The bottom line is that your body prepares for a potential pregnancy every cycle, whether or not you want to actually conceive. In essence, your hormones do not always confer with your heart. They just do their thing regardless of your intentions.*

Every cycle, under the influence of Follicle Stimulating Hormone (FSH), about 15 to 20 eggs start to mature in each ovary. Each egg is encased in its own follicle. The follicles produce oestrogen, the hormone necessary for ovulation to eventually occur. A race progresses for one follicle to become the largest. Eventually ovulation occurs when one ovary releases an egg from the most dominant follicle. (The other eggs that began to ripen disintegrate in a process called atresia.) It is fairly arbitrary which ovary ultimately releases the egg. Ovulation doesn't necessarily alternate between ovaries, as is often thought.

Although it averages about 2 weeks, this race to release an egg can take anywhere from about 8 days to a month or longer to complete. The primary factor that determines how long it will take before you ovulate is how soon your body reaches an oestrogen threshold. The high levels of oestrogen will trigger an abrupt surge of Luteinizing Hormone (LH). It's this LH surge that causes the egg to literally burst through the ovarian wall, usually within a day or so of its occurrence. After ovulation, the egg tumbles out into the pelvic cavity, where it is quickly swept up by the fingerlike projections of the fallopian tubes, called fimbria.

At this point you may be thinking, what is she talking about? How many hormones are we dealing with here? Actually, a tidy little way for you to remember the general order of the hormones is through the expression FELOP, which stands for:

Follicle Stimulating Hormone
Estrogen
Luteinizing Hormone
Ovulation
Progesterone

So the next time you're at a party and someone asks, you'll have a quick reply ready. Of course, things could get ugly if someone asks you for an even more detailed explanation of the menstrual cycle. For that, you should read the more comprehensive version of the cycle elaborated in Appendix E.

---

* Evolutionary biologist Margie Profet offers an altogether different theory as to why menstrual cycles occur. She believes the key function of menstruation is to rid the body of pathogens that are carried by the sperm and introduced into the woman's reproductive organs during sex. Her theory has caused considerable debate in the academic world, but she has maintained her sense of humor about it. "What they told you in kindergarten is true," she once told *Newsweek* (October 4, 1993), "boys really do have cooties."

THE FOUR PRIMARY REPRODUCTIVE HORMONES

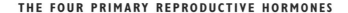

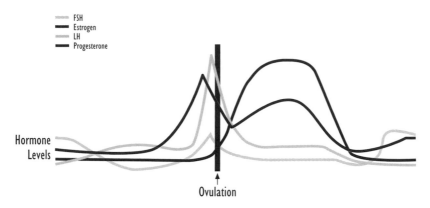

Once the egg enters the pelvic cavity, the fimbria reach over and draw it into the adjoining tube. Occasionally, the fimbria do not retrieve the egg, and therefore pregnancy would not be possible that cycle. This would be true even if intercourse occurred when the woman was at the height of her fertile phase.

Following the release of the egg from the ovary, the follicle that held the egg collapses on itself, becoming a yellow body, or "corpus luteum." The corpus luteum remains behind on the interior ovarian wall and starts releasing progesterone. The corpus luteum has a finite life span of about 12 to 16 days, with an average length just over 12 days. Rarely does it vary more than a couple of days within each individual woman, because its presence on the ovarian wall leaves it unaffected by the stresses of everyday life.

Thus, for example, if Myriam's luteal phase (the phase following ovulation) is normally 13 days, it may occasionally be 12 days, occasionally 14. Sometimes, luteal phases may be 11 or even 10 days. These are considered within a normal range, but phases less than 12 days can be *potentially* problematic if a couple is trying to get pregnant. (I discuss short luteal phases in greater detail in Chapters 11 and 12.)

Progesterone, the hormone released by the corpus luteum, is incredibly important for a woman's fertility because it does three things:

1. Prevents the release of all other eggs for that cycle.
2. Causes the uterine lining (endometrium) to thicken and sustain itself until the corpus luteum disintegrates 12 to 16 days later.
3. Causes the three primary fertility signs to change. These signs are waking temperature, cervical fluid, and cervical position.

In a small percentage of cycles, two or more eggs are released during ovulation, but always within a 24-hour period. This phenomenon, called multiple ovulation, is responsible for fraternal twins. The reason that more eggs cannot be released later that cycle is due to the powerful effects of progesterone mentioned above. *Progesterone quickly stops the release of all other eggs until the next cycle.* So a woman could not release an egg one day, get pregnant, than release an egg again weeks or months later. Her body protects that potential pregnancy by preventing her from being able to release more eggs following ovulation.*

❧ OVULATION: THE DIVIDING LINE

The first part of the cycle, from Day 1 of menses to ovulation, is the follicular (or oestrogenic) phase. Its length can vary considerably. The second phase of the cycle, from ovulation to the last day before the new period begins, is the luteal (or progestational) phase. It usually has a finite lifespan of 12 to 16 days. What this means is that, ultimately, it is the day of ovulation that will determine the length of your cycle.

For example, a woman could have an extremely delayed ovulation due to stress or other factors, not ovulating until Day 30 or so. This would result in about a 44-day cycle (30 plus 14). Thus, just because a woman is on Day 44 and hasn't gotten her period yet doesn't necessarily mean she's pregnant.

> *My brother Raymond was editing the manuscript for the first edition of this book when he got a call from his good friend Marcella, who lives in Los Angeles. She appeared mildly panicked about possibly being pregnant and was calling him for advice. (Ray was accustomed to his friends' inquiries, since he possessed a certain expertise on fertility that few men do.)*

---

* In the United States, about one out of every 50 to 55 live births produces a twin.(This figure is significantly higher than earlier generations because of the use of fertility drugs.) One-third of the time, they are identical twins, meaning that *one* fertilized egg splits in two. Two-thirds of the time, they are fraternal twins, meaning that *two* separate eggs are released and conceived within 24 hours of each other. Identical twins tend to be rare in nature in that there is no particular hereditary component involved. The birth of fraternal twins, on the other hand, may be influenced by heredity. What appears to be passed down is the propensity to release higher levels than average of FSH, which in turn may cause more than one egg to be released. In addition, older women may be more likely to release more than one egg, since FSH tends to increase as women get older.

Recent studies show that multiple ovulation may occur as often as 10% of all cycles, a much higher percentage than previously thought. While it is true that only about 1% of deliveries are fraternal twins, it must be remembered that most ovulations don't result in conception. In addition, research has shown many more fraternal twins are actually conceived than delivered, but that in the majority of cases, one of the conceptions is spontaneously miscarried or reabsorbed, resulting in a single baby. Scientists refer to this as the "vanishing twin syndrome." In any case, the fact that so many cycles may have multiple ovulations highlights the importance of the various FAM rules for avoiding pregnancy that you'll learn later.

She explained that she was worried because she was on Day 42 and had never had a cycle longer than 32 days. Clearly enjoying his role as supportive friend and menstrual detective, Ray proceeded to record all the relevant information. Sex with her boyfriend on Day 5. "Sloppy withdrawal." No cycles ever less than 25 days. And so on.

The data convinced Ray that pregnancy was extremely unlikely. He then went on to explain to Marcella that if she had been sick, or traveled, or had experienced a lot of stress before she ovulated, it was possible ovulation could have been delayed days or even weeks, thus causing the extended cycle. She was not terribly reassured. "You must have been stressed out about something," he said. Marcella insisted that all was basically uneventful in her life, and that the only unusual anxiety she was experiencing had crept in just a few days earlier, about a week after her last period was "due."

Beyond being a menstrual detective, Ray was also an amateur historian. He loved dates. He took out his calendar and stared at it. "Marcella," he said coyly, "let me just verify. Your last period started on January 6, so you normally would've ovulated around January 20, give or take a few days."

"Yeah, I guess," she mumbled nervously.

"So, I'm just curious, on January 17, did you just sleep through the earthquake, or what?"

There was a pause.

"Oh God, I forgot about that! That was one of the scariest things I've ever been through. 6.7 on the Richter scale! It was awful." Ray laughed and told her to relax, that she almost certainly wasn't pregnant. Three days later Marcella called back, delighted to inform him that she had just gotten her period.

Ray suggested that the next time a massive quake strikes, the mayor should go on citywide TV. That way he could assure the women of L.A. that if their periods are late, it's quite possible there's nothing to worry about. It could just be your garden-variety, seismically delayed ovulation.

It should also be noted that a woman may occasionally not release an egg at all. This is referred to as an "anovulatory cycle." These types of cycles may range from very short to exceedingly long, and are discussed further in Chapter 7.

❧ THE DRAMA OF CONCEPTION

When the egg bursts through the ovarian wall, it's usually picked up by the fallopian tube. Once it's released, it can take as little as 20 seconds for the fimbria to reach over and draw the egg into the tube itself. Assuming fertilization does not occur, the egg remains alive for a maximum of 24 hours, after which it simply disintegrates and either gets reabsorbed by the body or comes out in the menstrual flow. The egg is about the size of the period at the end of this sentence, hardly large enough to be seen reclining on the sanitary napkin.*

If fertilization does occur, it will take place in the outer third of the fallopian tube within a few hours of ovulation. (It does not take place in the uterus, as is popularly believed.) The lucky sperm may have journeyed up to several hours to reach its cherished date. The fertilized egg will then continue to be pulled toward the uterus by vibrating cilia, hairlike projections that line the fallopian tubes. After a week or so, it reaches its ultimate destination of the uterine lining, and begins the burrowing-in process. (See page 4 of color insert).

In order for conception to occur, though, there must be three factors present: the egg, the sperm, and a *medium* in which the sperm can travel to reach the fallopian tubes. The medium is the fertile-quality cervical fluid, which acts as a living conduit to direct the sperm through the cervix. Women produce cervical fluid under the influence of increasing levels of oestrogen in the first part of the cycle. Because the sperm can live up to five days in fertile-quality cervical fluid, it is actually possible to have intercourse on Monday and get pregnant from that act on Friday. So, without wanting to burst anyone's bubble, you could enjoy a deliciously romantic, snowy evening making love in front of the fire, but not actually *conceive* until five days later, while you're jogging, and your sweetheart is flying off to a meeting in Kalamazoo.

The body's response to conception is truly amazing. If you become pregnant, it would be disastrous for the endometrium to begin to disintegrate and shed in the form of menstruation, as it does cycle after cycle. So the pregnant body has a means of preventing that from happening. As soon as the fertilized egg burrows into the lining, it starts releasing a pregnancy hormone, HCG (Human Chorionic Gonadotropin), which sends a message back to the corpus luteum left behind on the ovarian wall. HCG signals the corpus luteum to remain alive beyond its usual maximum of 16 days, continuing to release progesterone long enough to sustain the nourishing lining. After several months, the placenta takes over, not only maintaining the endometrium, but providing all the oxygen and nutrients the fetus needs to thrive.

---

* A FAM instructor once told me that when she first began to menstruate, she would search her menstrual pads for a blue egg that resembled a robin's egg, and would continually be disappointed when she couldn't find it.

One of the reasons for "false negative" pregnancy tests is that the test is often done too soon, before the egg has had a chance to implant and start releasing HCG, or before the HCG has had time to reach a high-enough level to be detected in the urine or bloodstream. Of course, the occurrence of such misleading results could be decreased if women charted their cycles and could identify for themselves when ovulation, and therefore implantation, most likely took place.

I hope the last few pages have convinced you that your menstrual cycle is an amazing orchestration of biological events. Far from being only about menstruation, it is a continual hormonal chorus working together toward the ultimate goal of releasing and nurturing a healthy egg. And, as you will see in the next chapter, your body gives you conspicuous signs to help you understand on a daily basis what is transpiring within.

CHAPTER 5

The Three Primary Fertility Signs

I was completely ignorant of this bodily change every cycle. Boy, what my mother never told me. In fact, I learned about love and baby making from a neighborhood boy's declaration that a man puts his penis in a woman's "china."

—KELLEY HEIL, a *TCOYF* first edition reader

Ask the typical woman whether she is aware that her own body is a walking biological computer revealing the most enlightening information about her fertility, and you're likely to meet a blank stare. But the truth is, all women of reproductive age can easily learn how to observe and chart three primary fertility signs that their bodies produce. This information can then be used to tell them numerous things about their cycle, the most obvious being whether they can or can't get pregnant on any given day.

As you know, the three primary fertility signs virtually all ovulating women produce are:

1. waking temperature
2. cervical fluid
3. cervical position

Let's take each sign individually.

✌ WAKING (BASAL BODY) TEMPERATURE

The easiest sign to observe is the waking temperature, for the simple reason that it is usually very graphic and objective. Many women who have charted their fertility for a few months find that it becomes a fun challenge to predict the day their temperatures will shift.

A woman's preovulatory waking temperatures typically range from about 97.0 to 97.5 degrees Fahrenheit, with postovulatory temperatures rising to about 97.6 to 98.6 degrees. After ovulation, they will stay elevated until her next period, about 12 to 16 days later. If she were to become pregnant, they would remain high throughout her pregnancy.

Temperatures typically rise within a day or so after ovulation and are the result of the heat-inducing hormone, progesterone. Progesterone is released by the corpus luteum (the follicle that previously housed the egg before it burst out of the ovary, as discussed in the last chapter). So usually, by definition, the rise in temperature signifies that ovulation has *already* occurred. Waking temperatures within a cycle typically look like Chart 5.1 below.

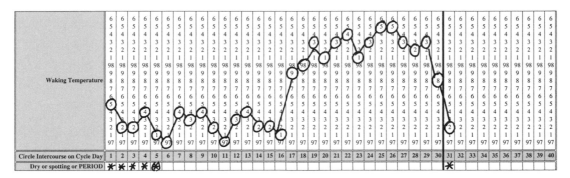

Chart 5.1. A typical waking temperature pattern. Note the rise in temperature starting on Day 17, which means that for this particular cycle, ovulation most likely occurred on Day 16.

When interpreting temperatures, it is important that you train your eyes to "see the forest through the trees." The key to doing so is to look for a *pattern* of lows and highs. In other words, you'll find that your temperatures before ovulation will go up and down in a low range, and the temperatures after ovulation will go up and down in a high range. The trick is to see the whole, and not focus so much on the day-to-day changes.*

---

* A very small percentage of women won't have biphasic temperature patterns even if they are ovulating. In such a case, contraceptors wouldn't be able to use waking temperatures as a fertility sign, but they would still be able to use the Billings Method, which relies on cervical fluid alone. This method, though, is not quite as accurate, and often requires more days of abstinence to be effective. Pregnancy achievers whose temperatures don't reflect a shift will need to initially use other means of determining whether they are ovulating, such as cervical fluid patterns (which are not as conclusive), ovulation predictor kits, blood tests, ultrasound, or endometrial biopsies.

I learned how helpful this concept is when I first taught at a women's clinic. Within a few weeks of the first class, I would inevitably start getting calls from clients who were convinced they must not be ovulating. But when they read me their temperatures over the phone, the pattern seemed perfectly evident. I couldn't understand why they didn't see what I saw. Then it dawned on me. They were not seeing the pattern, but were instead focusing on the fact that on Monday it was up, on Tuesday it was down, on Wednesday is was back up, and so on. Remember, stand back and see the whole picture. If you find that your temperatures are not obvious the first cycle, I would encourage you to chart for several cycles before you depend on FAM as a method of birth control.

The preovulatory temperatures are suppressed by oestrogen, whereas the postovulatory temperatures are increased by heat-inducing progesterone. In fact, one of the ways to remember that the second phase of the cycle is the "progesterone" phase is to think of it as the "pro-gestation" phase. In other words, this is the phase of the cycle that is warmer, as if designed to act as a human incubator to nurture an egg which may have just been fertilized.

I want to stress here that the rise in waking temperature almost always indicates that ovulation has already occurred. It does not reveal impending ovulation, as do the other two fertility signs, the cervical fluid and cervical position. In addition, you should also be aware that in only a minority of cycles will women ovulate at the lowest point of their temperature graph. Because a preovulatory temperature dip is so rare, women should not rely on its occurrence for fertility purposes. Rather, they should use the cervical fluid and cervical position to anticipate approaching ovulation.

You need to be aware of certain factors that can increase your waking temperature, such as:

- having a fever
- drinking alcohol the night before
- getting less than three consecutive hours sleep before taking it
- taking it at a substantially different time than usual
- using an electric blanket or heating pad that you normally don't use

However, as you will see in the following chapter, you needn't worry about the occasional erratic temperatures that may result. This is because you can discount them without compromising the accuracy of the method. In any case, FAM gives you two other signs to daily cross-check your fertility.

Temperatures, Stress, and the Dreaded Late Period

Waking temperatures can be extremely helpful in projecting how long a cycle will be, because they can identify if you've had a delayed ovulation that would cause your cycle to be longer than normal. Remember, once the temperature rises, it is typically a set 12 to 16 days until your period. And after you've charted for several months, you will be able to determine even more specifically what your particular postovulatory range usually is. (As previously discussed, for most women the phase after ovulation doesn't vary more than a couple of days.)

I myself experienced a classic delayed ovulation during a cycle when I was moving from one home to another. Three things were happening in my life that cycle, any one of which would have been enough to delay ovulation.

> *It was November of '86, and I had all the signs that I was approaching ovulation. My cervical fluid was getting very wet, and my cervix was rising and becoming more open and soft. On Day 16 of my cycle, though, I had to completely move out of my old home and into the new one, meaning every speck of dirt had to be washed off the walls of the apartment, and all of my boxes moved into my new home. In addition, I had to lecture at a midwifery school across town before catching a plane during rush hour to lecture at a conference in another state the next morning. So what was going on? I was moving, traveling, and totally stressed out.*
>
> *My body basically said, "Tell 'ya what. I think I'll just put your ovulation on hold until you're good and ready." In the end, as you can see from the chart below, I didn't even ovulate until about Day 24, and ended up with a 38-day cycle! Had I not been charting, I probably would have been completely panicked, thinking I was pregnant, since I had never in my life experienced such a long cycle.*

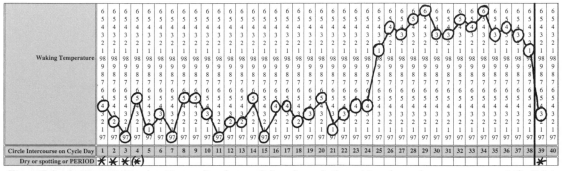

Chart 5.2. A temperature pattern showing a delayed ovulation. Note how the temperature shift didn't occur until Day 25.

This illustrates an important point. Women who don't chart are continually fearful when their periods seem "late," not realizing that long cycles are usually simply due to ovulating later. This is a phenomenon that is very easy to identify through waking temperatures.

I have used my own experience above to exemplify the point that there are numerous things that can delay (or even prevent) ovulation, including stress, travel, moving, illness, medication, strenuous exercise, and sudden weight change. But, by charting your temperature, you can accurately determine when you might be having a delayed ovulation. Whether you are trying to avoid or achieve pregnancy, knowing this information is invaluable, sparing you needless stress and confusion.

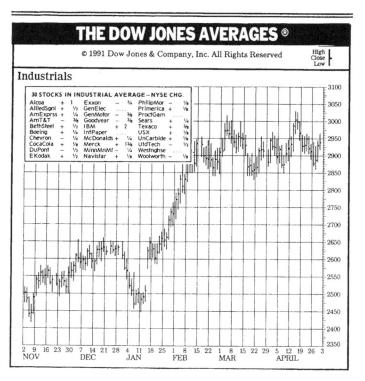

Dow Jones has a thermal shift!

✌ CERVICAL FLUID

One of the first things you'll probably be struck with when you start charting is the distinct pattern of cervical fluid throughout your cycle. And, if you are like most women who learn how to observe their fertility signs, the second thing you may experience is the sense of frustration and even anger when you realize how little you understood your body before. No, you were probably not experiencing recurring vaginal infections all the time. No, you were not dirty and in need of douching away the "discharge." In fact, the beauty of charting your cervical fluid is that you will be able to discern once and for all what is absolutely normal from the symptomatic secretions that result from a true vaginal infection. For this reason, I would suggest you never use the "*d*-word" to describe your healthy cervical fluid. After all, we don't refer to men's healthy semen as "discharge."

Cervical fluid is to the woman what seminal fluid is to the man. Since men are always fertile, they produce seminal fluid continually. Women, on the other hand, are only fertile the few days around ovulation, and therefore only produce the substance necessary for sperm nourishment and mobility during that time. It is fairly intuitive. Sperm require a medium in which to live, move, and thrive—otherwise they will die. Once the sperm travel from the penis to the vagina, they need an analogous substance to sustain them. But the only time it is critical for the sperm to survive is around the time the egg is released. It's for this reason that women produce the substance that resembles semen for only a few days per cycle.

In essence, the fertile cervical fluid functions exactly like the seminal fluid. It provides an alkaline medium to protect the sperm from an otherwise acidic vagina. In addition, it provides nourishment for the sperm, acts as a filtering mechanism, and functions as a medium in which to move.

In a nutshell, a woman's cervical fluid starts to develop and resemble a man's seminal fluid in a very predicable way. After the woman's period and directly under the influence of rising oestrogen, the cervical fluid typically starts to develop in the pattern shown on the next page.

In other words, right after your period, you may have a very dry vaginal sensation and observe *nothing* near the vaginal opening. Or you may notice a slight moisture similar to the way it would feel if you touched the inside of your cheek for a second. Your finger would have a dampness on it that would evaporate within a few seconds. This is the way the vaginal opening typically feels when there is no cervical fluid.

After perhaps a few days of this dryness, you may begin to develop a type of cervical fluid that is best described as *sticky,* like the paste you used in elementary school. Occasionally, it may even resemble drying rubber cement in that it is

CERVICAL FLUID PATTERNS

Cervical Fluid	Description	Accompanying Vaginal Sensation
(Menstruation)		
Nothing/dry	No cervical fluid present.	Dry
Sticky	Pasty, tacky, crumbly, gummy, springy, and dry like rubber cement. Usually white or yellow.	Dry or sticky
Creamy	Lotiony, milky, smooth. Usually white or yellow.	Wet, moist, gooey, or cold
Slippery and/or eggwhite	Slippery, will usually stretch. Clear, streaked, or opaque.	Wet, lubricative, slippery, or humid
Nothing/dry (or sticky)	No cervical fluid present.	Dry (or sticky)
(Menstruation)		

somewhat rubbery and slightly "springy," but the critical point is that it is *not wet.* The sticky and "rubber-cement" type of cervical fluid in themselves are not conducive to sperm survival, but for contraceptive purposes are considered possibly fertile if found *before* ovulation.

The next type of cervical fluid you may notice for several days is *creamy* or lotionlike. It tends to feel rather cold at the vaginal opening, just as hand lotion itself feels cool to the touch. Sometimes the cervical fluid is so wet or watery that it is hard to physically handle (with a consistency similar to skim milk), but the obvious clue to your fertility at that point is the very wet vaginal *sensation* you will feel.

The final and most fertile cervical fluid resembles raw *eggwhite.* It's extremely slippery and can stretch from one to even ten inches. (This ability to stretch is called spinnbarkeit, or "spin," for short.) It's usually clear or partially streaked, but it can be yellow-, pink-, or red-tinged, all indicating the presence of possible ovulatory bleeding. It could also be very watery. The critical determinant of this quality cervical fluid is the extremely wet and lubricative vaginal sensation you usually feel. It may even leave a fairly symmetrical, round pattern of fluid on your underwear due to its high water content.*

* Women in their early 20s may have as many as 4 or 5 days of eggwhite, but by their mid-30s, most will only have a day or two.

THE CERVIX WITH MAGNIFICATION OF SPERM IN INFERTILE AND FERTILE CERVICAL FLUID

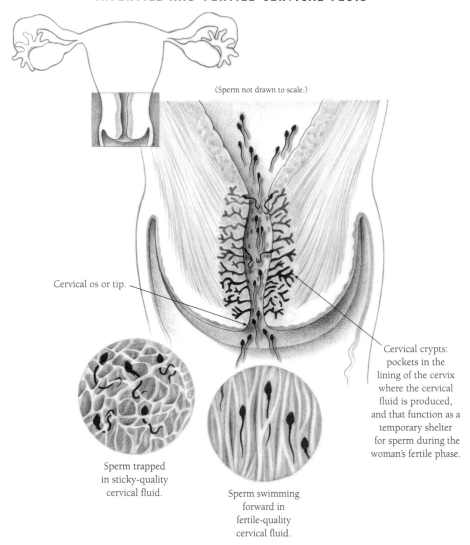

(Sperm not drawn to scale.)

Cervical os or tip.

Cervical crypts: pockets in the lining of the cervix where the cervical fluid is produced, and that function as a temporary shelter for sperm during the woman's fertile phase.

Sperm trapped in sticky-quality cervical fluid.

Sperm swimming forward in fertile-quality cervical fluid.

The most important feature of this extremely fertile cervical fluid is the lubricative quality. I cannot stress enough the importance of paying attention to the slippery sensation you will feel as you approach ovulation. You may even notice that the lubricative vaginal sensation continues a day or two beyond the actual stretchy eggwhite. *Pay close attention, because that sensation indicates that you are still extremely fertile.* Of course, vaginal sensation should not be confused with sexual lubrication. Vaginal sensation is something you simply feel throughout the day, without actually observing anything. In the end, quality is more important than quantity when evaluating the fertility of cervical fluid.

CERVICAL FLUID ON UNDERWEAR

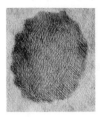

Very fertile-quality cervical fluid often forms a fairly symmetrical round circle, due to its high concentration of water.

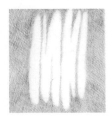

Nonwet-quality cervical fluid tends to form more of a rectangle or line on your underwear.

After oestrogen has peaked, the cervical fluid changes abruptly, often within a few hours. This is due to the sudden drop in oestrogen combined with the surge of progesterone following ovulation. In other words, it may take up to a week for the fertile-quality cervical fluid to build up, but then it will usually dry up in less than a day. This sudden drying of the cervical fluid is the best way to know that oestrogen has plummeted and that progesterone has taken over. The lack of wet cervical fluid will usually last the duration of the cycle. Note in the graphic on the next page that the phases of cervical fluid buildup and subsequent drying are usually not symmetrical.

Circle Intercourse on Cycle Day	1	2	3	4	5	6	7	8	9	10	11	12	13	14	15	16	17	18	19	20	21	22	23	24	25	26	27	28	29	30	31	32	33	34	35	36	37	38	39	40
Eggwhite																																								
Creamy																																								
Sticky																																								
Dry, Spotting or PERIOD	✱	✱	✱	✱	—	—	—	—	—								—	—	—	—	—	—	—	—	—	—	—	—	—	—	✱									
Fertile Phase and PEAK DAY																PK																								
Vaginal Sensation				dry	≈	≈	≈	≈	dry	dry	sticky	cold	wet	wet	lube	dry	≈	≈	≈	≈	≈	≈	≈	≈	≈	≈	≈	≈	≈								
Cervical Fluid Description																																								
Eggwhite Slippery, Will Usually Stretch Clear/Streaked/Opaque Lube, Wet or Humid Feeling											really wet, white cream	I" stretchy	4" clear eggwhite																										
Creamy Lotion, Milky, Smooth Usually White or Yellow Wet, Moist or Cold Feeling									a lot more, lotiony																														
Sticky Pasty, Crumbly, Opaque Rubber-Cement Dry or Sticky Feeling							scant sticky	scant sticky	little more, sticky																											

Chart 5.3. A typical cervical fluid pattern. There is usually a gradual progression from dry to sticky to wetter types, seen here in 2 days each of creamy and eggwhite. Also notice that the vaginal sensation generally corresponds with the cervical fluid ("lube" is used to signify a lubricative sensation at the vaginal opening). Finally, observe how she records Day 1 of the new menses on the same chart before repeating it again on a new chart. Every cycle is clearly delineated with a vertical closing line.

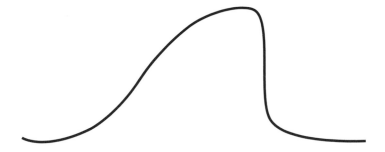

Finally, in the day or so before menstruation, women may occasionally notice a very wet, watery sensation, which in some women even resembles watery eggwhite. This is due to the drop in progesterone that precedes the disintegration of the lining of the uterus. The first part of the endometrium to flow out is typically water, hence the very wet sensation. Obviously, this wet fluid immediately preceding menstruation does not indicate a fertile time.

A trick to help you identify the actual quality of the cervical fluid is to notice what it feels like to run your tissue (or your finger) across your vaginal lips. Does it feel dry, impeding movement? Is it smooth? Or does it simply glide across? When you are dry, the tissue won't pass across your vaginal lips smoothly. But as you approach ovulation, your cervical fluid gets progressively more lubricative, and thus the tissue should just glide easily.

The concept of paying special attention to wet sensations is especially important for women who seem to have some type of cervical fluid almost every day. In other words, for some women, their Basic Infertile Pattern (BIP) on either side of their fertile phase is to have sticky-quality cervical fluid rather than being truly dry. It is even more important for these women to learn how to identify that change to a fertile-quality cervical fluid, which I discuss in further detail in Appendix B.

Knowing What's What

One of the saddest examples of a woman being misled about the nature of normal cervical fluid was a client I had a few years ago.

> *Brandy was a young woman who attended my class after having been on the Pill six years. Prior to my seminar she endured a traumatic, humiliating, and painful diagnostic test—all because she had never been taught to recognize the amazing signs her body produces every cycle.*

Brandy noticed that every now and then when she would have a bowel movement, she would feel a slippery substance when she used the toilet paper. She became quite concerned that perhaps something was wrong with her intestinal tract, because she only noticed it after using the bathroom, and only periodically. The doctor suggested she have a colonoscopy to rule out inflammatory bowel disease or polyps. She was required to fast a couple of days, have an enema, and then be subjected to one of the most painful experiences of her life. And why?

Because she was experiencing the absolutely normal and common occurrence of fertile eggwhite cervical fluid flowing from the vagina. Since that type is so slippery and profuse, it can easily be spread to the rectum with tissue paper. Of course, it is no wonder she only experienced this slippery substance every now and then, since she only produced eggwhite around the time of ovulation.

Such accounts of unnecessary and demoralizing tests are what have motivated me to educate women about the simple signs their own bodies tell them about their reproductive health. This is not to say that women don't occasionally have genuine infections or other problems and medical concerns. But the point is that women should be taught what is normal so that they can better detect problems themselves.

You should also be aware that as with the temperature, there are certain factors which can potentially mask cervical fluid, such as:

- vaginal infections
- seminal fluid
- arousal fluid
- spermicides and lubricants
- antihistamines (which can dry it)

In addition, women who have recently come off the Pill may notice one of two very different patterns. They may not produce much cervical fluid at all, since the Pill can temporarily compromise the ability of the cervical crypts to develop healthy cervical fluid. Or by contrast, they may tend to have continuous fertile-quality cervical fluid for up to several months. This is thought to be caused by excess synthetic oestrogen being released from the fatty tissue in the body.

Still another reason for the presence of this unusual pattern is that women on the Pill often develop cervical erosion, a condition in which the lining of the cervical canal grows out over the opening of the cervix, causing an irritation that leads to a type of wet cervical fluid. Some women may also experience midcycle spotting or bleeding during the first few cycles after going off it. Until all these conditions resolve themselves, women desiring to use FAM as birth control will need to be especially careful, as discussed in Chapter 9.

Finally, women often wonder how cervical fluid differs from seminal fluid and arousal fluid. Both are much thinner and typically dry quicker on the finger, whereas cervical fluid tends to remain on your finger until you wash it off. I will discuss this in greater detail in the following chapter. Of course, once again, because you have three fertility signs to rely on, you can have the peace of mind of knowing that you can still interpret your fertility by cross-checking the other two signs if there is any ambiguity.

🖋 CERVICAL POSITION (OPTIONAL SIGN)*

Have you ever noticed that intercourse can sometimes be fairly uncomfortable in certain positions? Maybe you have wonderful memories of a lazy Sunday morning with your partner. You woke up that day feeling pretty amorous, and slid on top of him. But a week later, when you wanted to relive that wonderful day, you noticed that, instead of experiencing the same delicious feeling, you felt a deep pain inside. What was going on? Why the discomfort this time?

Or have you ever noticed that there are times when it is quite easy to insert your diaphragm or cervical cap, but other times it seems almost impossible to find your cervix to insert it properly? Or worse yet, it seems like there is not even enough room to insert it? Or has your health practitioner ever commented on your appearing fertile during a pelvic exam, even though she had done nothing more than insert a speculum?

All of this has to do with the fact that your cervix, the lower part of the uterus that extends into your vagina, goes through some amazing cyclical changes throughout your cycle, all of which can be easily felt. Your cervix is actually a wealth of information about your fertility, literally at your fingertips.

---

* As you will read, "cervical position" as used in this book actually refers to more than just the height of the cervix in the vagina. However, it is easier to use this one term to describe the various cervical changes that occur in the cycle, particularly given that they're checked simultaneously, usually in a matter of seconds.

As with the cervical fluid, the cervix itself prepares for a pregnancy every cycle by transforming into a perfect "biological gate" through which the sperm can pass on their way to finding the egg. It does so by becoming soft and open around ovulation in order to allow the sperm passage through the uterus and on to the fallopian tubes. In addition, the cervix rises due to the oestrogenic effect on the ligaments that hold the uterus in place.

After your period and directly under the influence of oestrogen, your cervix typically starts to change. One of the easiest ways to remember how your cervix feels as you approach ovulation is the acronym SHOW, as seen in the following illustration.

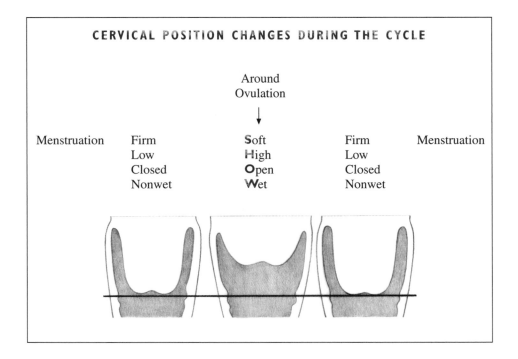

Let's take each facet in the order listed above. The cervix is normally firm like the tip of your nose, and only becomes soft and rather mushy, like your lips, as you approach ovulation. In addition, it is normally fairly low and closed, feeling somewhat like a dimple, and only rises and opens in response to the high levels of oestrogen around ovulation. And finally, it is the cervix itself that emits fertile-quality wet cervical fluid when the egg is about to be released. Chart 5.4 on the next page shows how to record your cervical changes.

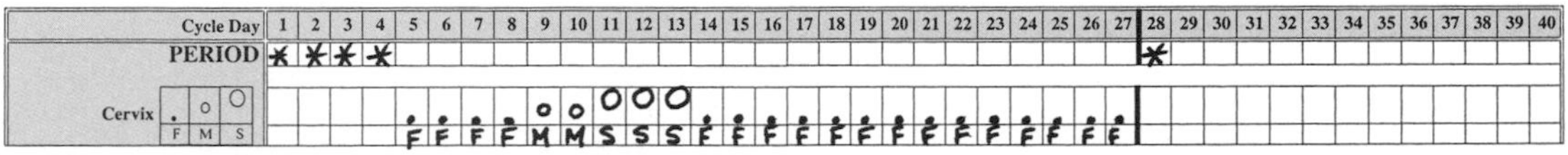

Cycle Day			1	2	3	4	5	6	7	8	9	10	11	12	13	14	15	16	17	18	19	20	21	22	23	24	25	26	27	28	29	30	31	32	33	34	35	36	37	38	39	40
PERIOD			✳	✳	✳	✳																							✳												
Cervix	.	o						✢	✢	✢	o o	o o	O O O																													
	F	M									M	M	S	S	S																											
		S						F	F	F					F	F	F	F	F	F	F	F	F	F	F	F	F	F													

Chart 5.4. A typical cervical position pattern. Note how the circles represent how open the cervix is and their position in the box represents how high it is. The letters below the circles stand for the firmness of the cervix—firm, medium, and soft.

◇ SECONDARY FERTILITY SIGNS

Many women are lucky enough to notice other signs on a regular basis, all of which are very helpful in being able to further understand their cycles. These signs are referred to as secondary fertility signs, because they do not necessarily occur in all women, or in every cycle in individual women. But they are still very practical for giving additional information to women to identify their fertile and infertile phases.

Secondary signs as ovulation approaches may include:

- midcycle spotting
- pain or achiness near the ovaries
- increased sexual feelings
- fuller vaginal lips or swollen vulva
- abdominal bloating
- water retention
- increased energy level
- heightened sense of vision, smell, and taste
- increased sensitivity in breasts and skin
- breast tenderness

The first sign listed above, midcycle or ovulatory spotting, is thought to be the result of the sudden drop in oestrogen just before ovulation. Because progesterone has not yet been released to sustain it, the lining often leaks a small amount of blood until the progesterone takes over. It can range from merely tingeing the slippery fertile cervical fluid to actually appearing bright red. Spotting is typically more common in long cycles.

Courtney represented the classic example of a woman not understanding the distinction between different causes of bleeding. She called saying she wanted to use FAM for birth control, but thought she might not be an appropriate candidate for the method because she had "such short cycles." When I questioned her about them, she said they were "literally every two weeks, but alternated heavy, light, heavy, light." Of course, what she was experiencing was a typical length cycle with classic ovulatory spotting. I encouraged her to take my Fertility Awareness class. I don't know if she still uses FAM for contraception, but she certainly understands her body a lot better than before.

As for the various pains that women often notice midcycle, there are several theories as to their causes. The important point is that you cannot say with certainty whether they are occurring before, during, or after you've actually ovulated.

Dull achiness:	This is thought to be caused by the swelling of numerous follicles in the ovaries as the eggs race for dominance and ultimate ovulation. It is typically felt as a general abdominal achiness, since both ovaries swell with growing follicles as the woman approaches ovulation.
A sharp pain:	This could be the actual moment that the egg bursts through the ovarian wall and is usually felt on only one side.
Crampiness:	This is probably the result of irritation of the abdominal lining caused by leakage of blood or follicular fluid released from the ruptured egg follicle. It could also be due to contractions of the fallopian tubes around ovulation.

Because there are several pains that may occur, none of them are considered primary fertility signs that can be depended upon independently. But ovulatory pain in general is an excellent secondary fertility sign to corroborate the three primary signs. The pain is usually referred to as *mittelschmerz* (midpain) and is felt by many women around their ovulation. It typically lasts anywhere from a few minutes to a few hours, and is usually felt on the side where ovulation occurs.

One of the more interesting secondary fertility signs is that of a swollen vulva just before ovulation. If women are especially attentive as their cervical fluid becomes slippery and wet, they may notice that their vulva becomes more swollen on the side on which they ovulate. In fact, there is another secondary fertility sign that can also help you determine on which side you will ovulate, as seen on the next page.

If you are especially attentive as you approach ovulation, you may be able to feel a small lymph gland swell to about the size of a pea. This is the Lymph Node Sign, and as seen in the illustration below, can be felt by lying down and placing your hand near your groin. By positioning your middle finger just over the pulsating artery of your leg, your index finger will hopefully be able to feel the tender and enlarged lymph gland. This sign is particularly intriguing since it usually indicates the side on which ovulation occurs.

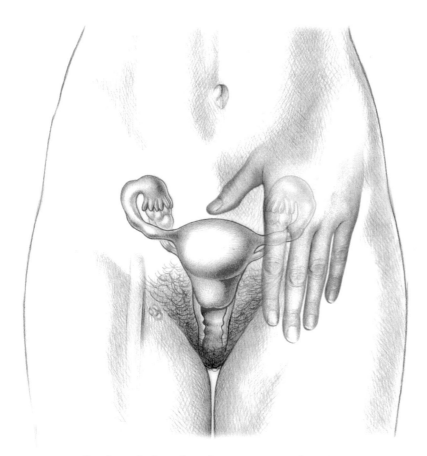

Checking the lymph node as you approach ovulation

In addition to those signs previously listed, you may find through charting that you yourself have some unique secondary fertility signs. I've certainly heard of many in my years of counseling women:

> *Sandy gets hiccups as ovulation approaches. The skin on Cindy's thumb actually cracks in a somewhat painful lesion every cycle around ovulation. But through learning to chart, she was able to at least identify what caused it. And Kendel develops such a heightened sense of smell around ovulation that, as she describes it, if her chef-husband cooks something in their house during her fertile phase, she can smell it for days after and no amount of open windows will relieve her of the nausea. Likewise, if she eats potato chips, or anything with mustard on it, she practically sterilizes her hands afterward, but unfortunately can still smell the residual effects. But if she is outside her fertile phase, he can whip up an onion-garlic casserole, and she's not the least bit affected by it.*

When women learn that all this is happening inside their body on a regular basis, they are often amazed. And to think that all they were taught about their menstrual cycles in the sixth grade was whether to opt for tampons or sanitary napkins during their periods!

CHAPTER 6

How to Observe and Chart Your Fertility Signs

*W*hen some women first hear about observing fertility signs, their reaction is typically:

"You've got to be kidding me. Too much bother."
"There's no way. Take my temperature every day?"
"What a hassle. Who'd do it?"

I, too, had a similar response when I first heard about charting the cycle 18 years ago. But once I learned how simple it really was, I was chagrined. Today, I have a different attitude. Quite simply: *Charting is a privilege rather than a burden.*

How could I have been so ignorant about such a fundamental aspect of my body before I learned to be so aware? A cynic might question the time involved in checking every day. But I think many would agree that it is infinitely more appealing to take one's temperature in the morning before getting up than to stop lovemaking to insert a diaphragm or cervical cap, or to contend with the numerous side effects and inconveniences of other methods. And for those frustrated in their desire to get pregnant, the time involved is minuscule compared to the inevitable office visits and procedures for those not educated in FAM.

To show how simple charting really is, let me make an analogy. If someone were to ask you to describe how to tie your shoelaces, you might begin:

Let's see. Well, you take your right shoelace, and place it over the left one. Then take the left shoelace and twist it under the right, pulling both shoelaces away from each other to form a twisted knot. Then make a loop with the right shoelace, which was originally the left. Take the left shoelace and . . .

I'm exhausted just trying to write the rest of the directions. If you had to learn something as simple as tying your shoes through following directions, you'd probably never get it right. Observing and charting your fertility signs is really no different. Once you learn the basic principles, it becomes second nature.

When reading this chapter on how to observe and chart fertility signs, refer to the sample birth control and pregnancy achievement charts on pages 72 and 73. (Trust me. It's not as involved as it may first appear.) Several versions of blank master charts are printed on the last pages of the book. Whichever you choose to use should be enlarged to about 125%.

The First Day of Charting

Although it may be easier to wait until the first day of your next period in order to start charting, you can begin on any day so long as it is, in fact, reflective of how long it has been since the first day of your last period. (See Chart 6.1 below.) Just remember that for closure, you should draw a vertical line in between the last day of your partially completed cycle and the first day of your new period. You will then be ready to begin charting your first complete cycle on Day 1 of a new chart.

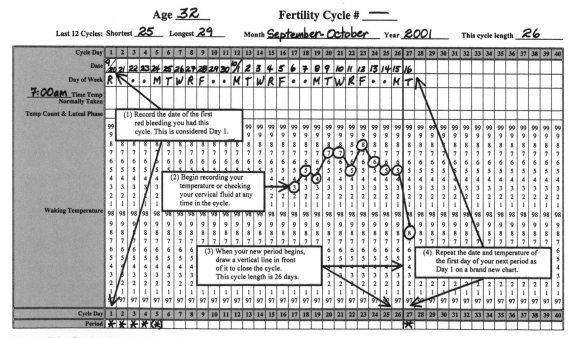

Chart 6.1. Beginning to chart in midcycle.

WHEN TO START CHARTING
FOLLOWING SPECIAL CIRCUMSTANCES

Coming off the Pill

There is no way of predicting how long it will take for your cycles to return to their former patterns before you were on hormones. Some women may ovulate within a couple of weeks while others may take several months or even years. Ideally, you should begin charting on the first day of the withdrawal bleeding you typically experience during your week off the Pill, recording Day 1 as the first day of that bleeding. If that is not possible, follow the directions on page 70 for beginning to chart midcycle.

Irregular Cycles

Unless you've been recording your period, it can be challenging to begin charting cycles that vary extensively from month to month. Assuming you have, follow the directions on the previous page. But if you haven't, just start recording your observations on Day 1 of the chart, acknowledging that the cycle day numbers don't reflect the true days of your cycle. Once you menstruate, that will become Day 1 of your first full cycle.

Miscarriage

The amount of time it takes you to resume cycling following a miscarriage will depend on a number of factors, including how far along you were when you miscarried. If you didn't have any major complications, you might resume ovulating shortly after, with your body perceiving the miscarriage as a period. This means that you could start charting within a few weeks, counting Day 1 as the first day you started bleeding. Of course, you should only start charting when you are emotionally ready.

Childbirth

How quickly you resume ovulating after giving birth will depend on several factors, with the most important being whether or not you breastfeed. If you don't, your cycles may resume very quickly, as soon as a month or so after you give birth. If you do breastfeed, it could take up to a couple of years, depending on how often you do so. In any case, charting during breastfeeding can be somewhat tricky, so I encourage you to read Appendixes B and C carefully.

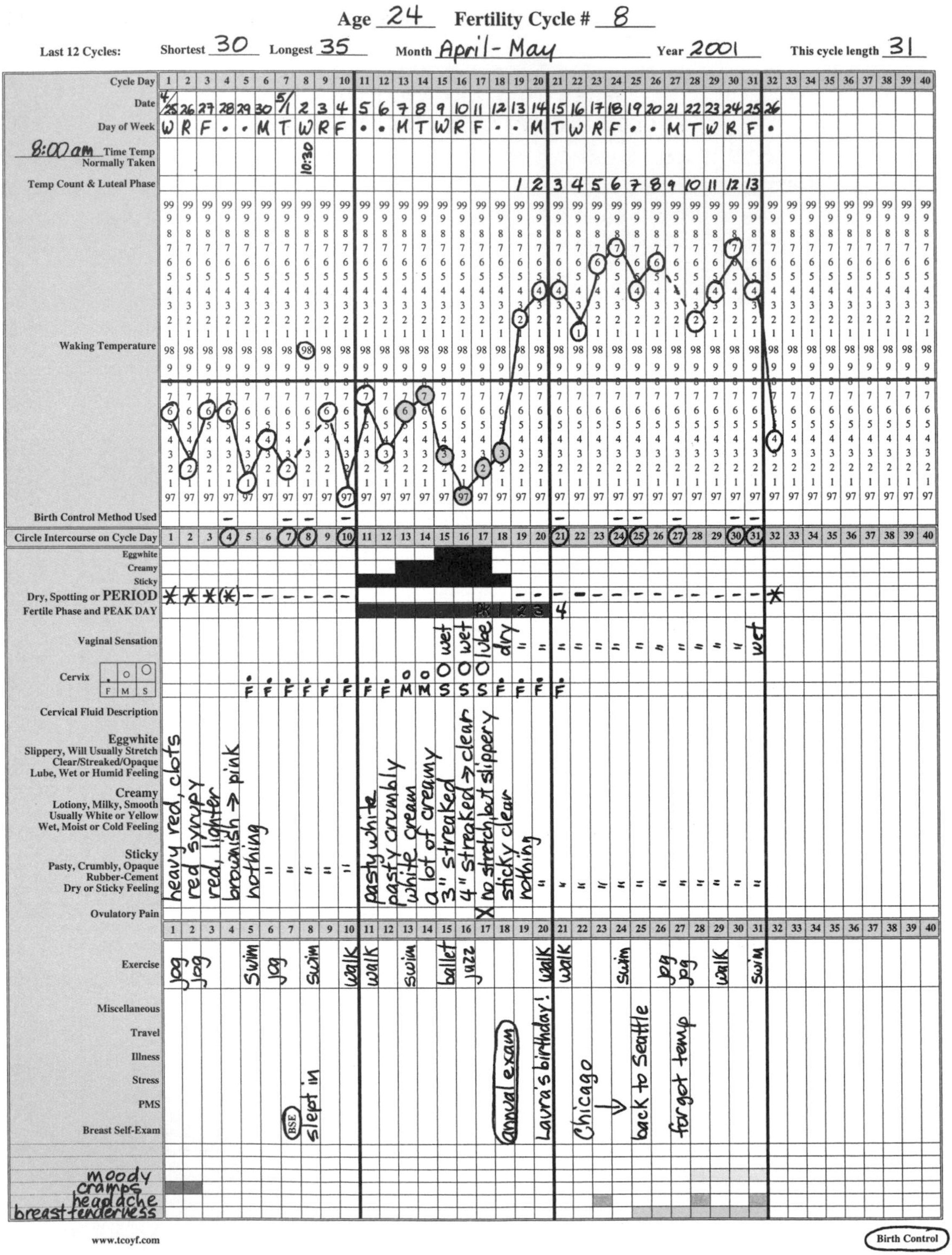

Age 24   Fertility Cycle # 8

Last 12 Cycles: Shortest 30   Longest 35   Month April-May   Year 2001   This cycle length 31

| Cycle Day | 1 | 2 | 3 | 4 | 5 | 6 | 7 | 8 | 9 | 10 | 11 | 12 | 13 | 14 | 15 | 16 | 17 | 18 | 19 | 20 | 21 | 22 | 23 | 24 | 25 | 26 | 27 | 28 | 29 | 30 | 31 | 32 | 33 | 34 | 35 | 36 | 37 | 38 | 39 | 40 |

Date: 4/25 26 27 28 29 30 5/1 2 3 4 5 6 7 8 9 10 11 12 13 14 15 16 17 18 19 20 21 22 23 24 25 26

Day of Week: W R F · · M T W R F · · M T W R F · · M T W R F · · M T W R F ·

Time Temp Normally Taken: 8:00 am   (10:30)

Temp Count & Luteal Phase: 1 2 3 4 5 6 7 8 9 10 11 12 13

Waking Temperature

Birth Control Method Used

Circle Intercourse on Cycle Day: 1 2 3 (4) 5 6 (7) (8) 9 (10) 11 12 13 14 15 16 17 18 19 20 (21) 22 23 (24) (25) 26 (27) 28 29 (30) (31) 32 33 34 35 36 37 38 39 40

Eggwhite / Creamy / Sticky

Dry, Spotting or PERIOD: X X X (X) - - - - - - - - - - - - - - - - - - *

Fertile Phase and PEAK DAY: PK 1 2 3 4

Vaginal Sensation: wet wet wet lube dry ... wet

Cervix: F M S

Cervical Fluid Description: F F F F F F F F M M S S O O S S F F F F

Cervical Fluid:
- Eggwhite: Slippery, Will Usually Stretch, Clear/Streaked/Opaque, Lube, Wet or Humid Feeling
- Creamy: Lotiony, Milky, Smooth, Usually White or Yellow, Wet, Moist or Cold Feeling
- Sticky: Pasty, Crumbly, Opaque, Rubber-Cement, Dry or Sticky Feeling

Notes (handwritten): heavy red, clots / red syrupy / red, lighter / brownish → pink / nothing / pasty white / pasty crumbly / white cream / a lot of creamy / 3" streaked / 4" streaked → clear / no stretch but slippery / sticky clear / nothing

Ovulatory Pain

Exercise: jog jog / swim jog / swim / walk walk / swim / ballet jazz / walk walk / swim / jog jog / walk / swim

Miscellaneous / Travel / Illness / Stress / PMS / Breast Self-Exam:
(BSE) slept in / annual exam / Laura's birthday! / Chicago / back to Seattle / forgot temp

moody / cramps / headache / breast tenderness

www.tcoyf.com   Birth Control

Chart 6.2. Natural Birth Control.   ▬ Fertile Phase

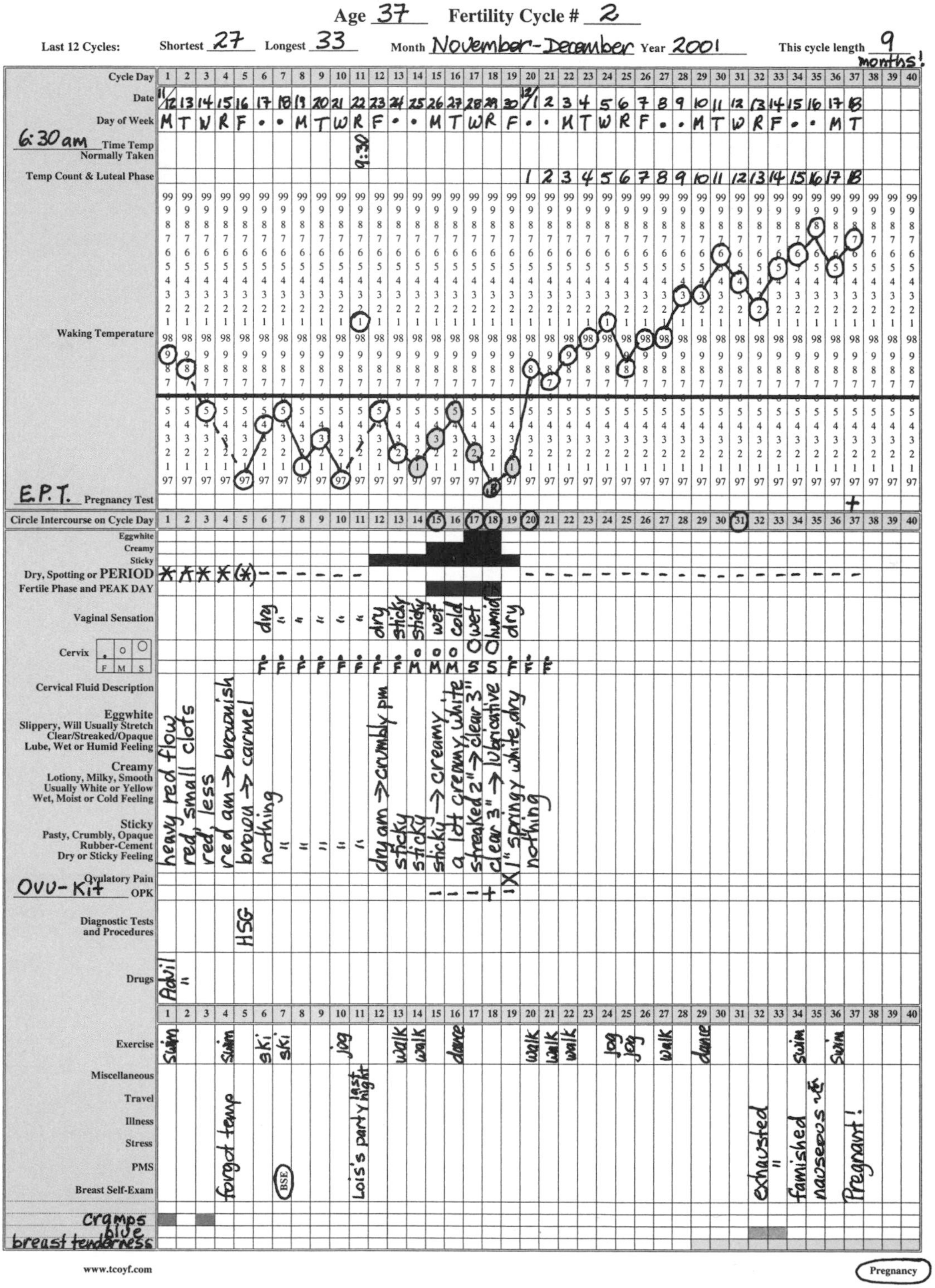

Age 37   Fertility Cycle # 2

Last 12 Cycles: Shortest 27 Longest 33   Month November-December Year 2001   This cycle length 9 months!

6:30 am — Time Temp Normally Taken

E.P.T. — Pregnancy Test

Ovu-Kit — OPK

Chart 6.3. Pregnancy Achievement. ■■■ Fertile Phase

www.tcoyf.com

Pregnancy

৯৯ WAKING TEMPERATURE

The first time I heard that FAM involved taking a temperature every day, I thought it wouldn't be worth it. But 6,575 temperatures later, I've lost sight of what the big deal was. In fact, it's nice to have an excuse to snuggle a minute, warm and cuddly—rather than feeling the need to bolt out of bed the second the alarm goes off.

Now granted, in order to get an accurate reading, you can't do fifty jumping jacks before taking it. Nor, for that matter, can you gab on the phone with your Aunt Maria, or even get up to urinate first thing upon awakening, even if you downed two pints of lemonade the night before.

But on the positive side, taking your temperature will provide you with a wealth of information about your body that, when all is said and done, will probably have taken about a minute of your day. To fully appreciate what I am saying, let me list the benefits of taking your temperature every morning. You will be able to identify:

- if you are ovulating
- when it would be safe to have deliciously natural intercourse without risk of an unplanned pregnancy
- when you are *no longer* fertile, if you desire to avoid a pregnancy, or when you are *still* fertile if you desire to achieve one
- when you will get your period
- if there are potential problems in your cycle

Taking Your Temperature

1. Take your daily temperature first thing upon awakening, *before any other activity* such as getting up to use the bathroom, brushing your teeth, or talking on the phone. It should be taken throughout the cycle, ideally during menstruation as well. (If you prefer, you may restrict temperature-taking to about one-third of the cycle, as discussed in Chapter 10 on "Shortcuts." However, I would strongly discourage you from using shortcuts until you have charted several cycles.)

2. If using a digital thermometer, wait until it beeps, usually about one minute. If using a glass basal body thermometer, leave it in five minutes. Digital thermometers should reflect a clear pattern of lows and highs. But if the temperatures seem confusing, see page 301 or use a glass thermometer.

3. Take your temperature orally. (If you find that you don't get a clear temperature pattern, you may want to try taking it vaginally. Just be aware that it's important to be consistent and always take it from the same opening throughout the cycle because vaginal temperatures tend to be higher than oral temps.)

4. Take it about the same time every day, within an hour or so. However, you don't need to be a slave to your thermometer. If you sleep in on the weekends, or for whatever reason take it later or earlier, just be sure to note the time on your chart. For every half hour you sleep in, the temperature tends to creep up about one-tenth of a degree. (For how to handle the outlying temperatures that may result, see the Rule of Thumb, page 78.)

5. Take your temperature after *at least three consecutive hours* of sleep which, for most women, is first thing upon awakening in the morning. Note that if you normally take it at 8 A.M., but one morning you wake up at 6 A.M. and have to go to the bathroom, it is better to take your temperature at 6 and then get up. Otherwise, you will have had only two hours sleep after getting up (from 6 to 8), which would make the reading inaccurate.

6. If you use a glass basal body thermometer, shake it down the day before. (This is because shaking the thermometer down upon awakening could raise your temperature.)

7. If you suspect you are getting sick, be sure to use a traditional fever or digital thermometer rather than the glass basal body type, since basal thermometers don't go above 100 degrees F. (Note that the high temperatures will be eliminated by the Rule of Thumb.)

Charting Your Temperature

1. It's a good idea to record your temperature sometime in the morning. If this isn't practical, it doesn't need to be done until the evening, since most digital and glass thermometers will remain accurate until read or shaken down. (Just be sure not to leave your thermometer roasting on a hot windowsill all day.)

2. If the temperature falls between two numbers on a glass thermometer, always record the lowest temperature.

3. Record and connect the temperatures with a pen.

4. Unusual events such as stress, illness, travel, or moving should be noted in the Miscellaneous row of the chart and taken into consideration when interpreting the temperature pattern. And temperatures taken earlier or later than usual should be noted in the Time Temp Taken row.

5. If you think a temperature is outside the normal range, wait until the next day to draw the connecting line. Omit any aberrant temperatures by drawing a dotted line between the normal temperatures. Record possible reasons for their aberrations (see Chart 6.5 on page 78).

A GUIDE TO THERMOMETERS

Digital Thermometers

For most women, the best type of thermometer is digital. It usually requires only about a minute to register, and typically beeps when it is ready. For charting purposes, it should have memory capable of storing the last temperature until you retrieve it at the time you record. Also, although it is imperative that it be accurate to within .1 degree F (for example, 97.4), do not use those that measure to within 1/100th of a degree (for example, 97.46), since the latter are unnecessary and confusing. Be attentive to the possibility of needing to change its batteries.

You can rely on digital thermometers as long as they clearly show the midcycle thermal shift that signals the passing of ovulation. If you are following all the FAM rules for birth control, using digitals shouldn't increase your risk of pregnancy, though it could force you to assume that you're fertile for more days than you really are. Thus, if your temperatures seem confusing, do not show a clear pattern of pre- and postovulatory lows and highs, or do not correlate closely with the other fertility signs, switch to a glass thermometer.

I personally prefer the BD basal digital thermometer. I like the fact that it beeps every four seconds to let you know that it is placed correctly, retains the temperature until recorded, and has a built-in light.

Glass Basal Body Thermometers

Glass thermometers are considered the most reliable thermometer for detecting your waking basal body temperature (BBT). However, they do require a full five minutes to register an accurate reading. It must specifically say "basal body" as opposed to "fever thermometer." A basal body thermometer is easier to read because the temperatures are shown in increments of .1 rather than .2 degrees F. But BBT thermometers only go up to 100 degrees F, so if you have reason to think you are developing a fever, be sure to use a fever thermometer during those days.

Ear Thermometers

Although I was quite optimistic when I wrote the first edition of this book, the general consensus in the Fertility Awareness community is that ear thermometers are still not reliable enough to be used for charting purposes (which is to say they don't clearly show a thermal shift).

Drawing the Coverline

Ultimately, the reason you are charting your temperature is to determine when you ovulated in any given cycle. Remember that after ovulation, temperatures quickly rise above the range of lows that preceded it. This thermal shift is often so obvious that you'll be able to spot it simply by glancing at the chart. However, in order to interpret accurately, you'll want to draw a *coverline* to help you differentiate between temperatures that are low (preovulatory) and high (postovulatory). The coverline is easily drawn using the following instructions:*

1. After your period ends, as you are charting your temperatures, always notice the highest of the previous six days.
2. Identify the first day your temperature rises at least two-tenths of a degree higher than that highest temperature.
3. Go back and highlight the last six temperatures before the rise.
4. Draw the coverline one-tenth of a degree above the highest of that cluster of six highlighted days preceding the rise. (Note that high temperatures during your period are irrelevant. It's not unusual to have high temperatures during menstruation due to the residual effects of progesterone lingering from the last cycle. Other aberrant high temperatures can also be discounted as seen by the Rule of Thumb on the following page.)

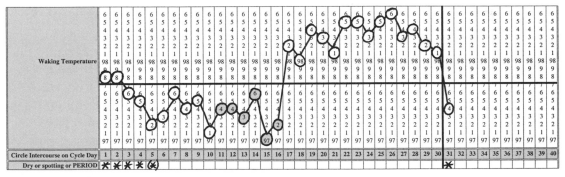

Chart 6.4. A standard temperature pattern with coverline. Note the cluster of six temps before the thermal shift on Day 17 is highlighted. (An alternative way of drawing the coverline is discussed in Appendix H.)

* An alternative way of drawing a coverline is discussed in Appendix H.

Outlying Temperatures and the Rule of Thumb

If you have an occasional temperature that is artificially high due to reasons such as fever, a restless night's sleep, or alcohol consumption the night before, you may cover the outlying temperature with your thumb when you are determining your coverline. Circle the outlying temperature as you would any other, but then draw dotted lines between the temperatures on either side, so that it doesn't interfere with your ability to interpret your chart. You essentially ignore the abnormal temperature, and thus still must count back the required six days, *not including the day eliminated,* to determine your coverline.

You should also be aware that temperatures tend to rise about two-tenths of a degree for every hour you sleep in, but again, you simply follow the guidelines above. See the box on page 80 for how to handle special circumstances such as Daylight Savings and night shifts, as well as page 312 in Appendix A for how to deal with fevers.

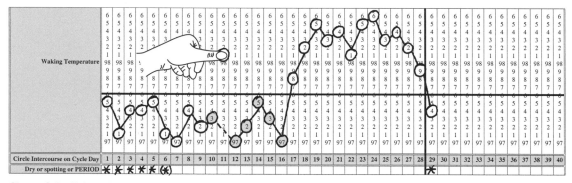

Chart 6.5. Using the Rule of Thumb for aberrant temperatures. Note the thumb covering the outlying temperature on Day 11. A dotted line should be drawn between the days on both sides of it. Also notice that Day 11 is not counted among the necessary 6 days to draw the coverline.

Types of Thermal Shift Patterns

Chart 6.4 on page 77 shows a coverline drawn with a *standard* thermal shift pattern. The standard pattern clearly shows the range of low temperatures, followed by a distinct thermal shift of at least two-tenths of a degree, followed by a consistent range of high temperatures that remain until the end of that cycle. Standard patterns are the easiest to interpret, and thus drawing their coverline is a breeze.

Most women tend to experience the same type of thermal shift patterns within their own cycles, although they may see variation now and then. While the standard shift is the most common, there are three other types that some women experience. They are shown in Chart 6.6 on the next page.

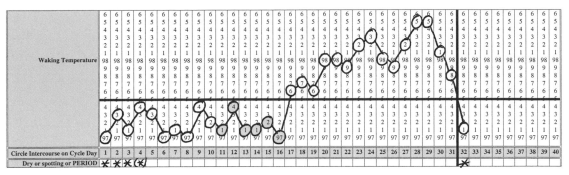

Chart 6.6a. The stair-step rise. Note how the temperature rises in an initial spurt of about 3 days on Day 17 before rising further on Day 20.

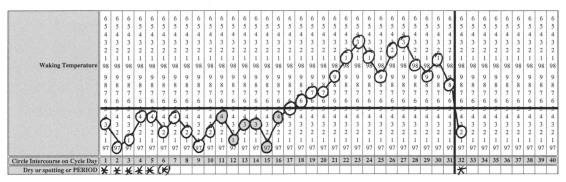

Chart 6.6b. The slow-rise. Note how the temperature rises one-tenth of a degree at a time, starting with Day 17 as the first temperature higher than the cluster of the six before it. Also notice that with this particular pattern, the coverline cannot be drawn using the standard instruction. (See page 308 for how you would do so.)

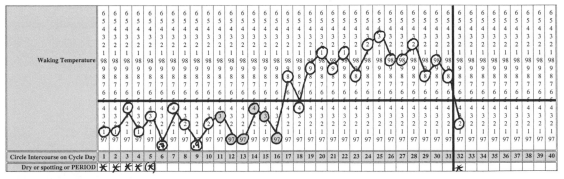

Chart 6.6c. The fall-back rise. Note how the temperature initially rises above the coverline on Day 17, but then falls back the next day before rising above again on Day 19.

While the above patterns can be a bit confusing initially, they are easy to interpret once you are familiar with them. Pages 307–309 in Appendix A give further explanation should you find that you have cycles that resemble them.

SPECIAL TEMPERATURE CIRCUMSTANCES

British Summer Time

While British Summer Time can be a welcome change, it can be a minor annoyance if it happens to occur right smack in the middle of your fertile phase. The time change has the same effect as taking your temperature an hour later than usual in the fall (and thus they may tend to be higher than normal) and an hour earlier in the spring (and thus they may tend to be lower than normal).

If you are one of the lucky women who don't seem to notice any effect on your temperature whether you awaken later or earlier than usual, then just skip this section altogether. Likewise, if you are already in your (postovulatory) luteal phase when British Summer Time occurs, you don't really need to do anything. Just be aware that your temps may tend to be a little higher or lower for the few days it may take until your body adjusts to the time shift.

If your body is sensitive to time differences, however, and especially if you are approaching ovulation, you may want to adjust your waking times for a few days leading up to the weekend. Using a 6 A.M. wake-up time as an example, take your temperatures as follows:

In the Fall

Friday	6:00 A.M.	British Summer Time
Saturday	6:20 A.M.	British Summer Time

(Set your clock back one hour before you go to bed on Saturday night.)

Sunday	5:40 A.M.	Greenwich Mean Time
Monday	6:00 A.M.	Greenwich Mean Time

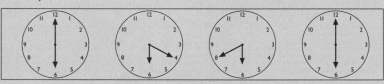

Fall

In the Spring

Friday	6:00 A.M.	Greenwich Mean Time
Saturday	5:40 A.M.	Greenwich Mean Time

(Set your clock ahead one hour before you go to bed on Saturday night.)

Sunday	6:20 A.M.	British Summer Time
Monday	6:00 A.M.	British Summer Time

Spring

Travel to Other Time Zones

If you travel to other time zones, think of it as going through British Summer Time changes for each time zone you travel through. So, for example, if you travel from West to East, the effect would be like taking your temp three hours earlier than usual. Likewise, if you traveled from east to west, it would be like taking your temp three hours later. The potential impact may last about as long as jet-lag, which can be about one day for every time zone you cross. As with the British Summer Time guidelines, if the travel occurs in your (postovulatory) luteal phase, it's no big deal. But if you are approaching ovulation, you may want to adjust your waking times for the few days leading up to the day you travel, in order to minimize the changes you would perhaps experience otherwise. Realistically, you should expect the temps to be higher or lower than they would be with just a one-hour time change.

Night-Shift Work

Working the night shift tends to come with many challenges, not the least of which is when to take your basal temperature. But remember, the definition of a basal temperature is the temp first thing upon awakening, which will not be the morning for those who work nights. (Of course, if your night job is really boring and you sleep through it, you've probably got bigger issues than when to take your temperature.)

The general rule in night-shift situations is still to take your temperature first thing upon awakening, but the difference is, it should be the first thing upon awakening from your longest, most restful sleep. For many of you, that will be late afternoon or evening.

If you work various shifts, you may find it more challenging to see a clear pattern of lows and highs. Depending on your work schedule, you may still be able to identify a clear thermal shift for every cycle, but if you cannot, you may need to rely on the other fertility signs discussed in this chapter.

A GENERAL NOTE ON SPECIAL TEMPERATURE CIRCUMSTANCES

While most of you will be able to recognize a thermal shift despite these challenges, you will want to be especially attentive to your cervical fluid and cervical position in order to clearly identify your fertile phase. And regardless, you should never use your temperatures for contraceptive purposes unless you can see a clear pattern of postovulatory highs above the coverline. If in doubt, wait until your next cycle or use a barrier.

How Temperature Patterns Predict Length of Cycles

The beauty of charting temperatures is that it can give you a sneak preview of how long your cycle will be simply by observing when the temperature rises. Remember that once your temperature shifts, it will remain basically the same length from the rise to your period. So, for example, if you experience a fever or a lot of stress during the first part of your cycle, you may experience a delayed ovulation that will be reflected in a late thermal shift. In such a case, you will still be able to count ahead to determine when you will menstruate.

Cassandra and Everett were clients of mine. They were a young couple who were very much in love with each other. They both attended college but still lived at home to save money for their future marriage. One weekend, Cassandra's family went out of town, and they took the opportunity to finally be together without her younger siblings barging in on them.

A couple of months later, I met with them for their private follow-up consultation. One of the first things that struck me about her charts was that she was having a long cycle with a delayed ovulation. When I asked her whether she was experiencing stress, the two of them glanced at each other and burst into nervous laughter. With a little prodding, I soon discovered that several days after her parents had returned, her mother called Cassandra into her bedroom to inquire what a whipped-cream cap was doing wedged between the mattress and the headboard. At least her charts would prevent her from worrying about a period that was sure to be late this cycle.

Chart 6.7 helps illustrate the point that the preovulatory phase can vary considerably both between women and within any one woman's pattern from cycle to cycle. The postovulatory phase, while varying somewhat from woman to woman, usually remains fairly constant for each individual woman (plus or minus a day or so).

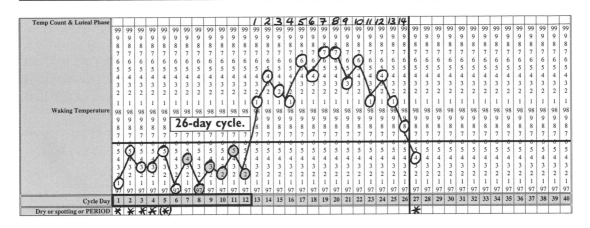

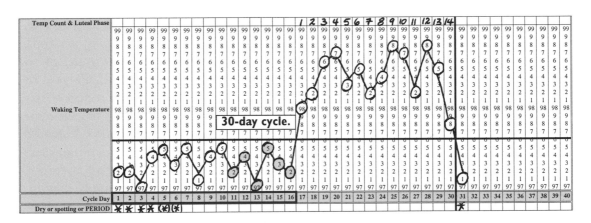

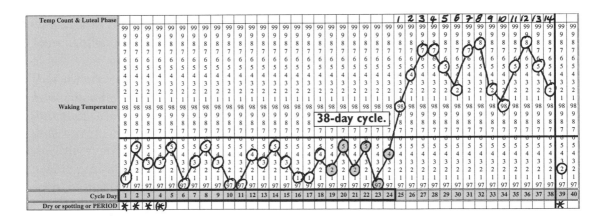

Chart 6.7. Temperature charts showing one woman's cycles of 26, 30, and 38 days. Note that the preovulatory phase varies in length, whereas the postovulatory (luteal) phase remains consistent from cycle to cycle.

ᵹᴀ CERVICAL FLUID

Virtually all ovulating women experience an observable pattern of changes in their cervical fluid throughout their cycles. Once they learn to recognize these subtle differences, they realize that interpreting the pattern is really very simple. When a woman is extremely fertile, her cervical fluid becomes wet and humid. You could say it gives a whole new meaning to "feeling hot and steamy."

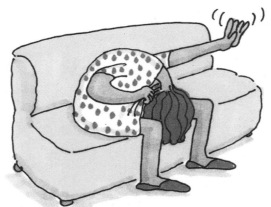

"Monica's been on this marvellous self-examination course"...

Indeed, as you approach ovulation, the eggwhite-quality cervical fluid most women experience can feel so slippery that you may have a sensation of slip-sliding on your underwear as you sit down.

Just as some women may initially balk at the idea of taking their temperature every morning, there are others who react similarly to the idea of checking their cervical fluid before urinating. But when you think about it, it only takes a second to touch the outside of your vagina, then feel its quality between your fingers.

For those of you who think of yourselves as too squeamish to do any of this, all I can say is that once you've checked a couple of times, you realize it's really no big deal. (And if you are even *considering* having a baby, I can assure you the world of diapers and infant regurgitation is a thousand times more traumatizing than cervical fluid!)

Observing Your Cervical Fluid

1. Begin checking cervical fluid the first day after menstruation has ended.

2. Focus on vaginal *sensations* throughout the day (i.e., Does the outside of the vagina feel dry, sticky, wet? Does it feel like you are sitting in a puddle of egg white?). Vaginal sensations alone are extremely helpful in identifying fertility.

3. Try to check cervical fluid every time you use the bathroom, doing vaginal contractions called Kegel exercises on the way. This will help to get the cervical fluid to flow down to the opening. Find creative times to do Kegel exercises throughout the day, such as while washing dishes, or waiting for an annoying red light to change. (See page 88 for more on Kegel exercises.)

4. Check cervical fluid at least three times a day, including the morning and night.

5. Be sure to check when you are not sexually aroused, since sexual lubrication can mask cervical fluid. (In other words, it would be highly ineffectual to whisper in your partner's ear after an hour of foreplay: "Let me just check my cervical fluid to see if I am fertile, hon.")

6. Learn to tell the difference between semen and cervical fluid. Semen sometimes appears as a rubbery whitish strand or slippery foam. It tends to be thinner, breaks easily, and dries on your fingers quicker. By contrast, eggwhite-quality cervical fluid tends to be clear, shimmering, and stretchy. Since the two are similar, though, it is imperative that you mark any ambiguity with a question mark in the Cervical Fluid row. Doing Kegel exercises to eliminate semen should minimize any potential confusion.

7. Separate your vaginal lips and check your cervical fluid at the lower opening closest to your perineum, either with tissue or your fingers. (If using tissue, wipe from front to back to avoid spreading bacteria.)

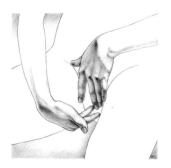

8. Glance away before looking at the cervical fluid. Focus on the quality as you rub your fingers together. Does it feel dry? Sticky? Creamy? Slippery or lubricative (like eggwhite)?

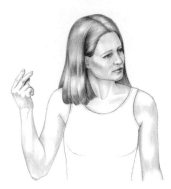

9. Feel your cervical fluid. Then slowly open your fingers to see if it stretches, and if so, how much before it breaks.

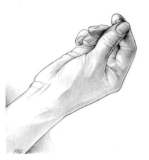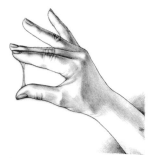

10. After urinating, focus on how easily the tissue slides across your vaginal lips. Does it feel dry, smooth, or lubricative?

11. Note your underwear throughout the day. Remember that very fertile-quality cervical fluid often forms a fairly symmetrical round circle, due to its high concentration of water. Nonwet-quality cervical fluid tends to form more of a rectangular square or line on your underwear.

12. Around your most fertile time, look in the water while you use the toilet. You would be surprised how often eggwhite-quality cervical fluid flows out so quickly that you could miss it if not paying attention. In addition, it's interesting to see how eggwhite-quality cervical fluid often forms a ball when it hits the water, appearing like a cloudy marble sinking to the bottom.

13. If you find it hard to differentiate between cervical fluid and basic vaginal secretions, remember that cervical fluid is insoluble. A little trick that can help you initially learn to tell the difference is the glass of water test. Take the sample between two fingers and dip it into a glass of water. If it is true cervical fluid, it will usually form a blob that sinks to the bottom. If it's basic vaginal secretions, it will simply dissolve.

14. Note the quality and quantity of the cervical fluid (i.e., color, consistency, and amount).

15. Pay special attention to cervical fluid after a bowel movement, since that is when it is most likely to flow out. Of course, to prevent infections while checking, you must always use two separate tissues, first wiping the vaginal opening from front to back.

16. If you find that it is difficult to detect any cervical fluid at your vaginal opening, you can check internally by using your index and middle fingers to draw out the cervical fluid from the cervix itself.

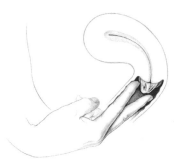 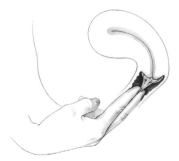

Keep in mind, though, that if you choose to check internally, you should be consistent in doing so. You shouldn't alternate external-internal checking. In addition, remember that you will always notice a moistness on your finger if you check internally. But this is different from actual cervical fluid, which does not dissipate within a few seconds the way natural vaginal moisture does.

KEGEL EXERCISES

Kegel exercises strengthen the vaginal muscles, which are usually referred to as pubococcygeus muscles or, thankfully, just PC muscles. Strengthening them serves many useful purposes, including aiding in:

    a. increasing sexual pleasure
    b. pushing cervical fluid down to the vaginal opening
    c. pushing semen out of the vagina (see SETs, below)
    d. restoring vaginal muscle tone following childbirth
    e. maintaining urinary continence in older women

How to Identify the PC muscles

Sit on a toilet and stop and start the flow of urine without moving your legs. Your PC muscles are what is turning the flow on and off.

The Exercises

When you are first learning to chart, you may want to do Kegel exercises at set times to get used to strengthening your vaginal muscles. But soon it will become such habit that you'll find yourself doing them throughout the day without even thinking about it.

Slow Kegels: Tighten the PC muscles as you do to stop urine flow. Hold it for a slow count of three. Relax. Repeat.

Fast Kegels: Tighten and relax the PC muscles as rapidly as you can. Repeat.

When to Do Kegels

You can do Kegels any time during your daily activities. Be creative and find times throughout the day, such as while driving your car, watching television, or washing dishes.

What You May Initially Experience When You Start Doing Kegels

When you first start practicing Kegels, you will probably notice that the muscles don't want to stay contracted during the slow exercises and that you can't do the quick ones as fast or evenly as you'd like. In addition, sometimes the muscles will start to feel a little tired, which is not surprising. You probably haven't used them much before. Take a few seconds and start again. In a week or two you will probably notice that you can control them quite well.

A good way to check how you are doing is to insert one or two fingers into your vagina and feel if you are able to tighten your PC muscles around your finger.

Semen Emitting Technique (SETs)

In order to determine daily fertility without confusing semen (or spermicide) with fertile cervical fluid, you should eliminate the semen as soon as possible. The first time you urinate following intercourse, push out as much of it as you can, absorbing the rest with tissue. The next couple of times, stop and start the flow with Kegels, wiping away the semen after each contraction. You will usually be able to get rid of it by the time you are through urinating. (Pregnancy achievers should wait at least half an hour after intercourse to assure enough time for the sperm to swim up through the cervical fluid before doings SETs.)

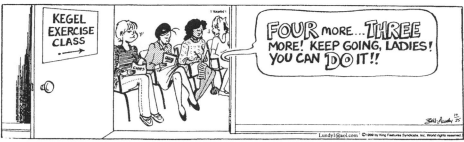

Charting Your Cervical Fluid

1. Day 1 of the cycle is the first day of red menstrual bleeding. If you have brown or light spotting in the day or two before the flow, it is usually considered part of the previous cycle. (See page 295.)

2. The graphic below shows how the various types of cervical fluid are recorded on your chart. Note that menses is marked by ✳, while spotting is marked by (✳) to show the latter is not red blood. For clarity, both should be marked in the "Dry, Spotting or Period" row.

Menses: Red blood flow.

Eggwhite					
Creamy					
Sticky					
Dry, Spotting or PERIOD	✳				

Spotting: Brown, pink, or discolored.

Eggwhite					
Creamy					
Sticky					
Dry, Spotting or PERIOD	✳	(✳)			

Nothing: Dry. No cervical fluid present. May feel dampness on finger that quickly dissipates after you check your vaginal opening.

Eggwhite					
Creamy					
Sticky					
Dry, Spotting or PERIOD	✳	(✳)	—		

Sticky: Opaque, white, or yellow, occasionally clear. Can
be fairly thick. Critical quality is its stickiness or
lack of true wetness. May be crumbly or flaky
like paste, or gummy and rubbery like rubber
cement. May form small peaks when you separate
your fingers.

	Eggwhite						
	Creamy						
	Sticky				■		
Dry, Spotting or PERIOD	✱	(✱)	—				

Creamy: Milky or cloudy, white or yellow. Creamy or
lotiony. Wet, watery, or thin. When separating
fingers, doesn't form peaks, but remains smooth
like hand lotion.

	Eggwhite						
	Creamy					■	
	Sticky				■		
Dry, Spotting or PERIOD	✱	(✱)	—				

Eggwhite: Usually clear but can have opaque streaks in it.
Very slippery and wet, like raw eggwhite. Often
causes extremely lubricative feel at vaginal
opening. May stretch from one to ten inches.
(Surprisingly, you may experience a completely
dry sensation after it slides out.)

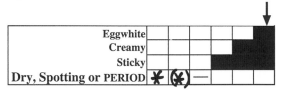

3. Record the most *fertile-* or *wet*-quality cervical fluid of the day, even if
you are dry all day except for one single observation. (Obviously, any spotting
should also be recorded.) The Cervical Fluid row will appear similar to Chart 6.8
on the next page.

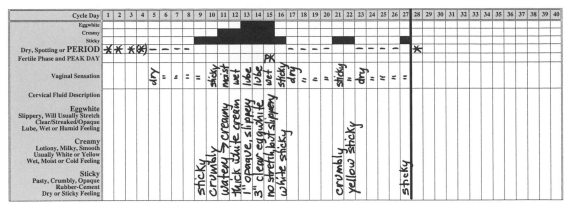

Chart 6.8. A typical cervical fluid pattern. Note how cervical fluid becomes progressively wetter as ovulation approaches.

4. Treat all signs of semen or residual spermicide as a question mark in the Cervical Fluid row, since they can mask cervical fluid. Remember, doing Kegels following intercourse will usually get rid of both.

5. The vaginal *sensation* you notice throughout the day is an extremely important indicator of your fertility. Don't be surprised if the cervical fluid seems to disappear a day or so before the slippery, lubricative vaginal *feeling* dissipates.

Identifying Your Peak Day

Once you have learned to chart your cervical fluid, you will want to use this information to determine your most fertile day. Generally speaking, this is considered the last day that you produce fertile cervical fluid *or* have a lubricative vaginal sensation for any given cycle. It is called the "Peak Day," because it denotes your peak day of fertility. It most likely occurs either a day before you ovulate or on the day of ovulation itself (the only way to know for certain would be to have an ultrasound). Practically speaking, this means that your Peak Day will usually occur one or two days before your temperature shifts.

You may have already noticed that *you will only be able to determine the Peak Day in retrospect,* on the following day. This is because you can only recognize it after your cervical fluid and vaginal sensation have already begun to dry up. This concept should become intuitive fairly quickly. Also be aware that the Peak Day is not necessarily the day of the greatest quantity of cervical fluid. In fact, the "longest eggwhite stretch" or greatest amount could occur a day or two before, as seen on page 93.

1. Your Peak Day is the last day of either:

* **eggwhite-quality cervical fluid** (which is slippery and usually stretchy)
* **lubricative vaginal sensation** (which is wet and slippery, but may not be accompanied by any cervical fluid), or
* **any midcycle spotting**

This means that if your last day of eggwhite is on a Monday, but you still have one more day of lubricative vaginal sensation (or spotting) on Tuesday, your Peak Day is Tuesday. Of course, the reverse applies as well.

2. If you don't have eggwhite cervical fluid, you would count the last day of the wettest-quality cervical fluid that you do have, which would probably be *creamy*. (Of course, once again, if your last day of creamy is on a Monday but your last day of wet or lubricative vaginal sensation is on a Tuesday, your Peak Day would be Tuesday.)

3. Some women will occasionally have a day of creamy cervical fluid after their last eggwhite day. Most fertility awareness instructors still consider the last day of eggwhite the true Peak Day.

4. Once you have identified the Peak Day, you should write "PK" in the Peak Day row of your chart. Chart 6.9 on the next page shows the most common cervical fluid patterns and how their corresponding Peak Days would be recorded.

ANOVULATORY CYCLES AND THE PEAK DAY

One of the reasons I stress charting your cervical fluid *and* temperatures is that if you only observe your cervical fluid, you could be misled to believe that you are ovulating when you are not. This is because your body may make attempts to ovulate by increasing its levels of estrogen in a seemingly consistent pattern, but if the estrogen doesn't make it over the hormonal threshold, the egg won't be released. By charting both, you will be able to observe the increase in fertile cervical fluid that indicates approaching ovulation, but the lack of a thermal shift can clarify that you have in fact not yet ovulated.

A trick to help you identify whether or not you are ovulating is to pay special attention to the concept of the Peak Day. If you do ovulate, the cervical fluid should dry up fairly abruptly, due to the release of progesterone following ovulation. In situations where your body may be unsuccessfully attempting to ovulate (for example, in long cycles, while breastfeeding, or experiencing PCOS) you would typically observe a pattern of increasingly wet cervical fluid, but instead of fully drying up under the influence of progesterone, it would likely return in sporadic patches, or simply remain somewhat wet. (Further discussion of anovulation appears in the following chapter.)

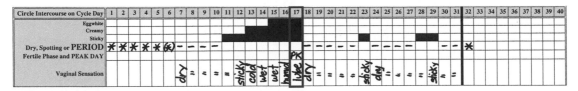

Chart 6.9a. The classic cervical fluid pattern, with the last day of eggwhite as the Peak Day. In this case, her Peak Day is Day 17.

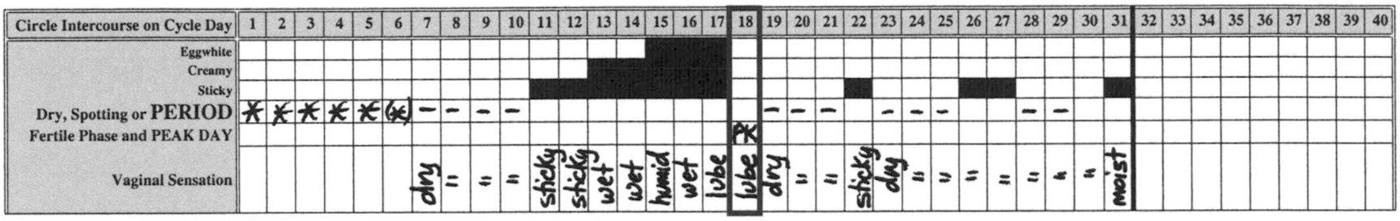

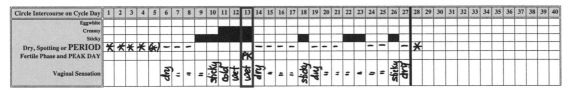

Chart 6.9b. The same basic pattern of cervical fluid as Chart 6.9a above, except she still has a lubricative vaginal sensation the day *after* her last day of eggwhite (recorded as "lube"). Thus, her Peak Day is Day 18.

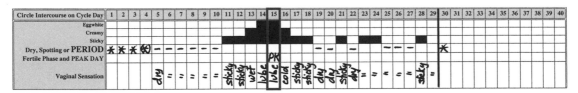

Chart 6.9c. A cervical fluid pattern in which eggwhite is never observed. Her Peak Day is therefore Day 13, the last day of wet, creamy cervical fluid.

Chart 6.9d. A cervical fluid pattern in which a day of creamy follows the last day of eggwhite. In this case, the Peak Day is still considered Day 15, the last eggwhite day.

Knowing how to accurately determine your Peak Day is critical if you are to correctly follow the rules for both birth control and pregnancy achievement, so be sure to carefully internalize the guidelines on the previous page as well as the sample charts above.

✢ CERVICAL POSITION (OPTIONAL)

The cervical position is the one fertility sign that often takes more than one cycle to grasp, since you probably haven't had experience feeling your cervix. It may take a few cycles to be able to tell the difference between high and low, soft and firm, or open and closed.

You should notice that as you approach ovulation, your cervix tends to rise, soften, and open. It progresses from feeling firm like the tip of your nose (when not fertile) to feeling soft like your lips as you approach ovulation. Your cervix will drop abruptly into the vagina when oestrogen levels fall, and progesterone becomes dominant after ovulation. By simply inserting your clean middle finger, you can detect these subtle changes.

The cervical position is an optional sign, but it is especially helpful if either of the other primary signs are confusing in any particular cycle. It should never be relied upon alone. The best time to observe dramatic changes are right around ovulation, when the cervix shifts the most abruptly.

Some women may be initially squeamish about checking the cervix. This is understandable, since it is not something they are accustomed to feeling. Simply breathe slowly and let your body relax. You'll probably find that it can be fascinating to observe how it varies throughout the cycle. And once you become familiar with the various changes, you can restrict your cervix checking to about a week per cycle. (See "Shortcuts," Chapter 10.)

Remember, the cervix is an optional sign, so you may decide you'd rather not check it at all, though I do recommend it for the following people:

1. Those women whose temperature patterns do not reflect a completely obvious thermal shift. The cervix in such cases would provide corroborating evidence of fertility.
2. Those whose cervical fluid or temperatures are not easy to interpret.
3. Those who are willing to take slightly increased risks in order to extend the time they consider themselves infertile.
4. Those women who absolutely cannot risk an unplanned pregnancy and want a third sign to confirm infertile days.

Observing Your Cervix

1. Begin checking your cervix once a day after menstruation has ended.

2. Always wash your hands with soap first.

3. Try to check about the same time each day. Checking just after a morning or evening shower is probably the most convenient.

4. The most effective position in which to check is squatting, since this pushes the cervix closest to the vaginal opening. However, some women prefer to check while sitting on the toilet, or putting one leg on the bathtub. The most important thing is to be consistent about the position you choose, since different positions will change the cervical height.

5. Use your finger as a convenient gauge. Insert your middle finger (nails should be trimmed) and remember the mnemonic device SHOW as you observe the following conditions of the cervix:

    a. **Softness** (firm, medium, or soft)
    b. **Height** in the vagina (low, midway, or high)
    c. **Opening** (closed, partly open, or open)
    d. **Wetness** (nothing, sticky, creamy, or eggwhite)
       (Technically, wetness is a quality of the cervical fluid and not the cervix, but it is included here since, when checking the cervix, you can't help notice whatever fluid there is.)

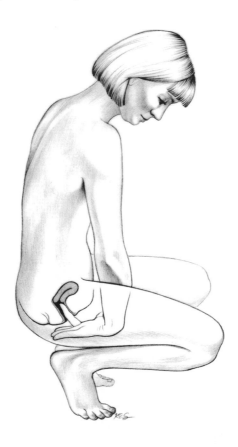

6. Note that women who have vaginally delivered children will always have a slightly open cervix. It will feel more oval and is usually shaped like a horizontal slit, so it is important to focus on the subtle variation throughout the cycle.

Woman who has never
vaginally delivered children

Woman who has
vaginally delivered children

7. The best time to begin observing cervical changes is when the wet-quality cervical fluid starts to build up in the days before ovulation. You should continue observing at least until the cervical fluid and cervix abruptly revert back to their infertile quality. Cervical changes will become easier to observe with practice.

8. Don't be surprised if you notice small firm bumps that feel like granules of sand under the skin of your cervix. These are called nabothian cysts, and typically come and go without treatment. (See illustration on page 227.)

9. Obviously, you should not check your cervical position if you have genital sores or vaginal infections.

Charting Your Cervix

1. Use a circle to represent the cervical opening (called the cervical os.)

= low, closed, and firm (F)

= midway, partly open, and medium (M)

= high, open, and soft (S)

2. The general cervical pattern will look like Chart 6.10, below.

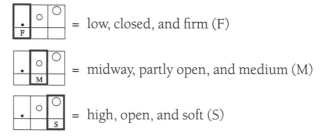

Chart 6.10. A typical cervical position pattern. Note that the cervix quickly reverts back from its Peak Day of fertility, and thus in this case is closed and low by Day 16.

SOME CHARTING LOGISTICS

Record almost everything except temps in fine-point pencil.

To record cervical fluid or color-coded signs, fill in the squares with any one of the following:

- thick marker such as a Marvy
- Staedtler Lumocolor 314 permanent marker
- calligraphy marker
- thick-leaded pencil

Put a question mark in the column anytime you forgot to observe signs.

If your temps fall below 97, write the correct temp just below it and circle that number (e.g., if your temp was 96.7, record 7 just below the 97, and circle the 7). Likewise, if your temps rise above 99, write the correct temp just above it and circle that number (e.g., if your temp was 99.3, record 3 just above the 99, and circle the 3).

If your preovulatory temps tend to be consistently in the 96s, you may prefer to write a 96 to the left of the tiny 97s, and 97 to the left of the tiny 98s in the Waking Temperature row. Then use that as your master chart, making copies from that modified chart from then on.

If you have artificial insemination, you may prefer to use a slash rather than a circle on the appropriate cycle day.

If your cycle extends beyond Day 40, cut and tape your charts together so that they look like one continuous, long cycle.

Keep your charts in a notebook with the most recent on top, for easy recording.

If you are faxing your charts to your health practitioner, be sure to put your name on the charts, and send them on high resolution.

Copy the annual exam master form onto the back of the chart for the cycle in which you get your exam. To easily access your annual exams in the future, you may want to use a little metal clip in the top right corner.

If you would prefer to chart your cycles on the computer, you can download the fertility software that accompanies this book at www.TCOYF.com.

❧ PUTTING IT ALL TOGETHER: A SUMMARY

The time it takes to actually check all three signs is negligible compared to the advantages to be gained. The following, then, is a summary of how to observe and chart the three fertility signs:

❧ TEMPERATURE

Taking Your Temperature

1. Take your daily temperature first thing upon awakening *before any other activity* and record throughout the cycle.
2. If using a digital thermometer, wait until it beeps, usually about a minute. If using a glass basal thermometer, leave it in 5 minutes.
3. Take your temperature orally or vaginally, but always *from the same opening* throughout the cycle.
4. Take it about the same time every day, within an hour or so.
5. Take your temperature after *at least three consecutive hours* of sleep.
6. If you use a glass basal body thermometer, shake it down the day before.
7. If you suspect you are getting sick, be sure to use a traditional fever or digital thermometer.

Charting Your Temperature

1. Try to record your temperature sometime in the morning, although it can be done later.
2. If the temperature falls between two numbers on a glass thermometer, always record the *lowest* temperature.
3. Record and connect the temperatures with a pen.
4. Note unusual events such as stress, illness, or fever in the Miscellaneous row. Temperatures taken earlier or later than usual should be noted in the Time Temp Taken row.
5. Omit any temperatures that are out of line by drawing a dotted line between the normal temperatures.

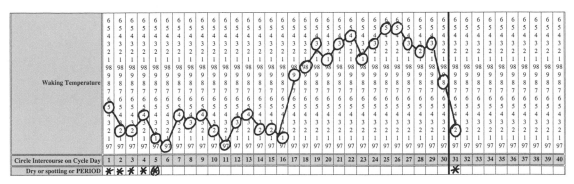

Chart 6.11. A typical waking temperature pattern.

Drawing the Coverline

1. After your period ends, as you are charting your temperatures, always notice the highest of the previous six days.

2. Identify the first day your temperature rises at least two-tenths of a degree higher than that highest temperature.

3. Go back and highlight the last six temperatures before the rise.

4. Draw the coverline one-tenth of a degree above the highest of that cluster of six highlighted days preceding the rise.

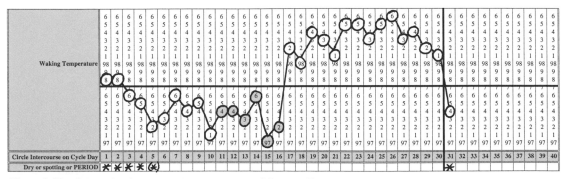

Chart 6.12. A standard temperature pattern with coverline.

CERVICAL FLUID

Observing Your Cervical Fluid

1. Begin checking cervical fluid the first day after menstruation has ended.
2. Focus on vaginal *sensations* throughout the day.
3. Try to check cervical fluid every time you use the bathroom, doing Kegels on the way.
4. Check cervical fluid at least three times a day, including the morning and night.
5. Don't check cervical fluid while you are sexually aroused.
6. Learn to differentiate between semen and cervical fluid (and learn to do Kegels to get rid of the semen, as discussed on page 88).
7. Separate your vaginal lips and check your cervical fluid at the opening either with tissue or your fingers.
8. Glance away before looking at the cervical fluid. Focus on the *quality*. Does it feel dry? Sticky? Creamy? Slippery or lubricative (like eggwhite)?
9. Feel your cervical fluid. Then slowly open your fingers to see if it stretches.
10. After urinating, focus on how easily the tissue slides across your vaginal lips.
11. Note your underwear throughout the day.
12. Around your most fertile time, look in the water while you use the toilet.
13. If you find it difficult differentiating between cervical fluid and basic vaginal secretions, do the glass of water test by inserting the cervical fluid in the water.
14. Note the quality and quantity of the cervical fluid (i.e., color, consistency, and amount).
15. Pay special attention to whether you see cervical fluid after a bowel movement, since that is when it is most likely to flow out.
16. If you find that it is difficult to detect any cervical fluid at your vaginal opening, you can check internally by using your index and middle fingers to draw out the cervical fluid from the cervix itself.

Charting Your Cervical Fluid

1. Day 1 of the cycle is the first day of true menstrual bleeding.
2. Use the following notation to record the Cervical Fluid on your chart.

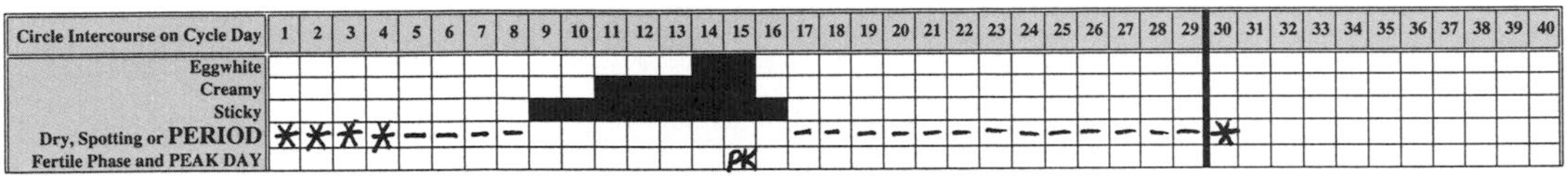

Circle Intercourse on Cycle Day	1	2	3	4	5	6	7	8	9	10	11	12	13	14	15	16	17	18	19	20	21	22	23	24	25	26	27	28	29	30	31	32	33	34	35	36	37	38	39	40
Eggwhite																																								
Creamy																																								
Sticky																																								
Dry, Spotting or PERIOD	✳	✳	✳	✳	—	—	—	—									—	—	—	—	—	—	—	—	—	—	—	—	—	✳										
Fertile Phase and PEAK DAY															PK																									

Chart 6.13.

3. Record the most *fertile-* or *wet-*quality cervical fluid of the day, as well as any spotting. Your cervical fluid will become progressively wetter as you approach ovulation.
4. Treat signs of semen or spermicide as a question mark in the Cervical Fluid row.
5. The vaginal sensation you notice throughout the day is an extremely important indicator of your fertility.

Identifying Your Peak Day

1. Your Peak Day is the last day of eggwhite cervical fluid or lubricative vaginal sensation, or midcycle spotting.
2. If you don't have eggwhite, you would count the last day of your wettest-quality cervical fluid or wet or lubricative vaginal sensation.
3. If you have a creamy day after your last day of eggwhite, that last day of eggwhite is still considered your Peak Day.
4. Once you have identified the Peak Day, you should write PK in the Peak Day row of your chart.

✤ CERVIX

Observing Your Cervix

1. Begin checking the cervix once a day after menstruation has ended.
2. Always wash your hands with soap first.
3. Try to check about the same time each day.
4. The most effective position in which to check is squatting.
5. Insert your middle finger and observe the conditions of the cervix (softness, height, opening, and wetness).
6. Women who have vaginally delivered children will always have a slightly open cervix that feels more oval.
7. The best time to begin observing cervical changes is when the wet quality cervical fluid starts to build up in the days before ovulation.
8. Don't be surprised if you feel nabothian cysts on the cervix.
9. Do not check your cervical position if you have genital sores or a vaginal infection.

Charting Your Cervix

1. Use a circle to represent the cervical opening.

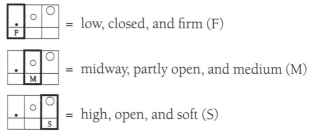

= low, closed, and firm (F)

= midway, partly open, and medium (M)

= high, open, and soft (S)

2. The general cervical pattern after menstruation will typically progress gradually from low, closed, and firm before ovulation to high, open, and soft around ovulation, before abruptly returning to its original position.

✤ NOW THAT YOU KNOW

Congratulations! If you understood this chapter, you are now ready to apply your newfound knowledge toward avoiding pregnancy naturally, achieving pregnancy, or simply taking control of and understanding your body.

CHAPTER 7

Anovulation and Irregular Cycles

one of us are Barbie dolls. As much as Madison Avenue tries to convince us that all women should be 5 feet 9 inches and thin as a rail, the reality is that there is tremendous variety among women. Even the conventional (not-so-wise) wisdom out there is that all women should have 28-day cycles and ovulate on Day 14. Of course, you know by now that's not true.

Not only can a woman have cycles that vary—but a woman's cycles may be different depending on whether she is an adolescent, just coming off the Pill, breastfeeding, or approaching menopause. Her cycles may also vary depending on other temporary factors such as illness, travel, stress, or exercise.

The beauty of charting your cycles, though, is that you can take control and understand what is transpiring in your body on a daily basis, regardless of your particular circumstances. You may find that you'll go through months or even years with only intermittent ovulation. If you are using FAM as birth control, it's important to realize that any time you don't ovulate, you need to treat each day as if you were in a *pre*ovulatory state. Thus the presence of any cervical fluid must be very carefully observed to see if it is potentially fertile.

There are differences in the way your fertility signs are reflected over time, depending on whether you are ovulating:

A typical cycle: In a normal cycle, your body prepares for the release of an egg in a fairly timely, predictable manner. After your period, under the influence of rising oestrogen, you'll usually have several days of no cervical fluid, followed by days building up to a progressively wetter fertile-quality cervical fluid. After the egg is released, your cervical fluid will rapidly dry up until you start the pattern over again the next cycle.

An anovulatory phase (low body weight, breastfeeding, pre-menopause, etc.): This refers to those periods of time when women take longer to release an egg. In such special circumstances, your body could theoretically take up to a year or longer to build up to a high enough level of oestrogen to trigger an ovulation. It's almost a one-step-forward, two-steps-back situation, in which your body may make many attempts to ovulate before it finally is able to do so, as seen in the graphic below.

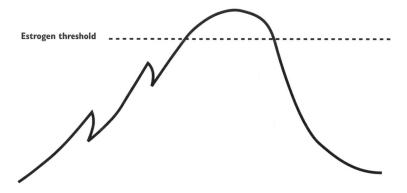

During this time, you may notice what are referred to as "patches of cervical fluid." Instead of the classic buildup typical of normal cycles, you may see a series of patches of wetness interspersed with drier days.

This chapter is devoted to what transpires in your body during these special circumstances when you don't ovulate. Appendix B discusses how to use FAM for birth control during such times.

𝒫 DIFFERENT PHASES OF ANOVULATION IN WOMEN'S LIVES

Adolescence

British girls typically start to menstruate between 12 and 16 years old with the average age being 13. But the onset of periods doesn't necessarily mean the release of an egg every cycle. In fact, one of the factors that characterizes menstrual cycles in teenagers is irregularity due to fluctuating oestrogen levels, and thus cycles don't automatically start out predictably. It is a gradual process that can take several years while the hormonal feedback system matures. During this time, then, an adolescent's cycles may vary considerably, with many anovulatory cycles dispersed throughout.

Pregnancy and Breastfeeding

If you were to take a survey of pregnant or breastfeeding women, one of the things they would probably tell you they enjoy about their condition is that their periods have stopped. Of course, it makes sense physiologically for the woman's body to be incapable of getting pregnant again following conception. Once a woman becomes pregnant, she won't ovulate until after the baby is born.

And if she is breastfeeding "on request," that is, virtually every time the baby cries to be fed, she may not resume ovulating again for many months after the baby's birth. This is because every time a baby suckles at the breast, it indirectly suppresses the hormones that trigger ovulation. But in order for breastfeeding to efficiently prevent the release of eggs, the baby must suckle consistently throughout the day and night.

A breastfeeding woman could go a year or more without a thermal shift and experience the same cervical fluid, whether it be dry, sticky, or a combination, day after day. The reason she usually won't see wet-quality cervical fluid initially is that the low oestrogen levels which are indirectly caused by the prolactin will also keep the fertile-quality cervical fluid from being produced. The trick is for breastfeeding women to be attentive to the *change* in the quality of cervical fluid that indicates that ovulation will be resuming soon. Because cycles while breastfeeding can be either nonexistent or quite confusing, you should read Appendixes B and C if you plan to use FAM for birth control during these times.

Premenopause

Menopause is the time in a woman's life when she ceases ovulating and having menstrual periods altogether. It typically occurs around age 51. But the time leading up to menopause can take several years. During this phase, her cycles may start appearing very different than anything she is used to. Cycle lengths tend to initially decrease due to more frequent ovulations combined with shorter luteal phases. Eventually, though, the cycles become longer and longer as the number of times an egg is released becomes less frequent. Finally, cycles cease altogether. A woman is generally said to have completed menopause if she's in her 40s or older and has gone for one full year without a period.

It used to be that the concept of menopause was taboo, shrouded in mystery and misinformation. Luckily, today much more is known about menopause, and women are reaping the benefits of such newfound knowledge. As with breastfeeding, though, cycles while approaching menopause can be fairly tricky. You should read Chapter 19 and Appendix B carefully for how to use FAM as contraception during the premenopausal phase.

✍ OTHER MAJOR CAUSES OF ANOVULATION

There is a huge difference between cycles in which the woman may ovulate but not get her period, and one in which she gets her period but doesn't ovulate. Stop and think. What is the difference? In the former case, the woman is almost certainly pregnant! In the latter case, she has had an anovulatory cycle. The two charts below show how very different these scenarios look on paper.

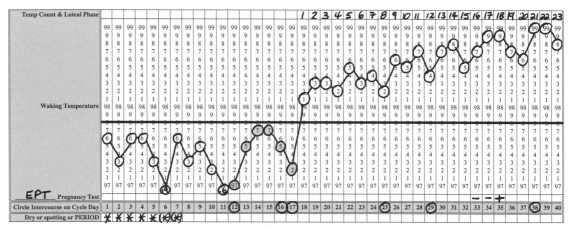

Chart 7.1. A typical temperature pattern for pregnancy. Note that Rena almost certainly ovulated by Day 17 as seen by the next morning's thermal shift. Her chart shows more than 18 high temperatures following the shift, thus confirming her pregnancy.

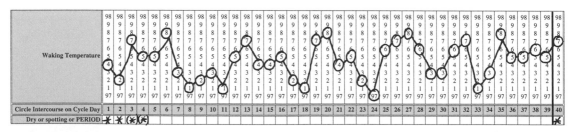

Chart 7.2. A typical temperature pattern with anovulation. Note that there is no thermal shift reflecting ovulation, and thus the "period" that follows on Day 40 is actually anovulatory bleeding, which is technically not menstruation.

In anovulatory cycles, noncharting women may assume they are menstruating normally. So why would they continue to experience bleeding if ovulation has not occurred? Such bleeding results when oestrogen production continues to develop the uterine lining without reaching the threshold necessary to trigger ovulation. In such a case, one of two things may happen that lead to what *appears to be* a menstrual period: (1) The oestrogen will build up slowly to a point below the threshold and then drop, resulting in "oestrogen withdrawal bleeding." Or (2), more commonly, the endometrium builds up slowly over an extended period of time, eventually to the point where the resulting uterine lining is so thickened it can no longer sustain itself. This is known as "oestrogen breakthrough bleeding."

In either case, if you weren't charting, you might think you were simply menstruating, though you may notice a difference in the type of bleeding. Specifically, the flow can be either unusually heavy or light, and of course, the timing can result in cycle lengths all over the map, or the chart, as it were.

The following are common reasons why women may not ovulate, either temporarily or for extended periods of time:

Illness

Being sick does not necessarily affect your cycle, but if it does, its impact is usually influenced by which phase you are in when you get sick. If your illness occurs before ovulation, it may delay it, or even prevent it altogether (see page 312). If it occurs after, it will almost never affect your cycle, because the luteal phase has a consistent life span of 12 to 16 days that is typically not affected by factors such as sickness, travel, or exercise. (For each individual woman, the luteal phase is even more consistent and will generally not vary more than a day or so.)

In any event, you needn't worry that a fever will affect your ability to interpret your chart. For one thing, you can usually depend on the other two fertility signs. In addition, the temperatures will indeed indicate if fever has affected your cycle by either delaying or preventing ovulation. Remember, if getting sick affects your cycle at all, it will depend on when it happens.

Travel

Traveling is notorious for affecting cycles. There's nothing like wearing a pair of crisp white walking shorts while strolling down the Champs-Elysées in Paris when . . . uh-oh, surprise, surprise. Although many women are blessed with cycles that continue like clockwork while vacationing, many others are faced with the challenge of trying to figure out if or when they will get their periods.

COMING OFF THE PILL OR OTHER HORMONES
SUCH AS NORPLANT OR DEPO-PROVERA

Women who discontinue hormones are often surprised that their cycles don't necessarily resume in the same clockwork manner that they had become accustomed to while taking hormones. But you must remember that cycles on hormones are artificially induced to be perfect. Ovulation doesn't necessarily resume immediately, usually because of the oversuppression of the feedback mechanism of the hypothalamus and pituitary gland.

The Pill can cause any of the following disruptions for up to several months after discontinuing:

Temperatures
- false high temperatures
- temperature that seems completely out of sync with cervical fluid

Cervical Fluid
- absence of typical ovulatory cervical fluid, leading to an unchanging Basic Infertile Pattern (BIP) even when ovulation occurs
- continuous seemingly fertile watery or milky cervical fluid
- erratic pattern of patches of varying types of cervical fluid

Luteal Phase
- short luteal phase indicating an unsuitable ovulation

Bleeding
- heavier and redder bleeding than you became accustomed to while on the Pill
- irregular preovulatory bleeding and spotting in the luteal phase
- poor menstrual flow following ovulation

When a woman comes off the Pill or other hormones, her cycles will eventually revert back to the way they were before. However, the length of time it takes varies tremendously among women. For some, it is almost immediate. But for most women, there is at least a short delay. For others, it could take many months to years. This variation is a function of the type and dosage of hormones used, as well as the basic physiology of the woman.

Those who tend to take longer to clear the drug from their systems, and therefore take several months to resume cycling after hormones, are often young or thin (especially those who lost weight while on hormones). Those who were irregular before hormones typically return to their irregular pattern after. In addition, you should be aware that once women do resume natural cycling, they may experience short luteal phases for the first few months. This will usually be reflected in high temperatures of fewer than 10 days after the thermal shift.

Once they discontinue hormones, but before their cycles start showing the classic buildup of fertile-quality cervical fluid, they may notice that it has a somewhat milky quality. Some experience a type that is a combination of both sticky and wet. Still others may discover that their cervical fluid doesn't attain classic fertile qualities because the Pill can damage the cervical crypts that produce it. Gradually, these abnormalities in their fertility signs disappear, and they can anticipate returning to cycles similar to what they experienced before starting the Pill.

It is clear that when coming off the Pill your cervical fluid can initially be confusing. Obviously, it is imperative that women who are just starting to chart do not rely on FAM as their sole method of birth control until they feel confident in being able to interpret their fertility signs.

As delightful as vacation may be for you, your body still interprets it as a type of stress. Many women find that their cycles become extremely long due to delayed ovulations. Others actually stop ovulating and getting periods altogether. Once again, charting your cycle can be very helpful in determining what is happening with your body. Keep in mind, though, that traveling is a time when it is especially helpful to chart all three signs in order to understand any ambiguities that result from the disruption in your life. In particular, always be on the lookout for factors that may affect your temperature.

Years ago, my college roommate seemed to redefine the limits of travel-related anovulation. Cathy spent her junior year in England. She had a period just before she arrived in London, then didn't menstruate for the ten months she lived there. But sure enough, the month she returned home, she got her period again.

Exercise

Strenuous exercise has the potential to delay or even prevent ovulation altogether. Although you may be tempted to use this as an excuse not to exercise, don't! It seems to affect mostly those who are competitive athletes with a very low ratio of body fat to total body weight. The women most affected are runners, swimmers, and ballet dancers. But what is somewhat inconclusive about studies of these athletes is that they have been unable to separate the effects of fat ratio from physical and emotional stress, diet, and even changes in thyroid metabolism. It appears that all of these can affect a woman's cycle.

Weight Gain or Loss

In order for the average woman to maintain normal ovulatory cycles, she should probably have a minimum of about 20% body fat. The purpose of the fat is to store oestrogen as well as convert androgens (another hormone) to a type of oestrogen needed for ovulation to occur.

Extremely thin women, particularly those with the eating disorder anorexia nervosa, often stop having periods altogether. It is thought this occurs because their bodies are unable to pass above the oestrogen threshold necessary to cause an egg to be released. In addition, women who lose 10 to 15% of their total body weight (or about one-third of their body fat) may also cease having periods. And as mentioned above, female athletes often stop menstruating because of the combination of lean body fat and stress caused by competition.

Among my clients was a French couple who had been trying to get pregnant for five years. They asked to meet with me privately rather than take a group seminar because he was a doctor and felt the class might be too elementary for them. When they arrived at my office, I sensed a potential fertility problem immediately.

The woman was tall and fit, but extremely thin. I asked her whether she would consider gaining a little weight to alter her cycles, but she said she was adamantly opposed to consuming any fat in her diet. They both claimed they were totally perplexed as to why she wasn't getting pregnant, since she took such good care of herself. But when I asked her to describe her cycles to me, she said there weren't any to describe—she hadn't had a period in five years!

I was stunned. Here were two educated people, one of them a doctor, yet they couldn't understand why she wasn't getting pregnant even though she wasn't menstruating. I questioned why they thought she was fertile if she hadn't had a period in all those years. Their answer amazed me. Years prior, when they were trying to avoid *pregnancy, her physician asked her what form of contraception she used. She said they didn't use birth control because she wasn't menstruating. Her physician at the time insisted that she protect herself anyway, since, as he rightly pointed out, she could still ovulate at any time. Based on that one comment, that she could ovulate at any time, she interpreted that to mean she was indeed fertile.*

I was able to explain to them that the odds of pregnancy must be seen differently, depending on the desires of the couple. From the contraceptive perspective, it's imperative that women protect themselves because ovulation always occurs before menstruation. But if a woman is trying to get pregnant and is not menstruating, then she is clearly not ovulating. Their experience taught me how easy it is to confuse the risk of an unwanted pregnancy with the slight possibility of one that is wanted. Unfortunately, I never did learn what happened to them because they returned to France shortly after we met, but I assume that they at least dealt with her anovulatory condition.

On the other end of the spectrum are women who tend to be overweight. They too may stop ovulating. At this point, you may be thinking, "Wait a second. She said that it could be problematic if the woman is too thin, and now she's saying it could be a problem if she's too heavy." Such is the nature of women's bodies! With obesity, excess fatty tissue can cause too much oestrogen, disrupting the hormonal feedback system that tells the egg follicles to mature.

Stress

One of the most likely causes of occasional long cycles is stress, both physiological and psychological. If stress affects a cycle at all, it tends to delay ovulation, not accelerate it. As you know, the timing of ovulation will determine the length of the cycle—the later it occurs, the longer the cycle will be. Sometimes, if stress is severe, it can actually prevent ovulation from occurring altogether (see page 178).

Medical Conditions

In addition to the various temporary factors listed above, a variety of medical conditions may cause women to stop ovulating indefinitely. These include elevated prolactin levels and other pituitary gland problems as well as polycystic ovarian syndrome (a condition which is discussed on page 204). One of the most common and useful ways of determining the cause of your anovulation is through a Progesterone Withdrawal Test (see flow chart on the next page). In any case, many of these conditions can be treated, but all will require consultation with a physician.

PROGESTERONE CHALLENGE OR WITHDRAWAL TEST

To determine whether irregularity or lack of menstrual flow is hormonal or uterine

Oral dose of progesterone tablets (Provera) for 5 to 10 days or one progesterone injection.

Within 2 to 14 days after stopping the progesterone:

You Bleed
Your ovaries make enough estrogen to build your uterine lining and your uterus is capable of responding to progesterone. The fact that you bleed after the supplementation suggests that you are anovulatory.

You Don't Bleed
You may not have enough estrogen to build the uterine lining.

Estrogen supplements, followed by a second progesterone withdrawal test.

Within 2 to 14 days after stopping the progesterone:

You Bleed
You lack estrogen, which suggests you are anovulatory or perhaps menopausal.

You Don't Bleed
There is some type of obstruction of the uterine outflow tract.

AN ADDITIONAL WORD ABOUT IRREGULAR CYCLES

What defines an irregular cycle? As you know by now, cycles that vary between about 24 and 36 days are considered normal, unless you have other troubling symptoms. In general, you should have your cycles diagnosed if they fall outside of that range or are accompanied by varying amounts of bleeding. The quality of menstruation following ovulation is usually fairly consistent, and thus if your cycles are irregular with bleeding that is sometimes light, sometimes heavy, sometimes red, sometimes brown, sometimes with clots, and sometimes without, it is often an indication that you are not ovulating normally, if at all.

Whether you are trying to avoid or get pregnant, I would encourage you to be examined. If you are trying to conceive, highly irregular cycles can reflect a fertility condition requiring treatment. And if you are trying to avoid pregnancy, they can make the method a bit more difficult to use effectively.

In any case, your doctor will probably want to examine you for a number of conditions, including those below:

Excessive prolactin	Page 202
Polycystic Ovarian Syndrome	Page 204
Premature Ovarian Failure	Page 206
Thyroid disorders	Page 305

৯৯ PUTTING ANOVULATION IN PERSPECTIVE

As you have seen, there are many reasons why women don't necessarily ovulate every cycle. Some involve particular phases in a woman's life, such as adolescence, pregnancy and breastfeeding, or menopause. Others are due to more transitory factors such as coming off the Pill and other hormones, stress, illness, exercise, body weight, and travel. And finally, some are caused by more serious physiological conditions. The important point is that anovulatory cycles should be understood in the right context. At times, they are completely normal and even predictable. But if you think you have a serious medical problem, your charting may help your doctor to diagnose it.

✏ FERTILITY AWARENESS AND ANOVULATION

If you plan to use Fertility Awareness for contraception during periods of anovulation, you need to be aware that the rules are somewhat more involved than the normal ones you will be learning in Chapter 9. Remember that while you are, ironically, less fertile, you need to treat every day as if you were in your preovulatory phase. Depending on your own particular anovulatory pattern, this may or may not be difficult. I suggest that you finish reading the normal rules discussed in Chapter 9, then, if you have determined that you are in an anovulatory phase of your life, you should carefully read Appendix B.

PART THREE

NATURAL BIRTH CONTROL

CHAPTER 8

Practicing FAM Responsibly

*B*efore you use Fertility Awareness as a method of birth control, you must take the appropriate precautions needed to eliminate the risk of AIDS and other sexually transmitted diseases (STDs). In particular, I must state what I hope is obvious: As a form of contraception, Fertility Awareness is only advisable for those people involved in a monogamous relationship in which neither partner has an STD.

I have talked to many people who have told me that as wonderful as Fertility Awareness is, they aren't sure its promotion is compatible with today's essential "safe sex" message. As a woman's health educator, my primary concern is that women are given the information they need to take control of their own health and well-being. Certainly, this includes developing the knowledge and self-esteem necessary to minimize the risk of contracting the various STDs that now exist. However, it does not mean that Fertility Awareness is irrelevant given the realities of today's world. Simply put, FAM *is* compatible with safe sex, as long as the sex in question is *with a safe partner.* I would like to spend the rest of this chapter discussing the real-world decisions that this last statement suggests.

Before entering into a new sexual relationship in which you would like to use Fertility Awareness as your method of contraception, it is best to act as if your new partner were HIV-positive until proven otherwise.* This means using condoms every time, to protect both you and him. The condoms should be made of latex, and come with a spermicidal lubricant such as nonoxynol-9. Be sure you both know how to use them correctly.

After an appropriate amount of time, you might be considering a long-term relationship. If you feel intimate enough to trust your partner, you may be ready to take the most important step. Note again that for the purposes of Fertility

---

* HIV stands for human immunodeficiency virus, the virus that causes AIDS. If a person is HIV-positive, they have the virus in their blood, though they may have no symptoms of illness, and in fact they may not get sick for years. If a person is HIV-negative, they do not have the virus in their blood, and therefore there is no threat of passing it on to another person.

Awareness, trustworthiness is critical, because as has often been noted, "cheating" today means more than risking just the other person's feelings. Thus, at a minimum, monogamy is necessary if you're going to use FAM. And before every new sexual relationship, both you and your partner should consider undergoing an HIV-antibody test. Clinics generally recommend that you wait three months from the time of a possible risk before taking an antibody test as antibodies usually take between two and three months to appear in your blood.

There are numerous reasons to verify HIV-negative status before giving up condoms. Perhaps most important, the HIV-antibody test is accurate, inexpensive, and can be taken anonymously. Tests are not just inexpensive, but free if you use a NHS clinic. You will have to pay if you go private (usually anything between £20 and £70); however many people go to NHS GUM (genito-urinary medicine) clinics because they routinely offer pre- and post-test counselling which may not be offered in a private clinic.

If you test at a GUM clinic, you test confidentially. The clinic will be bound by legal confidentiality rules under the VD Act. If you go to a GP for testing, the test will go on your medical records. GPs may be asked to disclose details of test results to insurance companies and others making health checks on an individual. You do not need to be referred by your GP to have a test at the GUM clinic.

Even if both partners find themselves in a relatively low-risk group, I would still recommend the test for each. It's true that the highest-risk partners for women are those men who have engaged in homosexual acts, have used intravenous drugs, or received a blood transfusion between the late 1970s and 1985. Yet it is also true that risk is always a *relative* concept. A male partner may never have had sex with other men, but if he's slept with numerous women and only used condoms sporadically, he still poses a greater risk than a virgin. You should also be very aware that the danger of HIV transmission from women to men appears to increase substantially when other cofactors exist, most important, the presence of other STDs. This is because the open genital sores caused by certain STDs allow an easier pathway for HIV to get into a man's blood.

With all this in mind, the slight chance of receiving a false-positive scare is worth taking in order to minimize any possibility of spreading the HIV virus. This is hardly a controversial position given that the virus in question can cause a fatal disease for which there is still no known cure. It signals a sense of responsibility and seriousness on the part of each partner to the other, and thus confirms qualities that one would hope are present in any monogamous relationship in which you would find yourself. In addition, testing allows you to solidify the closeness of a developing relationship by giving both of you the medical confirmation to move beyond condoms to the more natural and enjoyable lovemaking Fertility Awareness allows.

This is not to say that if one partner were to test positive for HIV that a completely loving and full relationship could not blossom, but only that HIV-positive status requires taking very real precautions to protect the health of the other partner. And for those couples who test HIV-negative, a relationship can begin anew in which the fear of AIDS is put behind them, freeing them to look forward to the benefits of effective and completely natural contraception.

Assuming you decide to take the test, the next big decision is when to do so. If people who are HIV-positive take the test too early, they may get a false-negative result. Scientific studies have shown that a large majority of HIV-positive people develop antibodies within three months of exposure, but it is generally recommended that you wait six months before relying on an HIV-negative result. This is particularly true if the person's last exposure falls into what is considered one of the high-risk activities.

All pregnant women in the UK should be offered and recommended an HIV test as part of their routine antenatal care. If infection is diagnosed, there are a number of steps that can be taken to help reduce the likelihood of passing the infection to their baby. These include the use of antiretroviral drugs for the mother and her newborn baby, giving birth by Caesarean section and avoiding breastfeeding.

There are two forms of the HIV antibody test widely used; the ELISA (Enzyme Linked Immuno-Sorbent Assay) and the Western Blot method. The ELISA (a similar test is called the EIA, or Enzyme Immune Assay) is a reliable blood test that is simple to administer. It is offered at health department clinics, HIV testing and counseling centers, and some private doctors' offices. Depending on where the test is performed, results are given back in anywhere from a day to a couple weeks. Many clinics will offer free, anonymous testing. Private doctors may charge £30 or more, but usually get you the results more quickly. If an ELISA test were to turn up HIV-positive, another ELISA would be performed to check for false positives. After two ELISA tests in which the results are HIV-positive, a different and final test called a Western Blot will usually be performed in order to absolutely verify HIV-positive status.

As of this writing, a new generation of HIV-antibody tests is starting to be used in the USA with greater frequency. A so-called rapid HIV test that produces results in as little as 5 to 30 minutes is available in some clinics, and a variety of urine and oral fluid HIV tests are also gaining in popularity. In the UK, same-day testing is available by appointment in selected GUM clinics from the NHS.

Normally the test would take place in the morning session, and the client or patient would return in the afternoon to pick up the results.

There is also one other type of HIV test that you may have heard of, called the Polymerse Chain Reaction (PCR). Unlike the others, it is designed to detect parts of the virus itself, and not just HIV antibodies. The great advantage of this test is that it reveals HIV in the blood almost as soon as the HIV enters the body, thus eliminating the need for a waiting period between the last exposure and the time of testing. It is also considered an extremely accurate test in which an HIV-negative result virtually guarantees that you are indeed HIV-negative. Unfortunately, though, PCR testing in the United States is still limited to select circumstances. This is because its heightened sensitivity has made it a fairly expensive and impractical test to administer. In addition, it has also produced a somewhat greater number of false positives than the ELISA. In the UK PCR testing is not used in the standard HIV testing of adults although it is increasingly used to detect HIV infection in children before maternal HIV antibodies clear.

Of course, before taking any type of HIV test, it is necessary that you and your partner be physically and emotionally prepared. You should never feel pressured to take it, but if you don't, you obviously should continue using condoms. In addition, I suggest that you only undergo HIV testing where your anonymity is protected, and where counseling services are available should they be needed.

Finally, if the two of you have arrived at the point where your commitment to each other results in a decision to undergo HIV testing, you have probably reached a level of communication where open and honest discussion about all aspects of your sexual health is possible. That is both good and necessary, because the reality is that for the vast majority of you, the risk of contracting several other STDs is much greater than contracting AIDS.

Before giving up condoms, you should discuss with your partner all possible symptoms of any sexually transmitted diseases that either you or he may have acquired. Anything suspicious may merit a trip to a health clinic for some quick testing, or at minimum a review of the latest informational pamphlets available there. Of particular concern is chlamydia, which although not as well known as syphilis or gonorrhea, is the most common STD today. It is easily treated, but if left undetected can cause infertility in both men and women. This is important to keep in mind, since its usual symptoms, burning or an oozing when urinating, are occasionally so mild that people are not even aware that they have it.

There are two other prevalent STDs of which you should definitely be aware: genital warts, which are caused by the human papilloma virus (HPV), and genital herpes. There are two particular types of HPV that could lead to cervical cancer. This simply gives you another reason to get an annual Pap test, for if caught early, the disease is highly curable. (It's worth pointing out that the vast majority of HPV strains do not lead to cancer, and in fact the majority of infections will disappear on their own.) You should also know that in certain cases herpes can be dangerous to a developing embryo, so if you get pregnant and have it, you should inform your doctor.

Those risks aside, HPV and herpes are usually more of a nuisance than a real medical danger. Today, warts are easily removed through laser surgery or by freezing them off with liquid nitrogen. Herpes is more treatable than in the past, in that the occasional outbreaks of genital sores associated with the disease can often be reduced in severity and frequency with various drugs. For both genital warts and herpes, risk of sexual transmission to a partner is dramatically reduced if surface warts are removed or open sores are in remission. However, the risk is never completely eliminated, a fact worth keeping in mind given the prevalence of both in the general population. If you suspect that you or your partner has either of these viruses, you should discuss the situation with a doctor before giving up condoms.

I would like to conclude by stating that although I have been talking about the danger of AIDS and other STDs when *beginning* a new relationship, one certainly needs to be aware that the risk could exist for all couples, no matter how long they have been monogamous. The obvious question is whether either partner had contracted HIV or something else before the present relationship began (or by nonsexual transmission at any time in the past).

Clearly many of you reading this will be in a situation where you have been in a long-term relationship, and you may be desiring to use FAM instead of your old method, which might have been any number of other methods such as the Pill or diaphragm. The fact is that probably most of you are not in a high-risk group for HIV infection, and given your previous decision not to use condoms, I can't honestly say I believe you should immediately run out and get an HIV antibody test. That's a decision you can best make yourself, but it is important that every person intelligently analyze the risks, however small they may be. It's also worth remembering that for those who plan to use FAM as a method of pregnancy achievement, there is the danger of an HIV-positive mother passing on the virus to her baby.

All of this information is important to know so that each individual can make those decisions that are most advisable for their emotional and physical well-being, particularly as related to one's reproductive health. I have no doubt that using Fertility Awareness is consistent with a lifestyle that is both empowering and healthy, but for it to truly be either of these, it simply must be practiced responsibly.

Natural Birth Control Without Chemicals or Devices

Contraceptives should be used on every conceivable occasion.
—Spike Milligan

*T*here are certain clients I will never forget. One particular couple was given my seminar on natural birth control as a wedding gift by the woman's parents. Although they seemed thoroughly absorbed in the class, I was soon to discover that they failed to internalize the most fundamental concept of the method. A month after the seminar, I met with them for their follow-up consultation. Everything seemed to go just fine. Her charts looked great. She recorded her fertility signs perfectly.

But I noticed that even though they had had intercourse throughout her cycle, they didn't record what method of birth control they used in the "method" column of the chart. In other words, they didn't record whether they used condoms, for example, during her fertile phase. So as they were getting up to leave, I casually reminded them to be sure to record what contraceptive they use every time they have intercourse during her fertile phase. She gave me a completely puzzled look, quizzically glanced at her husband, then looked back toward me with a blank stare.

Silence.

I said, "In other words, every time you have intercourse, just be sure to record whether you specifically choose not to use birth control because you are infertile at the time, or record what method you used while you were fertile." Again, the glazed-over look.

And again, more silence.

"What do you mean, 'what method'? I thought this was a method of birth control." The hair stood up on my arms. It was only then that I realized that this couple actually thought that by merely recording her fertility signs, they were using a reliable method of birth control!

Needless to say, the Fertility Awareness Method only works as a contraceptive if you choose either to postpone intercourse or use a barrier method when you are fertile. Statistically speaking, though, you should be aware that the method is much more effective if you choose to abstain at that time. The reason for this is:

1. If a barrier method is going to fail, it's going to fail when you're in your fertile phase. And all contraceptives have a failure rate.
2. Using barriers with spermicide during the fertile phase can mask cervical fluid. (This is one of several reasons why I recommend condoms if you are not going to abstain.)

Ideally, then, the method would be most effective if you only have intercourse when you're infertile. Actually, while it may seem difficult to do, many users of natural birth control feel that this creates a "courtship and honeymoon" effect. This is to say that every cycle there is a phase when the couple finds creative ways to sexually express themselves, knowing that within a few days, they can resume intercourse again. By choosing to postpone sex rather than use a barrier method during the fertile phase, people often feel they're living in harmony with their fertility, rather than fighting it.

Much of this is simply learning to understand how your body works. A way to conceptualize the length of a woman's fertility is to remember that it is totally dependent on the man's fertility. In a vacuum, a woman would only be fertile a maximum of 24 hours, or 48 hours if two or more eggs were released at ovulation. But think of fertility in terms of a range that combines the viability of both sperm and egg. The only reason a woman is fertile for longer than 24 to 48 hours is because sperm can live up to 5 days.

In essence, then, the first part of the woman's fertile phase is determined by the survival of the sperm, the second part by the viability of the egg. When FAM is used for birth control, this typically adds up to about 9 or 10 days, during which abstinence or a barrier method of contraception is called for. This fertile phase includes a significant safety margin on both sides of the woman's fertile phase.*

---

* The maximum ova viability of 2 days is calculated by assuming a 24-hour life span for each egg, the last one being released a full 24 hours after the first. In reality, this is highly unlikely in that ova probably live closer to 12 hours, and multiple ovulations probably occur closer together. And while you must count on sperm survival of 5 days, 2 to 3 is much more probable. Sperm viability of longer than 5 days has been documented, though this is extremely rare, and in any case would not affect the contraceptive principles of FAM given that sperm without cervical fluid present will live at most a few hours.

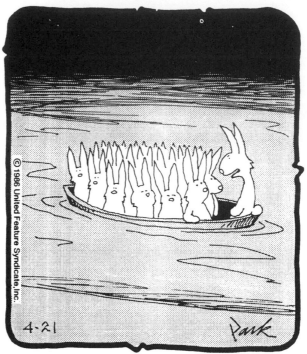

"I'm only gonna say this one more time:
Our only chance is self control."

By thinking of female fertility as a range, you should see that even experienced FAM users can only identify when their fertility begins and ends, and not the exact day of ovulation. To use the method effectively, though, it isn't necessary to pinpoint the precise moment that the egg is released.

For most women, the cycle can basically be divided into three parts. Note that the four FAM rules identify the beginning and end of the fertile phase, which is the time that unprotected intercourse can result in pregnancy.

THE THREE PHASES OF THE CYCLE		
Preovulatory Infertile Phase	**Fertile Phase**	**Postovulatory Infertile Phase**
	The Four FAM Rules	
1) First 5 Days Rule		3) Temperature Shift Rule
2) Dry Day Rule		4) Peak Day Rule

What follows are the contraceptive rules you must employ to use the Fertility Awareness Method with maximum safety. While they may be a bit tricky to internalize on a first reading, they should become intuitive if you've understood the basic biological principles presented earlier in the book. I suggest you read this section slowly and several times, as well as carefully review all of Chapter 6. It's basically easy, but as with any new process, it requires a little patience.

To be safe, I also strongly suggest that you chart at least two full cycles before relying on these rules for birth control. This especially applies to women coming off the Pill, since their bodies may take quite a few months to resume normal ovulatory cycles with clear fertility signs. The peace of mind you'll gain will be more than worth it. If you still find you need further clarification, I would encourage you either to take a class on the Fertility Awareness Method or meet with a qualified instructor. Finally, a guiding principle is that if you encounter any ambiguity, be conservative. All four rules should indicate that you are infertile before you consider yourself safe. If in doubt, don't!

🙊 THE FOUR FAM RULES

Preovulatory Infertile-Phase Rules

> ### 1. FIRST 5 DAYS RULE
>
> You are safe *the first 5 days* of the menstrual cycle *if* you had an obvious temperature shift 12 to 16 days before.

Circle Intercourse on Cycle Day	1	2	3	4	5	6	7	8	9	10	11	12	13	14	15	16	17	18	19	20	21	22	23	24	25	26	27	28	29	30	31	32	33	34	35	36	37	38	39	40
Dry, Spotting or PERIOD	✳	✳	✳	✳	✳		✳	(✳)																									✳							

Chart 9.1. The First 5 Days Rule.

The First 5 Days Rule applies to the first 5 days of the cycle, *regardless* how many days you actually bleed. Any bleeding after the 5th day of the cycle should be considered fertile, since it could mask your ability to check cervical fluid.

By noting an obvious thermal shift 12 to 16 days before you bleed, you have strong evidence that ovulation occurred that previous cycle. This confirms that the bleeding within the first 5 days of the new cycle is true menstruation and not ovulatory spotting or abnormal bleeding unrelated to menses.

This rule is highly effective because the combined risk of ovulation occurring on Day 10 or earlier and sperm living long enough to fertilize the egg is, statistically speaking, extremely rare. Remember, sperm can generally survive a maximum of 5 days, and even that is only in fertile-quality cervical fluid. Still, the rule should be modified for women with a recent history of very short cycles, and it should not be relied upon for women with premenopausal signs:

1. If any of your last 12 cycles have been 25 days or shorter, you should only assume that the first 3 days are safe. This extra precaution is taken because of the increased risk of a very early ovulation. If cervical fluid were to develop while you were menstruating, you would be unable to detect it through the blood, and thus sperm could theoretically survive the few days necessary to fertilize the egg. There is some disagreement in the FAM community over the necessity of this conservative guideline, but I would personally recommend it.*

2. Women approaching menopause with such signs as hot flashes and vaginal dryness should not rely upon this rule at all. This is because premenopausal women are subject to major hormonal changes which could result in dramatically early ovulations (see Chapter 19).

---

2. DRY DAY RULE

Before ovulation, you are safe the evening of every dry day.

Circle Intercourse on Cycle Day	1	2	3	4	5	6	7	8	9	10	11	12	13	14	15	16	17	18	19	20	21	22	23	24	25	26	27	28	29	30	31	32	33	34	35	36	37	38	39	40
Eggwhite																																								
Creamy																																								
Sticky																																								
Dry, Spotting or PERIOD	✗	✗	✗	✗	—	—	—	—	—	—							—	—	—	—		—	—		—	—		—	—	—	✗									
Fertile Phase and PEAK DAY																PK																								
Vaginal Sensation				dry	=	=	=	=	=	=	dry	sticky	wet	wet	WET	LUBE	dry	=	=	=	=	=	=	=	=	=	=	=	=	=										

Chart 9.2. Dry Day Rule. Note that she is safe the evening of every preovulatory dry day, which in this chart occurs on Days 5 to 10.

---

* Unlike the other three rules in this chapter, a part of the First 5 Days Rule admittedly relies on past cycles to estimate a possibly increased risk of present fertility. However, there is a fundamental difference between this particular guideline and the Rhythm Method. The likelihood of conception occurring from intercourse on Day 5 or before is very remote, whereas the chances of ovulation varying widely from Day 10 onward is extremely high. The principle here is to simply add one more buffer for women who may have a somewhat higher risk than the statistical average.

For the record, it is likely that the vast majority of women who truly conceived from sex during their period had intercourse at the end of a long menstruation, on Day 6 or after. There is also a definite possibility that what was perceived as sex during menses was actually sex during ovulatory spotting.

1. Before ovulation, you are safe for unprotected intercourse the evening of every dry day (after 6 P.M.).* Dryness is determined by checking throughout the day and observing that no cervical fluid or wetness is present at any point during the day. But as soon as you see *even sticky*-quality cervical fluid, you should consider yourself potentially fertile.

It may surprise you that you must consider sticky cervical fluid as potentially fertile before ovulation. It's true that it's very difficult for sperm to survive in it. However, the rules are extremely conservative, and take into consideration the fact that a woman may not be able to differentiate between sticky cervical fluid and the beginning phases of the wetter, creamier quality. In addition, this eliminates the risk of wetter fluid dripping down from the cervical tip in time to save the few hearty sperm that may have survived. But if you only experience one or two consecutive days of sticky cervical fluid and then revert back to dry days, you are considered safe again the evenings of each dry day.

To reiterate, then, before ovulation, the only days that are considered safe are those dry days in which there is no cervical fluid present. (Note that women will always notice a slight dampness or moistness at the vaginal opening, which quickly dissipates from the finger. These days are still considered dry if you have no cervical fluid.)

2. The day after intercourse is marked with a question mark if semen or spermicide is present, because they can mask the presence of cervical fluid. The evening of a "Semen Day" is considered fertile since there is no way to prove that day is indeed dry. (For recording semen, see Chart 9.3 below. Better yet, for an efficient way to eliminate semen, refer back to page 88 on SETs.)

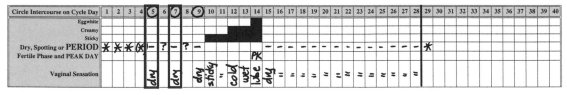

Chart 9.3. When semen masks cervical fluid. Note that she is safe on the evenings of preovulatory dry days, but any day with residual semen must be recorded with a question mark, as she did on Days 6 and 8. These days are considered potentially fertile.

If, by the end of the day after intercourse, you are dry all day, you are safe for unprotected intercourse again that evening. There are two reasons why you can have peace of mind using the Dry Day Rule before ovulation:

---

* If you are tempted to have sex before 6 P.M., see page 352.

a. Sperm can't survive if there's no cervical fluid present to sustain them. At longest, they will live a few hours. And because the sticky-quality cervical fluid that develops before wetter types is just about as inhospitable to sperm as a completely dry vaginal environment, the risk of conception is extremely low.

b. If you don't have cervical fluid, it's an indication that your oestrogen levels are so low that you're not near ovulation. Remember that ovulation is preceded by a buildup of wet-quality cervical fluid.

The above two reasons should reduce fears that you might have regarding the issue of sperm surviving long enough for an egg to pop out. To exaggerate the point, even if sperm could live *10* days in ideal conditions *and* ovulation occurred the day after intercourse, it's extremely unlikely you would get pregnant if your lovemaking was on a dry day. Of course, this scenario would probably never happen, but I want to stress the concept of sperm needing fertile cervical fluid in order to survive and move.

Finally, you should realize that because sperm can survive for five days if fertile-quality cervical fluid *is* present, you absolutely cannot rely on ovulation predictor kits, which only give about one day's warning of impending ovulation. And just for the record—no, arousal fluid and lubricants don't provide the necessary environment for sperm survival.

3. After a couple of cycles of charting, you may notice that immediately after your period ends, you don't have any dry days, as occurs in Chart 9.4 on the next page. Rather, you have a sticky- or even gummy-quality cervical fluid that starts just after menstruation and continues day after day until you see the *change* into a wetter quality. Since this could be an indication of cervical inflammation, you should probably have it checked when you first start charting. But assuming you are healthy, this pattern just means that your Basic Infertile Pattern (BIP) during your infertile phase is *sticky* rather than dry. If this is the case, you may be able to apply the Dry Day Rule on those days of sticky cervical fluid, treating the sticky days as if they were dry. Of course, the first sign of wet cervical fluid is considered fertile.

This exception, though, applies only to those who never experience dry days pre-ovulatory. And even then, you should be aware that you are taking a somewhat increased risk in following this modified guideline. Because of this, I suggest that if you are using FAM with a sticky BIP, you verify that there is no wet cervical fluid at your cervical tip before having intercourse (See Chart 9.4 and Appendix B for further clarification.)

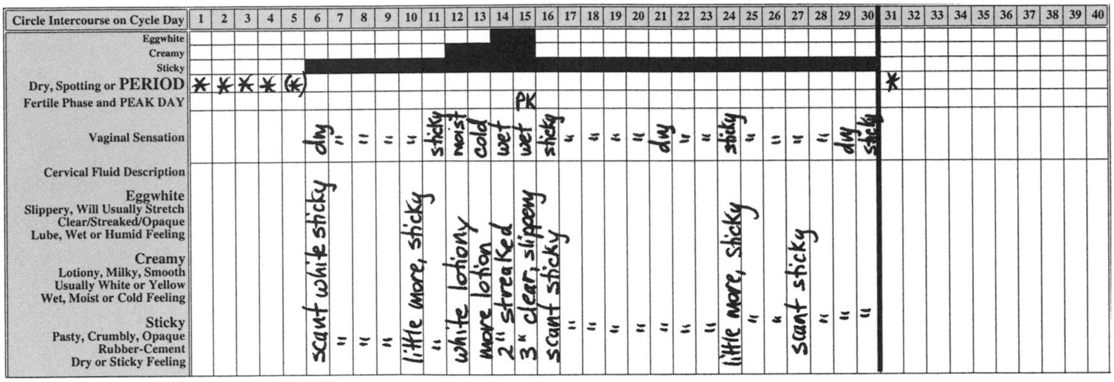

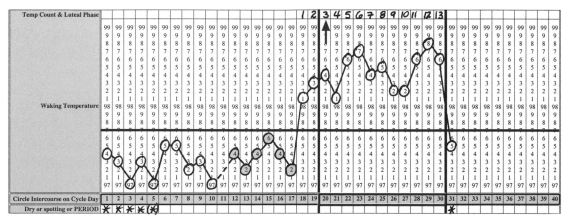

Chart 9.4. Basic Infertile Pattern of sticky cervical fluid. After charting a couple of cycles, Kelly notices that her Basic Infertile Pattern is sticky rather than dry immediately following her period. Because this is her pre-ovulatory pattern, she may treat Days 6 to 11 above as if they were dry, and follow the Dry Day Rule. In order to minimize the risk of pregnancy, she verifies that no *wet* cervical fluid is present at her cervical tip before having intercourse.

Postovulatory Infertile-Phase Rules

3. TEMPERATURE SHIFT RULE

You are safe the evening of the third consecutive day your temperature is above the coverline.

Chart 9.5. Temperature Shift Rule. Note that she had a thermal shift on Day 18, and then drew the appropriate coverline. She then recorded 1,2,3 in the Temp Count row and started her infertile phase the evening of Day 20 after three consecutive high temperatures above the coverline.

The Coverline and Your Thermal Shift

You may want to review how to draw a coverline on page 77. The following rules assume that you have already internalized that information.

1. You are considered infertile starting at 6 P.M. the third *consecutive* night that your temperature remains *above* the coverline. Record the 1, 2, 3 in the Temp Count row of your chart. Draw a vertical line between Days 2 and 3 of high temperatures to indicate that you are safe from the third evening on. (See Chart 9.5 on previous page.)

2. If a temperature falls *on or below* the coverline during the 3-day count, you must start the count over again once it has risen back above the line (I know, I know, boo, hiss). However, you don't have to draw the coverline again.

3. If you are sick, you should not consider yourself safe until you have recorded three consecutive normal temperatures above the coverline without having a fever. (Page 312 explains how illness can affect fertility.)

4. If your thermal shift is not obvious, you may prefer to use a more conservative rule. In this case, you would only consider yourself safe the evening of the third consecutive day your temperature is above the coverline, provided one temperature is at least three-tenths of a degree above.

Assuming that you are also following the Peak Day Rule described on the next page, this conservative approach is not necessary to maintain high contraceptive efficacy, but I still recommend it for those couples who want even further peace of mind. In reality, the majority of women will have thermal shifts in which the criteria for this modified rule are usually met anyway. (For a further discussion on how to handle ambiguous thermal shifts, see page 301.)

You should review the Rule of Thumb on page 78 to see how to handle outlying preovulatory temperatures caused by such factors as alcohol consumption and lack of sleep (as well as fever). Remember that the resulting temperatures can be discounted, but in order to determine your coverline, you must count back six low temperatures, not including the days eliminated. Also remember to compensate for any possible temperature rise caused by Daylight Savings or travel to another time zone.

If you notice that your temperature has risen either higher than normal or earlier than you would expect, pay close attention. This is an important time to observe your other fertility signs as well. Ovulation is virtually always preceded by a buildup of wet cervical fluid and changes in the cervix. If you didn't observe the fluid changes, you shouldn't assume that you've already ovulated.

4. PEAK DAY RULE

You are safe the evening of the 4th consecutive day after your Peak Day.

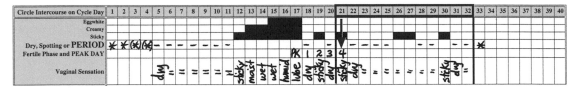

Chart 9.6. Peak Day Rule. Her last day of wet cervical fluid was Day 17. She marked "PK" (for "Peak") under it, then recorded 1,2,3,4 on the subsequent days in the Peak Day row. She considered herself safe the fourth evening after her Peak Day, on Day 21. Note that even though she had sticky cervical fluid on the fourth day, she is still considered safe as long as wet cervical fluid does not reappear during the 4-day count.

1. Identify your Peak Day (the last day of wetness, as described on page 91). Mark "PK" below it, in the Peak Day column. Subsequent days should be labeled "1,2,3,4" in that same row, but it is best to record them only in the evening after having observed your cervical fluid each day. You will only know it is the peak the following day, when your cervical fluid and lubricative vaginal sensation have already started to dry up.

Remember that if your last day of eggwhite is on a Monday, but you still have one more day of lubricative vaginal sensation (or spotting) on Tuesday, your Peak Day is Tuesday. Of course, the reverse applies as well.

2. You are considered safe after 6 P.M. the evening of the 4th consecutive day following the Peak Day. Draw a vertical line between Days 3 and 4 to indicate that you are safe from the 4th evening on. (Note that you are still considered infertile even if you have sticky days after you've drawn the vertical line.)

3. If you have a cervical fluid pattern in which you have a day of creamy after your last day of eggwhite (most women have nothing or sticky), your Peak Day is still considered that last day of eggwhite.

However, if you cannot identify an obvious thermal shift by the second morning after the last eggwhite day, or your creamy days continue, you should be conservative and consider the last creamy day that you have as your Peak Day.

4. Usually, any wetness will dry up until the next cycle, but if wet cervical fluid or vaginal sensations reappear during the 4-day count, as in Chart 9.7 on the next page, wait until the wetness ends to reestablish the Peak Day. Begin the count over again. This type of recurring pattern is sometimes referred to as a "split peak" and is often caused by stress or illness. A delayed thermal shift will ultimately confirm when you have finally ovulated.

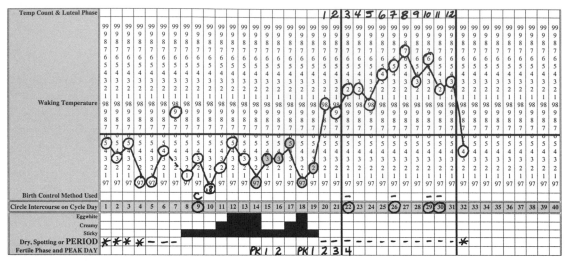

Chart 9.7. Split peaks. Note that she had what is referred to as a split peak. Her body prepared to ovulate by producing fertile-quality cervical fluid starting on Day 11, but then stress or some other factor delayed her ovulation. In this case, it appeared that her Peak Day was Day 14, but after only a couple days, she started producing wet cervical fluid again, so she had to start the count over. Her true Peak Day was then Day 18, after which she counted 1,2,3,4, and considered herself safe starting on the evening of Day 22. While these split peaks can be confusing, a thermal shift will clarify the picture and allow you to determine whether ovulation has actually occurred.

A Word About Vaginal Infections

Almost all women will experience real vaginal infections at various points in their lives. True infections will usually cause symptoms that can mask cervical fluid. For this reason, you should abstain from intercourse during an infection, since the signs may be too ambiguous to be reliable. Regardless, you should abstain anyway to allow your body a chance to heal and to avoid passing the infection back and forth. (For a more detailed description of true vaginal infections, see page 222.)

A Word About Your Cervical Position

As discussed in Chapter 5, the changes in your cervix can also help you determine if you are fertile. However, it is considered an optional sign since it is generally only used to confirm the changes in temperature and cervical fluid. For this reason, there are no specific rules about the changes in your cervix presented in this book. But I do encourage you to observe your cervix if you want one more fertility sign to corroborate with the others.

A Word of Caution About Ovulation Predictor Kits and Other Fertility Monitoring Devices

With the continuing proliferation of ovulation predictor kits and related devices that are designed to interpret your fertility signs, you may be tempted to solely rely on them as a form of birth control. While the kits are usually quite accurate and thus can be useful in helping you to *get* pregnant, they would almost always warn you too late to be of any contraceptive value. And while most of the other devices, such as those fertility monitors that rely on salivary ferning tests, are useful ways to *corroborate* the information that you have learned in this chapter, I don't think they are reliable enough yet to use by themselves. (See page 146 for a more thorough discussion of all of these products.)

🇧 PUTTING IT ALL TOGETHER

You should be aware that the Peak Day of cervical fluid typically occurs a couple of days before the rise in temperature. This pattern has an advantage in that cervical fluid usually dries up quickly the day after the Peak Day, and thus most women can predict their temperature rise the day before it appears.

In addition, note that *before* ovulation, the cervical fluid is the critical fertility sign to observe, because it is the one that reflects the high oestrogen levels indicating the impending release of the egg. But *after* ovulation, the temperature is the critical fertility sign, because it confirms that ovulation has indeed occurred.

The rules that apply to after ovulation will often work in harmony with each other, so that the third evening of high temperatures will coincide with the fourth evening after the Peak Day. However:

1. If there is a discrepancy between the two postovulatory rules, *always wait until both signs indicate infertility* to be most conservative (i.e., until the evening after the vertical line farthest to the right). This assures that all the signs have coincided before you consider yourself infertile.
2. *If in doubt, don't take a risk!* If your fertility signs don't make sense in any given cycle, it's not worth risking unprotected intercourse if it's critical that you avoid pregnancy.

The next two pages summarize the rules that you have learned in this chapter, as well as show you how they would typically appear on your chart.

NATURAL BIRTH CONTROL AT YOUR FINGERTIPS . . .

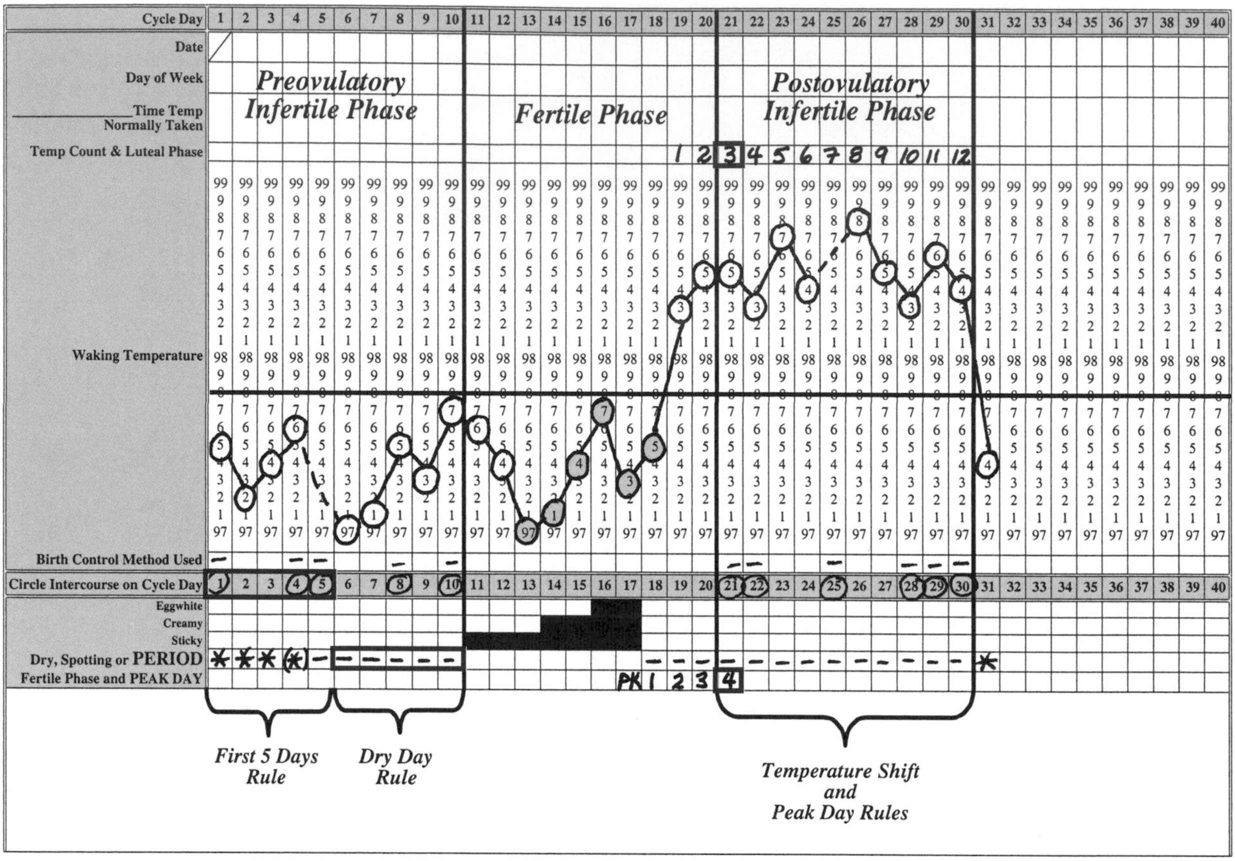

Preovulatory Infertile Phase

Fertile Phase

Postovulatory Infertile Phase

Cycle Day

Date

Day of Week

Time Temp Normally Taken

Temp Count & Luteal Phase

Waking Temperature

Birth Control Method Used

Circle Intercourse on Cycle Day

Eggwhite / Creamy / Sticky

Dry, Spotting or PERIOD

Fertile Phase and PEAK DAY

First 5 Days Rule

Dry Day Rule

Temperature Shift and Peak Day Rules

Chart 9.8. The fertile and infertile phases as defined by the four standard FAM rules.

SUMMARY OF THE FOUR FAM RULES

The basic biological principles are italicized below each respective rule.

I. FIRST 5 DAYS RULE
You are safe *the first 5 days* of the menstrual cycle *if* you had an obvious temperature shift 12 to 16 days before.
For most women, the combined risk of ovulation occurring on Day 10 or earlier and sperm living long enough to fertilize the egg is extremely remote.

2. DRY DAY RULE
Before ovulation, you are safe the evening of a dry day.
Sperm cannot survive in a dry vaginal environment, and the lack of cervical fluid indicates that estrogen levels are too low for ovulation to occur.

3. TEMPERATURE SHIFT RULE
You are safe the evening of the 3rd consecutive day your temperature is above the coverline.
The rise in temperature due to the release of progesterone indicates that ovulation has occurred, and waiting 3 days allows for the remote possibility of two or more eggs being released over a 24-hour period, with each one living a full day.

4. PEAK DAY RULE
You are safe the evening of the 4th consecutive day after your Peak Day.
The last day of wet cervical fluid or vaginal sensation indicates the imminence of ovulation, while allowing 4 days for drying up assures that any eggs released are already gone, and that the return of a dry vaginal environment is inhospitable to sperm survival.

A CAUTIONARY NOTE

While this box is a useful summary, you must clearly understand all the guidelines for each rule described in this chapter before using FAM for birth control. It is also critical that you don't consider yourself safe unless *all* the rules indicate that you're infertile. If you have any doubts, don't take the risk.

Finally, you should know that these rules are a highly effective form of contraception if they are consistently and correctly followed. However, the relative risks of natural birth control should be understood by the user. I therefore urge you to read Appendix D before relying on what you have learned in these last few pages.

CHAPTER 10

Shortcuts: Minimum Charting with Maximum Reliability

> For those of you who just skipped ahead to this page, don't even *think* of using the rules in this chapter until you've charted several complete cycles.

*A*lthough the Fertility Awareness Method is really very simple once you've learned it, even experienced users don't necessarily want to chart every day to achieve maximum reliability. With a little experience under your belt, you can restrict charting to only about a third of the cycle and still attain all the information necessary to apply this method, without compromising contraceptive efficacy.

The reason you can have peace of mind using the shortcuts explained on these pages is that once you have ovulated, your body won't release an egg again until the following cycle. So once you've identified when the egg is dead and gone, it's unnecessary to continue charting until your next period.

It is my recommendation, though, that you chart without using shortcuts. I personally think it's easier to do it everyday than to have to think about where you are in your cycle. As you've seen, charting is also about much more than just detecting when you can and can't get pregnant. And finally, by charting your complete cycle, you will often benefit from one of its most practical aspects: being warned often hours before you get your period by the drop in temperature that most women experience on the first day of the flow.

But if you still prefer to take shortcuts, you can use the modified guidelines discussed below. Contraceptive efficacy won't be compromised, as long as your fertility signs have confirmed that ovulation has already occurred for that particular cycle.

❧ WAKING TEMPERATURE

It's unnecessary to take your temperature during your period, since these temperatures tend to be somewhat high or erratic anyway. In addition, once you've established the occurrence of a thermal shift by counting at least three high temperatures above the coverline, you needn't take your temperature again until your period from the next cycle is over (Chart 10.1, below).

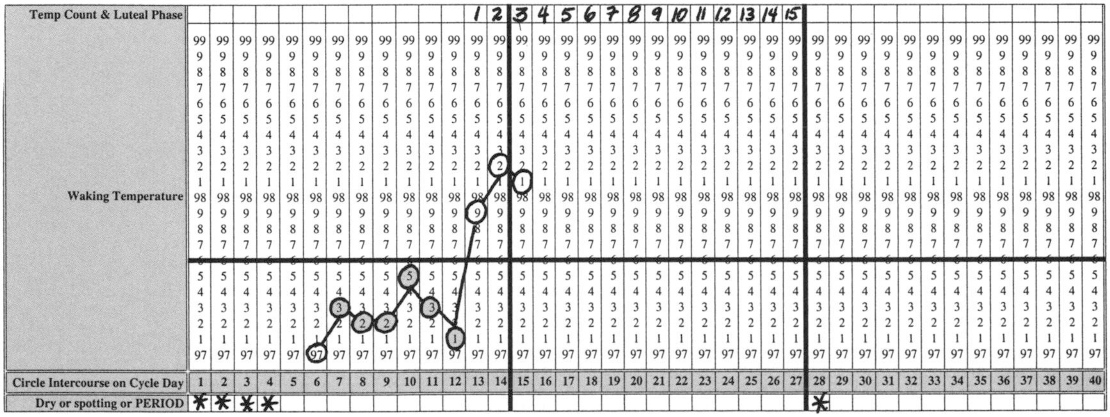

Chart 10.1. Temperature Shift Rule with minimum charting. Once she had her third high temperature above the coverline by Day 15, she no longer needed to chart her temperature until the next cycle because she had already established that ovulation has passed.

❧ CERVICAL FLUID

You never have to check your cervical fluid during your period. In fact, there is no point in checking while menstruating since the bleeding will mask it. And once you've established the first safe day under the Peak Day Rule, you needn't chart your cervical fluid again until your next cycle.

Circle Intercourse on Cycle Day	1	2	3	4	5	6	7	8	9	10	11	12	13	14	15	16	17	18	19	20	21	22	23	24	25	26	27	28	29	30	31	32	33	34	35	36	37	38	39	40
Eggwhite																																								
Creamy																																								
Sticky																																								
Dry, Spotting or PERIOD	✗	✗	✗	✗	✗	−	−						−	−	−												✗													
Fertile Phase and PEAK DAY											PK	1	2	3	4																									
Vaginal Sensation						*dry*	*=*	*=*	*wet*	*wet*	*lube*	*sticky*	*dry day*	*dry day*	*dry day*																									

Chart 10.2. The Peak Day Rule with minimum charting. She started to check her cervical fluid as soon as her period stopped, in this case on Day 6. Once she established that she was 4 days past her Peak Day on Day 15, she could be fairly certain that she had already ovulated and would therefore not have to continue charting her cervical fluid until the next cycle. (However, in order to rely on this shortcut, it is imperative that she confirm ovulation through the Temperature Shift Rule.)

A cautionary note: *If you intend to rely on the shortcut version of the Peak Day Rule, it is critical that you establish that ovulation has passed by observing three high temperatures above the coverline.* This is because you may have a delayed ovulation in which your cervical fluid could mislead you into thinking you had already ovulated. If you were no longer charting that cycle, you would perhaps not notice the return of fertile cervical fluid. By observing a true thermal shift, your chances of being misled in this way are virtually eliminated. Still, you should continue to check your cervical fluid throughout the cycle if the accuracy of your temperatures could have been compromised due to illness or other factors. As always, be conservative (see Chart 10.2).

❧ CERVICAL POSITION

The position of the cervix is considered an optional fertility sign. This means that it's not necessary to check the cervix in order for the method to be effective. However, the cervical position is an excellent sign to cross-check the other two signs if there is ever a discrepancy between them.

Since checking the cervix is not altogether necessary, there are two shortcuts you could take at this point. You could choose not to observe the cervix at all, or you could merely check the cervix about a week per cycle. The time to start checking it would be at the first notice of wet-quality cervical fluid, continuing to check through to the 3rd day after the cervix has begun to revert back to becoming firm, low, and closed. However, to use this shortcut, you may need to chart the cervix for several cycles to be able to detect the subtle changes that occur with it (see Chart 10.3 on the next page).

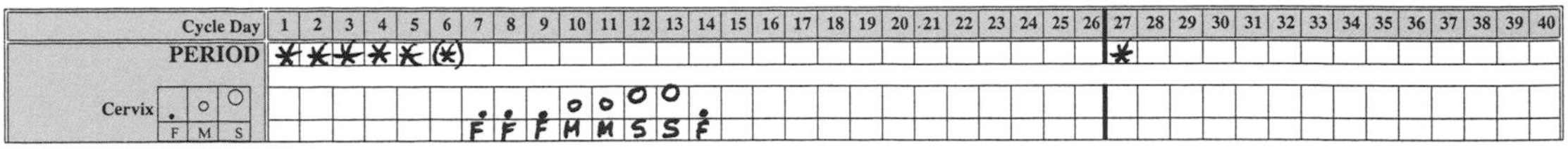

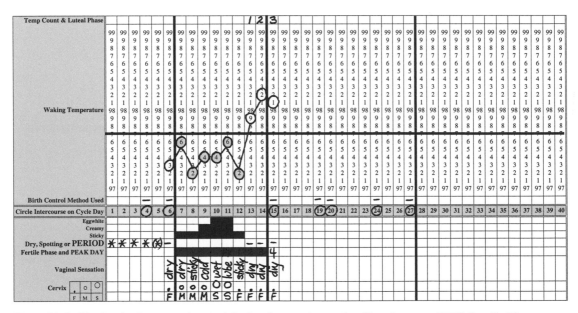

Chart 10.3. Observing the cervix with minimum charting. Because she wanted to chart the minimal number of days necessary while still being as conservative as possible, she recorded her cervical position to verify that ovulation had passed.

𝒫 A NOTE ON THE PREOVULATORY RULES

It should be obvious that if you choose to use these shortcuts, the preovulatory rules still apply. Thus, you can only assume you're infertile during the first 5 days of your cycle if you meet the criteria of the First 5 Days Rule, which states that you must have had an obvious temperature shift 12 to 16 days before. In addition, you must always follow the Dry Day Rule, and therefore must begin to chart no later than Day 6.

Chart 10.4. The basic shortcut chart with the three primary fertility signs. ▬ **Fertile Phase**

🙚 THE FALLACY OF THE I-JUST-KNOW-WHEN-I'M-FERTILE MENTALITY

One word of warning about taking shortcuts: Once you decide not to chart every day, it can be very tempting to slack off and either chart even less than recommended or stop altogether, convincing yourself that you just *know* when you're fertile. I cringe when women claim they don't need to record because they always know when they're fertile. Ironically, experienced women who have charted for years often feel that they, too, can become lax in charting because they "just know." But even if your cycles have always been regular and your charts easy to interpret, there's always the chance that the next cycle will be different from all others. Like any other birth control method that "fails" because of improper use—such as leaving the diaphragm in the drawer—FAM must be used correctly to work.

Simply intuiting when you are or aren't fertile is not a reliable method of birth control. In fact, it's no method at all. You need to chart your temperature and cervical fluid, even if it's for just a third of your cycle. Otherwise, it can be too easy to forget what transpired on any given day. In the end, you may find that charting becomes so second nature that you won't even be tempted to take the shortcuts described above.

PART FOUR

PREGNANCY ACHIEVEMENT

CHAPTER 11

Maximizing Your Chances of Getting Pregnant

Literature is mostly about having sex and not much about having children; life's the other way round.

—DAVID LODGE, British author

If you're like most people trying to get pregnant, you probably remember the years of hassling with birth control and all that entailed—the diaphragms that flew across the room when you attempted to insert them, the condoms that broke at the peak of lovemaking, or the Pill that caused you to balloon in weight. In fact, you may have even experienced sleepless nights worrying about whether you had accidentally become pregnant, even though you used birth control consistently.

Yet here you are, years later, perhaps bemoaning the fact that you spent so much time and energy trying to *avoid* pregnancy, only to discover that it may not have been so easy to get pregnant after all. For some couples, getting pregnant may indeed be difficult. But for many, it can be as simple as learning how to optimize your chances of conception by identifying when your combined fertility is at its greatest. Surprisingly, the chances of a typical couple of proven fertility conceiving in any one menstrual cycle is thought to be no higher than about 25%. But you can increase the chances dramatically by identifying the optimal time to try.*

While most would acknowledge the great benefits derived from advances in medical technology, there are drawbacks. One is that people are often led to believe that the most efficient and only way they will be able to get pregnant is through invasive procedures. Not only is this often untrue, it can also be counterproductive. Modern methods can ironically impede or delay the very pregnancy they were designed to aid (for example, Clomid tends to dry up cervical

---

* Of course, the odds of a successful pregnancy begin to steadily decrease as women age into their mid-30s and beyond, and thus if possible, you should try to conceive before this becomes an issue (see pages 177 and 216).

fluid, and artificial insemination may be inappropriately timed). Today, there are countless ways to diagnose and treat so-called infertility. But if you think you might face a fertility problem, FAM should always be the *first* step in the pursuit of pregnancy.

When trying to get pregnant, dispense with all the misinformation that well-meaning friends and clinicians seem to perpetuate. If you've read this book in sequence, and didn't sneak a peak at this chapter first, you should already know that there are a number of truths about fertility which differ from the myths you've heard.

One of my couples illustrated the benefit of knowing you are still fertile even though it would appear that you are well beyond the day of ovulation. Carrie and Jake were extremely demoralized when I met them. They had been trying to get pregnant for nearly two years since the tragic death of their baby. Since they didn't have any trouble conceiving the first time, they were perplexed by why it was taking so long to get pregnant again.

In their particular case, what helped them to conceive again after those two years was the realization that if Carrie's temperature hadn't shifted yet, they were still considered fertile. She said that she was almost relieved when her temperature was still low on Day 22, because it meant they still had an opportunity to get pregnant that cycle. So rather than feeling anxious, she felt much more in control. They knew to continue having sex each day that she had wet cervical fluid and the temperature remained low. They had intercourse and conceived on Day 22. Sure enough, her temperature rose the next day, confirming that they had timed it just right.

৯৯ FERTILITY TRUTHS

1. A normal cycle is not necessarily 28 days; it ranges from about 24 to 36 days. It varies from woman to woman as well as within individuals.
2. You can ovulate as early as Day 8, and as late as Day 22 or beyond. The point is that women do not necessarily ovulate on Day 14.
3. Your most fertile day cannot be determined by your temperature. In fact, most women don't even experience the "temperature dip" that they've often been told to look for.
4. You are *not* most fertile the day of the rise in temperature, either. In fact, by the time the temperature rises, it's usually too late—the egg is already gone.

5. The key to identifying your most fertile phase is through cervical fluid, and not waking temperatures.

6. You don't need to stand on your head for half an hour after making love in order to get pregnant! If you are timing intercourse at the most fertile time, the sperm will swim up through the cervical fluid rapidly, regardless of what position you are in.

7. How often you should have intercourse during your fertile phase (i.e., every day or every other day) is a function of the combination of your partner's sperm count and your cervical fluid. It's not a hard-and-fast rule that applies to all couples alike.

8. Both men and women are equally likely to have a fertility problem.

℘ WHY SOME WOMEN ARE MORE FERTILE THAN OTHERS

Even being armed with accurate knowledge doesn't necessarily guarantee a timely pregnancy. If it is taking longer than you had anticipated, probably the last thing you want to hear are the annoying clichés of well-meaning women about themselves:

"They just call me Fertile Myrtle."

"He just has to look at me and I get pregnant."

"I've gotten pregnant on every method of birth control [giggle, giggle]. I guess I was just destined to be a mom."

Actually, there are several reasons why such women do indeed tend to be more fertile than others. In addition to the obvious fact that their reproductive organs are healthy, they may have a long phase of extremely fertile-quality cervical fluid, providing them more opportunities to get pregnant. Also, women with short cycles tend to ovulate more often, which means that they have more fertile days in a given year. But even though these women have a biological head start, you can certainly level the playing field by charting your cycle.

> *Vanessa and Max were a charming couple who had taken my class initially to avoid pregnancy. After two years of using FAM successfully, they decided it was time to try to get pregnant. But a trip to Mexico delayed their plans by several months while they allowed the malaria medications to dissipate from their bodies. So the first month in which they were able to try was March. Then a little detail looked like it was going to interfere. Max had just had major surgery on a shoulder that had eroded from years of playing basketball. He spent several days in the hospital after the operation.*

His first night back home he was in a lot of pain, and was completely drugged to help him handle it. Vanessa walked in and proudly announced, "Tonight's the night." The eggwhite was too obvious to miss. As Max recounted. "Trust me, sex was the furthest thing from my mind. Here I was, with my shoulder and arm taped to my torso to immobilize it, flat on my back, pumped with painkillers, and my wife walks in and says: 'It's time. I'm fertile.' Needless to say, I explained to her that I was hardly in a position, so to speak, to have sex, when she reminded me that she could take care of everything herself. So with me half out of it, she proceeded to do what was necessary to allow conception to occur. Sure enough, from that one single act of sex that cycle, we conceived our little boy Don."

You may take a lot longer to get pregnant, of course. The point is that knowing when you are most fertile will expedite the process. If, after 4 to 6 cycles of timing intercourse on your most fertile days, you still haven't gotten pregnant, you should probably pursue diagnostic testing or fertility treatments. (Some couples may want to get a semen analysis even earlier, given how easy it is to have done.)

❧ A WORD ABOUT OVULATION PREDICTOR KITS

Before getting to the crux of how FAM can help you get pregnant, I want to say a few words about ovulation predictor kits, since so many of you will no doubt be tempted to use them. While they can in fact be quite useful, you should know by now that your own body usually provides you with as much valuable information as the kits, with less hassle and certainly at less cost. Still, if you do choose to use them (either exclusively or with Fertility Awareness), you should be aware that they can be misleading for the following reasons:

1. The kits test only for the occurrence of the luteinizing hormone (LH) surge that precedes ovulation. They don't indicate whether the woman has definitively ovulated afterward. In fact, women may occasionally experience a condition called LUFS (Luteinized Unruptured Follicle Syndrome) in which they have an LH surge but the egg never actually pops out of the ovary. This condition is further discussed on page 206.

2. A woman may experience false LH surges in which she has mini-peaks of LH before the real one, causing her to potentially time intercourse too early for the sperm to survive long enough for the release of the egg. In addition, if the woman has PCOS (see page 204), her body may continually produce false LH surges, not indicative of impending ovulation.

3. The kit does not indicate whether the woman has suitable cervical fluid to allow sperm a medium in which to travel to the egg. In addition, by the time the kit does show a surge, the cervical fluid could already be starting to dry up.

4. The kits are only as accurate as the individual using them. There are typically many steps involved, any one of which can be performed improperly, rendering the test invalid. In addition, their accuracy can be compromised if exposed to excessive heat during delivery and storage.

5. The kits are only accurate if they test a woman's fertility right around the time of ovulation. This is a very significant point, because often the type of woman who purchases them is one who, by definition, has irregular cycles. Therefore, the typical kit, which has only 5 to 9 days' worth of tests, will often not have enough to cover the range necessary for her to determine ovulation.

For example, if Mary has cycles that are between 29 and 42 days, then her ovulation will generally vary between Days 15 and 28, which is a range of 13 days. Since the kits last 9 days at most, it could be quite a challenge for the woman with irregular cycles to know on what day of the cycle to begin testing. What this means is that women with irregular or long cycles should not start testing their urine until they notice their cervical fluid start to get wet, so as to test at the most appropriate time around ovulation.

6. Women with short luteal phases may not realize that the kits instruct them to test for ovulation based on an average length luteal phase. This may lead a woman to test much earlier than she is actually ovulating. Therefore, the test results may reflect anovulation, when in reality, ovulation has probably not yet occurred (see page 174).

7. Some fertility drugs such as Pergonal, Danol, or injections containing HCG (e.g., A.P.L. or Profasi) can invalidate the results of these kits. Clomid does not have this effect.

8. Women over 40 and approaching menopause can have elevated levels of luteinizing hormone that are not indicative of ovulation. A kit should only show a surge of one day. If it shows more than one day, there is an increased chance it is invalid.

9. Finally, you should be aware that if you happen to be pregnant already, the kit will simply imply that you aren't ovulating. Of course, this is true, but this tells you nothing of your real condition (whereas charting would, as you'll soon learn).

OTHER METHODS OF OVULATION DETECTION

Aside from the standard ovulation predictor kits (OPKs) just discussed on the previous pages, there are now several other ways to predict ovulation. Here is a brief description of some of the more widely used devices that are currently available:

Clear Plan Easy Fertility Monitor

This is a palm-sized electronic system that works with a standard urine test to monitor your cycle. By analyzing both estrogen and LH within the urine, a computer is able to tell you if you are currently in a low, high, or peak phase of your cycle. If used correctly, it can effectively predict ovulation about 1 to 2 days before it occurs. The whole system costs about £120, including 20 urine test sticks.

Cue II Saliva Monitor

This is a device that measures the level of electrolytes in your saliva. By placing a probe in your mouth for a few seconds each morning, a "saliva reading" registers on a digital screen. The probe is used every day from the first day of your cycle until the computer signals you are within 7 days of ovulation. If you are trying to get pregnant, you would then begin having intercourse every day or every other day, while continuing to use a small accompanying vaginal sensor, which eventually confirms that ovulation has occurred. The Cue II costs over £210, though it may be possible to rent the base unit for much less while paying for just the sensors, which cost about £50.

Salivary Ferning Tests

Just as your cervical fluid will show a distinct ferning pattern as you approach ovulation (see page 3 of color insert), your saliva will often do the same thing. Although brands will vary, these tests generally come with several acrylic slides and a specially designed microscope through which to view the results. Each morning, before doing anything else, you put some saliva on one of the slides by licking it or using your fingertip. Perhaps not surprisingly, it is now widely accepted that there is a high correlation between salivary ferning and the approach of ovulation. Unfortunately, though, reports in the medical literature also suggest that it can often be difficult to interpret the slides. Prices vary by company, but they typically cost at least £30 for a microscope and several slides.

Bioself Fertility Indicator

Unlike the others, this computerized device is based exclusively on basal body temperature. You enter the date of the first day of your current cycle, then use the attached temperature probe. After you record your temps each morning, the system automatically calculates if you are pre- or postovulatory, based on the same temperature principles that you have learned in this book. It also projects when you have entered your most fertile phase, but since this is based on a statistical analysis of the length of your *past* cycles, its accuracy is questionable if you do not have consistent cycle lengths. It costs about £60.

A Brief Comment on These Ovulation Detection Devices

Like OPKs, these new technologies may be able to assist you in determining your most fertile days each cycle, but be aware that each one generally has at least a few of the same weaknesses that I noted for the kits.

And regardless, while they can do an excellent job of corroborating your charting, none will give you the comprehensive information that your own BBT and cervical fluid will give you directly every day.

✌ THE ROLE OF FAM IN PREGNANCY ACHIEVEMENT

I wish getting pregnant were always as easy as making love when the mood strikes. Yet for many people, it requires more knowledge than we were typically taught while growing up. And unfortunately, people can be incredibly educated and well-read and still require high-tech procedures to get pregnant. But for a lot of people presumed to have a fertility problem, FAM can help fulfill their desire to get pregnant in many ways.

Infertility can have many causes. FAM allows couples to hone in on them more quickly, thus helping their doctor determine if they require medical intervention. Conventional medical wisdom is for a couple to have intercourse for a full year before seeking help for pregnancy achievement. What an unnecessary waste of time and emotional energy that is for most people! Using FAM, couples often discover that getting pregnant simply involves optimizing their chances with newfound knowledge about their combined fertility, rather than simply trying haphazardly. In timing intercourse precisely with the most appropriate frequency, one should be able to tell if there is a problem within only a few months of trying.

Anne is a 36-year-old woman who almost never menstruated from the age of 28 on. Naturally, she suspected that it would be a real challenge to get pregnant. A fertility doctor prescribed the ovulatory drug Clomid for 6 months. During that time, although she ovulated, she experienced a number of unpleasant side effects, the most serious being vision problems so severe that they caused her to see in quadruple. In addition, the Clomid exacerbated her problem of poor cervical fluid production. So after several months of frustration on the drug, she decided to discontinue it. In fact, she and her husband, Jay, a physician, were so discouraged with the experience that they welcomed the break from feeling obligated to get pregnant.

One morning, about 4 months after stopping Clomid, she woke up "swimming in eggwhite," as she says. Since she hardly ever ovulated, she rarely experienced such fertile cervical fluid. They knew that if they had any hope of getting pregnant, they had to take advantage of that moment. Sure enough, she conceived that day, without the aid of anything but the knowledge of Fertility Awareness that they both possessed. Little Lena was born at home 9 months later.

Fertility Factors You Can Detect Through Waking Temperatures

As you saw from the couple above, cervical fluid is the critical fertility sign to chart when trying to get pregnant. But basal temperatures can be equally beneficial, for altogether different reasons. One of the most common mistakes couples make is trying to time intercourse by the waking temperature. Remember, temperatures are useful to determine if you are ovulating, and how long your luteal phase is. But they are not helpful for identifying impending ovulation, which is the most fertile phase of the cycle. So waiting for either the dip or rise in temperature is virtually useless for timing sex. The dip only occurs in a very small percentage of cycles, and by the time the temperature rises, it's usually too late.

However, I want to reiterate that taking your waking temperature is very useful for several reasons besides timing intercourse. Using the typical cycle in Chart 11.1 on page 152 as a standard of comparison, you can see how temperatures can reflect numerous things about your fertility.

Your waking temperatures show whether:

- you are ovulating at all (Charts 11.1 and 11.2)
- your luteal phase is long enough for implantation (at least 10 days), thereby preventing the need for painful and unnecessary diagnostic tests such as an endometrial biopsy. Note that a luteal phase is determined by the number of days between the rise in temperature and the first day of true menstruation, and not premenstrual spotting (Chart 11.3; also see box on the next page)

- your progesterone levels are high enough in your luteal phase (Chart 11.4)
- you are still fertile any given cycle as reflected by low temperatures (Chart 11.5)
- you may have gotten pregnant, as reflected by more than 18 high temperatures (Chart 11.6)
- you may have gotten pregnant, as reflected by more than 18 high temperatures, even though you have menstrual-like bleeding at about the time of your expected period (Chart 11.7)
- you may be in danger of having a miscarriage, as determined by a sudden drop in temperatures (miscarriages occur as often as one in three pregnancies) (Chart 11.8)
- you were pregnant before having what seemed to be just a "late period" (Chart 11.9)

HOW TO DETERMINE THE LENGTH OF YOUR LUTEAL PHASE

Technically, the luteal phase is defined as the time from ovulation until your next period. The most practical way to determine how many days that comprises is by counting the high temperatures above the coverline. Do not include the day of the new period.

There are two situations in which you might need to modify this slightly:

1. If your temperature drops below the coverline a day or two before you start your period, you simply include those low temperatures in the count. (See page 311.)
2. If your thermal shift consistently occurs more than two days after the Peak Day, it probably means that your body reacts slowly to the heat-inducing progesterone released after ovulation. In such a case, it may be more accurate to count the second day after the Peak as the first day of the luteal phase rather than waiting for a thermal shift. (See page 314.)

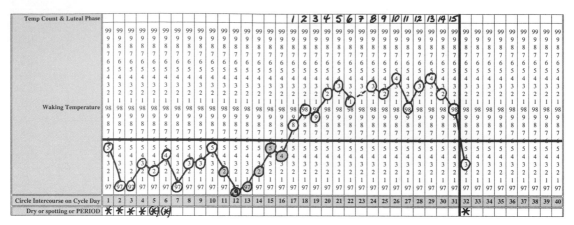

Chart 11.1. A typical ovulatory temperature pattern. Note that ovulation had almost certainly occurred by the thermal shift on Day 17. Her luteal phase was 15 days, determined by counting the high temperatures from Day 17 through to the last day before her period on Day 32.

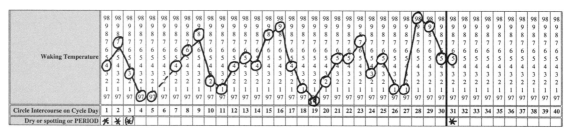

Chart 11.2. An anovulatory temperature pattern. Her temperatures indicate that she didn't ovulate because there was no thermal shift from a range of lows to a range of highs. The bleeding she experiences on Day 31 of her cycle is technically not menstruation but anovulatory bleeding. For charting purposes, it should still be treated as Day 1 of a new cycle.

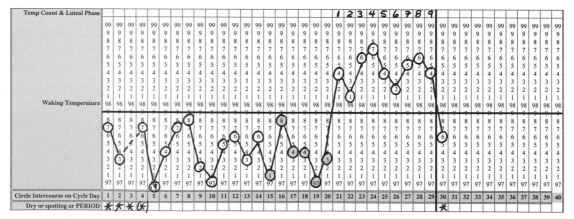

Chart 11.3. A short luteal phase. Note that while her 29-day cycle length is normal, her nine postovulatory high temperatures indicate a short luteal phase (counting Days 21 to 29). In order for implantation to successfully occur, it is believed that a woman should have a postovulatory phase of at least 10 days.

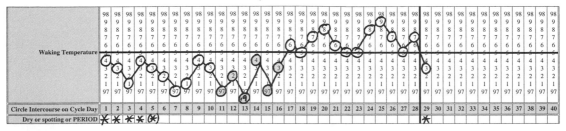

Chart 11.4. Low postovulatory progesterone. Note that her high temperatures do not remain above the coverline following ovulation. This could be an indication of low progesterone levels.

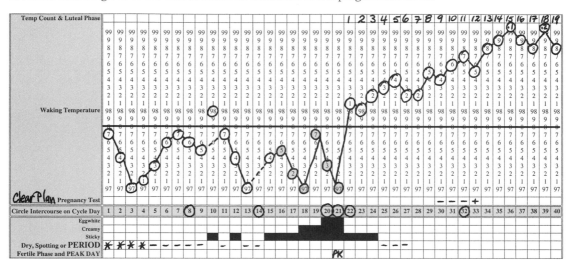

Chart 11.5. A delayed ovulation. Sabrina was able to determine that she was still fertile as late as Day 21, because her temperature had not yet risen and her cervical fluid was still wet. Therefore, she timed intercourse accordingly and got pregnant.

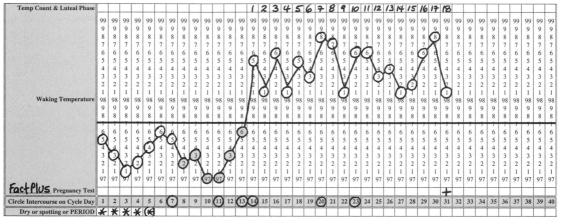

Chart 11.6. A pregnancy chart. Sandy could tell she got pregnant by Day 31, because she then had 18 high temperatures after ovulation. (The postovulatory phase is rarely more than 16 days if a woman is not pregnant).

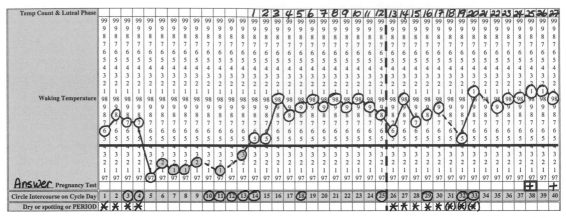

Chart 11.7. A rare and confusing pregnancy chart. On Day 26, Lynn assumed she started her period but was baffled when her temperatures remained high well into the next cycle. After 13 days of continued high temps, she took a pregnancy test, only to discover that she was indeed pregnant. Were she not charting, she would never have thought to take it. (See her story on page 157.)

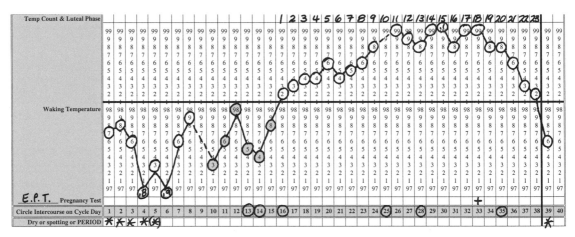

Chart 11.8. Pregnancy followed by a miscarriage. This woman was almost certainly pregnant, as seen by the fact that she had her 18th high temperature on Day 33, she confirmed her suspicion with a positive pregnancy test, but she then got a warning that she was probably about to miscarry by the pattern of falling temperatures starting about Day 36.

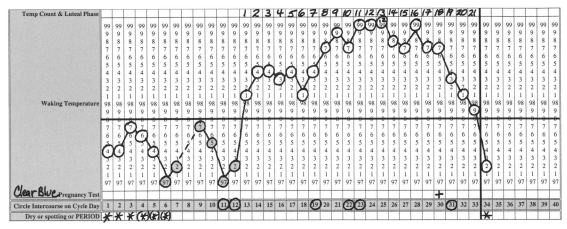

Chart 11.9. Miscarriage that would have seemed like a late period. Note that if she had not been charting, she wouldn't have been able to observe the 18 high temperatures, and thus she might have thought that her bleeding on Day 34 was simply a late menstruation, rather than a miscarriage.

How Charting Temperatures Can Indicate Conception and Prevent Unnecessary Interventions During Pregnancy and Delivery

As you can see, one of the most practical benefits of recording your temperature is to determine if and *when* you got pregnant.

> *One of the couples who took my class had been trying to become pregnant for exactly a year when they heard about my seminars. They returned for their follow-up consultation the succeeding month after "completing" one full cycle. I use "completing" loosely here, because the day they came in, something seemed suspiciously different. As I welcomed them into my office and set Zoey's chart on the desk, my heart skipped a beat. Rather than seeing the typical 12- to 16-day luteal phase most women experience, I noticed that Zoey's was awfully long. After having observed charts for over 13 years, I could usually spot such things immediately, without needing to count. But not wanting to give either of them a false sense of hope, I tried to discreetly look at the chart and count in my head . . . 12, 13, 14, 15, 16, 17, 18 . . . Yes, sure enough, she was pregnant. Today was the 18th day of her luteal phase.*
>
> *When I finally looked up, my eyes caught Zoey's, and both of us started laughing. Alex just didn't get it. She said, "Toni, are you laughing for the reason I think you're laughing?" I said, "Well, do you have any other explanation for today's eighteenth high temp?" The lightbulb finally went off, and he understood. At last, after a year of trying, they got pregnant the first cycle they charted.*

Of course, the most important reason to know the date of conception is to determine when the true due date will be, and not the one based on the pregnancy wheel's assumption of a Day 14 ovulation. Knowing this will prevent inappropriately timed tests such as amniocentesis. In addition, it may allow you to avoid an unnecessarily induced labor due to a miscalculation of the due date. (This is especially problematic in women who tend to have long cycles.) While it's true that ultrasound clarifies many of these ambiguities, many couples still prefer to avoid such procedures.

If you are charting and prefer not to use ultrasound, there is a simple mathematical formula for calculating your approximate due date. Simply add 9 months to the day of your thermal shift and then subtract 7 days from that date. Thus, for example, if your temperature shift was on January 20, you would jump ahead to October 20, and then subtract 7 days, for an approximate due date of October 13. If you ovulated about Day 14, the estimated due date will be about the same for both the formula and pregnancy wheel. But if you ovulated well after Day 14, the formula will be substantially more accurate. (Regardless how you calculate the due date, remember that they are still, at best, approximations.) *

---

* When clinicians measure a pregnancy by its *gestational age,* they assume a Day 14 ovulation based on the first day of your last menstrual period. A more accurate approach is to determine the *fetal age,* which is measured from the day of conception, as ascertained by either the thermal shift, Peak Day, or ultrasound.

I'm pretty sure that I am....
but what if I'm not.... what if
it's negative ... or nerves... or
imagination. Actually, I'm
positive I am. I'll phone
for a checkup. But what
if they tell me I'm not....
better wait another week
to make sure ..... No. Why
wait if I'm POSITIVE!...
Then again... what if I'm not....
On the other hand...
maybe.........

LYNN

More on How to Use Your Temperatures to Determine If You Are Pregnant

One of the more interesting examples of temperatures alerting a woman to a potential pregnancy was that of Lynn, a woman who was trying to conceive after 8 cycles of charting. Up until then, she had completely normal ovulatory cycles of between 24 and 27 days. This time, though, when she got her period on Day 26, she was naturally disappointed, but assumed they would try again the next month. Her period lasted longer than normal, but that was not the only thing that concerned her. Her temperatures simply did not drop as they should by the end of menstruation. Finally, on Day 13 of the following cycle, with her temps still well above the coverline, she took a home pregnancy test and, much to her amazement, discovered that she was pregnant (see Chart 11.7, page 154).

She never did learn what caused the bleeding, because she didn't realize the relevance of the high temperatures until about a week after it stopped. By then, it was too late for the doctor to determine why. But two doctors she consulted said that her HCG levels were so high that it could have been "vanishing twin syndrome." Today, she and her husband, Paul, are the delighted parents of a little girl named Jordan, conceived during Cycle 8.

As you've seen, a general rule is that 18 high temperatures mean you are pregnant (see Chart 11.6, page 153). And you can determine this without spending a dime on a pregnancy test (though it is advisable to confirm it with a clinician). In addition, you can usually tell even *before* 18 high temperatures whether you are pregnant by two means:

1. You can be fairly confident you are pregnant if your temperatures remain high three days beyond your longest luteal phase to date. For example, if your luteal phases are typically 12 days, and if your longest one has been 13 days, but one time it is 16 days, it is likely you conceived that cycle (see Charts 11.10 and 11.11, on the next page).

2. If you notice a *third* level of temperatures beyond the typical biphasic pattern you experience every cycle, you are almost certainly pregnant. This third level of high temperatures is thought to be due to the extra progesterone circulating in pregnant women. (Unfortunately, not all pregnant women experience such a triphasic pattern, and even when they do, the third set of high temperatures is often more subtle than the second set.) (See Chart 11.12, page 159.)

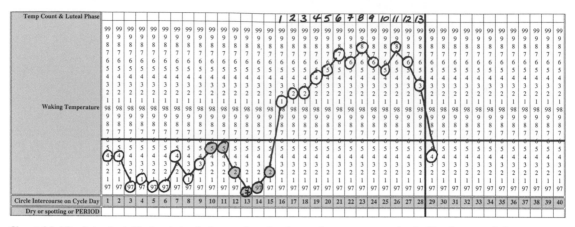

Chart 11.10. A typical 13-day luteal phase. Sara has been charting as a method of birth control about a year. Her luteal phases have always been 12 or 13 days, never more.

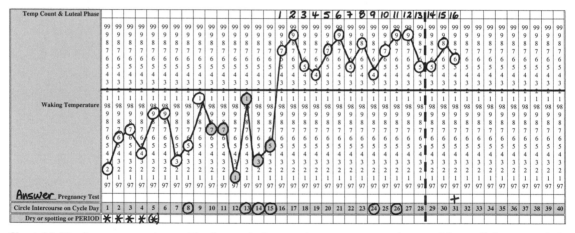

Chart 11.11. A pregnancy chart. The first cycle Sara tried to get pregnant, she was able to tell she succeeded as soon as her 16th postovulatory high temperature (by Day 31), because she knew that her normal luteal phase never extended beyond 13 days.

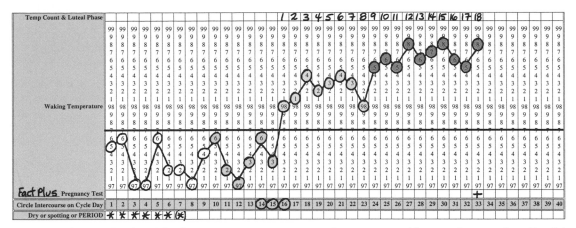

Chart 11.12. The classic triphasic pregnancy pattern. Note that Jenny was able to predict as early as Day 24 that she was probably pregnant because she was starting to observe a third level of high temperatures reflecting additional progesterone at the time of implantation. The fertilized egg burrows into the uterine lining about a week after ovulation.

℘ USING A COVERLINE

In order to interpret your chart, you'll want to draw a coverline to help you differentiate between low and high temperatures. You should review page 77 if you have not already internalized how to draw one. While the coverline is not as critical for pregnancy achievement as it is for contraceptive purposes, it is still a useful tool that will allow you to see more easily when you ovulated in any given cycle.

℘ MALE FERTILITY

You now understand why basal temperatures are so revealing for pregnancy achievement. And of course you already learned how critical cervical fluid is for conception to occur. But before you combine this information into an efficient strategy to use with FAM, you should at least know some basic information about male fertility and the standard semen analysis.

It's important to remember that in determining sperm count, the analysis of your partner's semen must do more than simply measure the number of sperm per ejaculate. It should also tell you what percentage of those sperm are of normal shape and size (morphology) and what percentage are rapidly moving forward (motility). It is a complete analysis of these three factors that actually tells you whether your partner's count is normal, low, or infertile, thus allowing you to strategize accordingly. In reality, this is quite intuitive, for what ultimately defines male fertility is the number of sperm that have the capacity to fertilize an ovum.

As of this writing, his sperm count would probably be considered normal if his ejaculate contains at least 20 million sperm per millimeter, and if the total number of sperm is at least 40 to 50 million. In addition, the percentage of those sperm that are of normal morphology and motility is a critical factor, but because sources vary so greatly as to what is considered an adequate percentage, it is best if you discuss this with your doctor.

The simple fact is that the standards by which semen analysis is judged vary from lab to lab and evolve over time. Therefore, when your partner gets his sperm analyzed, you should insist that his physician answer two questions as clearly as possible:

1. Is his sperm count considered normal, low, or infertile?
2. How did the lab reach this conclusion?

If a man's sperm count is subfertile, the analysis will be repeated at least one or two more times within a few weeks of each other. This is because different factors may impact sperm, and an occasional low sperm count may be an inaccurate reflection of his normal sperm.*

&a OPTIMIZING YOUR CHANCES OF GETTING PREGNANT

If you are just starting to try to get pregnant, there's no particular reason for your partner to rush out and get a semen analysis. *Unless you have reason to think otherwise, you should tentatively consider his sperm count normal and follow the guidelines listed below for normal counts.* However, for those who have been trying at random for a year, or have been timing intercourse by charting for about four cycles, I would encourage you to get a sperm analysis as soon as possible. It is a simple enough procedure and it's probably worth doing soon, since its results will help you know how best to time intercourse. Remember, fertility problems are *equally* divided between men and women.

---

* One of the troubling realities of contemporary life is that men's sperm counts have plunged by about 50% since the 1930s. It's unclear what is causing this, but some theorize that it may be due to modern environmental toxins.

And now you are ready for the nuts and bolts of maximizing your chances of pregnancy. This is the most practical part of the chapter on getting pregnant. The bottom line is that when deciding how to best time intercourse, the frequency with which you make love should be a function of your combined fertility. That is, it should be determined by your partner's sperm count and the timing of your fertile cervical fluid.*

If the Man's Sperm Count Is Normal

Under these circumstances, you should have intercourse every day that you have wet cervical fluid or vaginal sensation, through to and including the day of the first rise in temperature. Of course, the closer you time intercourse to your Peak Day (the last day of wetness as described on page 91) the more likely you are to conceive.

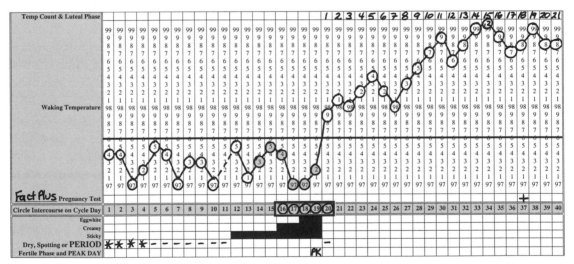

Chart 11.13. When to time intercourse with normal sperm count. Note that this couple started timing intercourse the first day she noticed wet (creamy) cervical fluid on Day 16, and continued every day through to the morning of the rise in temperature on Day 20. They were able to confirm that they succeeded 18 high temperatures later, by Day 37.

* Reread Chapters 5 and 6 if you don't remember how to identify the fertile cervical fluid necessary for conception to occur.

If the Man's Sperm Count Is Low

You should have intercourse every *other* day that you have eggwhite cervical fluid *or* a wet vaginal sensation, through to and including the day of the first rise in temperature (if you don't have eggwhite, follow this guideline with the wettest cervical fluid you have). The reason you should have intercourse less frequently is because men with low sperm counts may need the extra day to build up to higher, more fertile levels (Chart 11.14 below). In fact, ideally, you should abstain from intercourse until your cervical fluid becomes slippery, enabling the sperm count to reach an optimal level just before ovulation.

Another way to further your chances if the man's sperm count is low is the following: If you can, observe how many days you tend to have the most fertile-quality cervical fluid each cycle. For example, if you notice that you tend to have only two days of creamy cervical fluid (with no eggwhite) and your partner's sperm count is low, wait until the *second* day of creamy to have intercourse. This optimizes your chances the most, because the last day of creamy is considered the most fertile day of your particular cycle. By waiting until that day, you have allowed the sperm count to build up enough to maximize your chances of pregnancy (Chart 11.15).

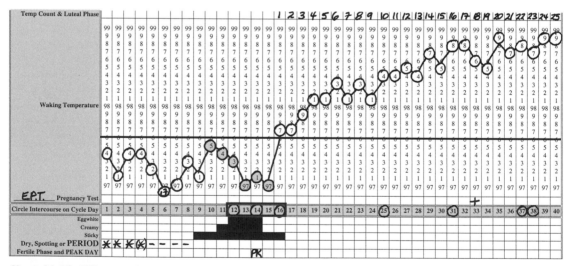

Chart 11.14. When to time intercourse with low sperm count. Note that this couple started having intercourse the first day she noticed eggwhite on Day 12, but then had sex only every other day through to the morning of the rise in temperature on Day 16. This allowed the sperm count to build up on the "off days." They were able to confirm that they succeeded 18 high temperatures later, by Day 33.

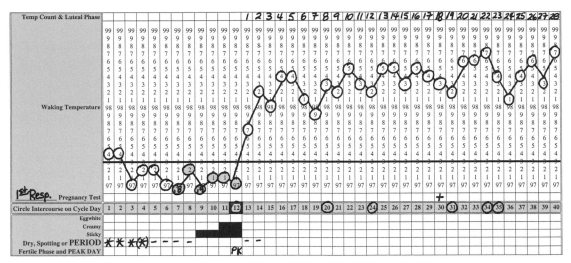

Chart 11.15. Maximizing your chances of conception when your partner's sperm count is low and you have minimal fertile cervical fluid. Note that she only has about 2 days of creamy cervical fluid per cycle. Since his sperm count is low, they chose to time intercourse on the second and last day of her creamy cervical fluid, optimizing their chances of pregnancy by reserving the highest number of sperm for her Peak Day of fertility. They were able to confirm that they succeeded 18 high temperatures later, by Day 30.

The table on the next page will summarize what is likely to be the best strategy for getting pregnant, assuming two conditions:

a. You tend to observe a fairly consistent number of fertile days each cycle (i.e., creamy or eggwhite cervical fluid or lubricative vaginal sensation).

b. Your partner has a low sperm count.

It requires a certain amount of discipline to be able to pass up an opportunity to have sex on a day of eggwhite, knowing full well that eggwhite is the most fertile-quality cervical fluid on the continuum. But the principle is to consider the combined fertility of the two of you. If your partner's sperm count is low, you'll want to increase your chances by making sure that it is high enough on the *last* day of the most fertile cervical fluid or vaginal sensation, since that day is the closest fertile day to ovulation.

BEST STRATEGY FOR GETTING PREGNANT IF YOUR PARTNER HAS LOW SPERM COUNT

Typical Number of Fertile Days You Have Each Cycle (i.e., creamy, eggwhite, or lubricative vaginal sensation)	Strategy
1 fertile day	Only day—Have intercourse
2 fertile days	1st day—Abstain 2nd day—Have intercourse
3 fertile days	1st day—Have intercourse 2nd day—Abstain 3rd day—Have intercourse
4 fertile days	1st day—Abstain 2nd day—Have intercourse 3rd day—Abstain 4th day—Have Intercourse

If the Man's Sperm Count Reveals Infertility

The good news is that with today's advanced technologies, there is still hope for a pregnancy. See Chapter 14 for high-tech treatments.

Tips That Apply to Men with Both Normal or Marginal Sperm Quality

A tip that may help men with either type of sperm count is to abstain from any ejaculation for at least a few days just before your cervical fluid begins to appear fertile. Of course, you may think this is like telling your mate to get off the bus at the stop before you. How would he know ahead of time when that is? But if you are really in tune with your body, you will be able to anticipate when it just begins to become slightly fertile. He should try to abstain from any type of ejaculation for those few "barely fertile sticky" days to build up a high enough count to take advantage of your ideal cervical fluid.

If you still haven't gotten pregnant after several months of trying this strategy, you may want to modify it slightly. In other words, those who had intercourse every day should try having intercourse every *other* day during your fertile cervical fluid. And those who had intercourse every 48 hours may want to try it every 36 hours instead.

Finally, most of the sperm is in the first spurt of ejaculate. Therefore, the man should try to penetrate deeply and remain still while ejaculating so that the majority of sperm will be deposited at the cervix, allowing easy access to the cervical opening.

A Note About the Semen Emitting Technique (Kegels)

In order to time intercourse most effectively, you should eliminate residual semen so that it won't mask your cervical fluid in the following days. This is easily done by doing Kegels a few hours after sex. Those sperm with potential to fertilize will then have had all the time they need to swim beyond the cervix (see page 88).

Why to Include the Day of the Rise in Temperatures for Intercourse

Given that you have already learned it is generally too late to conceive after the thermal shift has occurred, you may be wondering why I still suggest intercourse up through that very day. This is because there is still a small chance of conception due to several factors. A multiple ovulation may allow for another egg to still be viable, and there is even a slight possibility of a single ovulation occurring right after the shift. There is also a decent chance the egg is still alive if ovulation occurred within the previous 12 hours. While the odds are not good, it's still worth trying, particularly if you have intercourse the *morning* of the rise.

Sexual Frequency: Maximizing Your Odds

The number of days per cycle that you should have intercourse will be a function of your combined fertility. A woman will generally have fertile cervical fluid for 2 to 4 days. Depending on the man's fertility, you should take advantage of each of those days or just every other one. *The critical point is to include the Peak Day, which is the last day of eggwhite or lubricative vaginal sensation.* This day is considered the most fertile because it generally occurs either on the day you ovulate or the day before. Note that if you don't observe eggwhite, you should try for the last day of the wettest-quality cervical fluid you do have.

What that means, practically speaking, is the following: if you see eggwhite on Monday and take advantage of it by having intercourse that day—great. But, if you still see eggwhite the following Wednesday, have intercourse again because the ovum has probably not yet been released, and you are still extremely fertile. (Of course, Tuesday would have also been a good day to try, assuming your partner's sperm count is normal.)

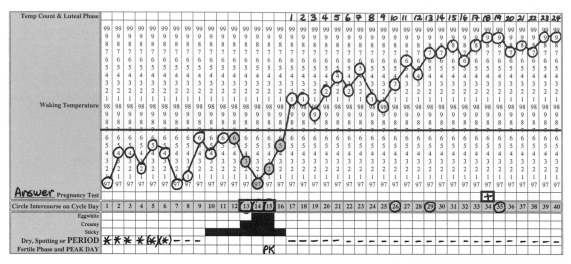

Chart 11.16. Going for the gold . . . got it!

WHEN THE LONG-AWAITED PREGNANCY OCCURS

Once your temperatures remain above the coverline for at least 18 days and you have not gotten your period, you are almost certainly pregnant.*

Pregnancy Symptoms

Beside the obvious 18 high temperatures above the coverline (or even the triphasic pattern that some women get), there are often other signs of pregnancy, including:

- tender breasts or nipples
- nausea
- fatigue
- excessive urination
- implantation spotting (light, brownish bleeding about 8 to 12 days after ovulation)

---

* The one rare exception when 18 high temperatures may not reflect a pregnancy is in the case of a corpus luteum cyst, as discussed on page 316.

A Few Words About Pregnancy Tests

If you can't wait 18 days because the suspense is killing you, you could get a blood test 7 to 10 days after your thermal shift that has a high degree of accuracy. Of course, blood tests are somewhat inconvenient and expensive. You could also do a home pregnancy test of your urine, but they are not quite as accurate, and usually cannot detect the presence of the pregnancy hormone (HCG) until about the time of your missed period or even later, depending on the sensitivity of the test.

Be aware that if you have been given an HCG shot to aid in ovulation induction, you may observe a false positive. And whether you get a blood test or urine test, you may occasionally have a false negative, meaning that you are in fact pregnant, but the test indicates that you aren't. The most common reason for false negatives is that they are performed too early, before the egg has had a chance to implant and start producing HCG. In some cases, implantation may have occurred, but it may still be too early for the HCG to be detected. Obviously, if your temperatures continue to remain above the coverline beyond 18 days, simply repeat the test a week later, and it will almost certainly reflect a positive result.

Or, if all else fails, you could always utilize the foolproof method that Skip Morrow so eloquently describes in his greeting card below:

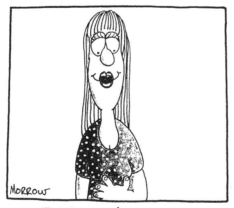

CONCLUDING REMARKS ON GETTING PREGNANT

As you've read, couples are usually told to see a physician if they haven't gotten pregnant within a year of trying. By now you should realize how unnecessary it is to wait a full year if you've been timing intercourse precisely. So if you have not gotten pregnant after 4 to 6 cycles of intercourse during your most fertile days, you should carefully read Chapter 14 to see what diagnostic tests and treatments to consider.

If, however, this chapter helps you to attain your dream of a healthy pregnancy, then congratulations! The joy that you'll receive will no doubt bring you bittersweet rewards to last a lifetime. As Elizabeth Stone once said, "Making the decision to have a child . . . is to decide forever to have your heart go walking around outside your body."

SUMMARY OF WAYS TO OPTIMIZE CHANCES OF GETTING PREGNANT

1. The most important tip for getting pregnant is to have intercourse on the Peak Day, which is the *last day* of eggwhite cervical fluid or lubricative vaginal sensation. (If you don't observe eggwhite, try for the last day of the wettest cervical fluid you have.)
2. If your partner's sperm count is normal, have intercourse every day you have fertile cervical fluid. If his sperm count is low, have intercourse every *other* day that you have fertile cervical fluid and, ideally, abstain from intercourse until your cervical fluid becomes slippery. In either case, try to have sex through to and including the first morning of your rise in temperature.

•••••••••••••••••••➤   NOW THROW THE CARD AWAY, IT'S YUCKY.

WAIT NINE MONTHS.

IF YOU HAVE A BABY, YOU WERE PREGNANT AT THE TIME OF THE TEST.

Practical Tips Beyond Fertility Awareness

*B*eyond using the principles of Fertility Awareness to time intercourse most efficiently, there are a number of tricks that can help you conceive. Most are things to avoid, but some are positive things you can do. All of them should be considered in light of your own personal situation. Because so many of the tips deals with the interplay between diet and conception, you may want to explore this topic more thoroughly in Marilyn Shannon's book, *Fertility, Cycles, and Nutrition* (Couple to Couple League International, Inc., 2001.)

ℬ LUBRICANTS

The bad news is that virtually all artificial lubricants, vegetable oils, glycerin, petroleum jelly, and even saliva can kill sperm. And though there have been recent studies that show canola oil (not available in the UK) and baby oil have minimal impact on sperm, I would be hesitant to use these since oil-based lubricants can increase the risk of vaginal infections.

Until recently, there really wasn't a viable option to use during the one time in your life that you probably would have appreciated it most. Luckily, though, a revolutionary new vaginal moisturizer has recently been developed that is specifically designed to mimic natural body secretions and provide an optimal environment for sperm. It is called Pre~Seed, developed by Bio~OriGyn, and works by delivering a pH balanced semen-like fluid. You can learn more about it at www.BioOriGyn.com.

✍ POSITIONS DURING INTERCOURSE

Although no definitive studies appear to have been done, there is considerable speculation that if the man has a marginal sperm count, the best position for intercourse is the traditional missionary position. This allows for deepest penetration, and will thus deposit the sperm closest to the cervix. Some clinicians also believe that if your cervical fluid is not that fertile, or the sperm quality is marginal, it may be advantageous for you to remain lying down for up to half an hour in the basic position in which you had intercourse. The theory is that this will help assure the sperm time to travel up.

✍ HEALTHY DIET, WEIGHT, AND EXERCISE

You've probably heard it a million times before, but I'll repeat it again. When trying to get pregnant, your body should be as healthy as possible. This may mean limiting consumption of refined foods, excess sugar, caffeine, and products with additives. (In other words, basically restricting yourself to nuts and twigs.) All of these can impede the liver's ability to metabolize hormones. Eating a well-balanced diet of wholesome foods can eliminate such potential problems. In addition, there is some speculation that heavy milk consumption may adversely affect fertility.

In order to ovulate, most women probably need at least 20% body fat. But just as being underweight can prevent ovulation altogether, being overweight can also alter your cycles by causing excessive production of oestrogen, which interferes with the normal feedback system of the hormonal cycle. Some of the signs of excessive oestrogen are prolonged periods of fertile cervical fluid buildup, delayed ovulation, and irregular cycles. To eliminate hormonal imbalances due to being under or overweight, you should try to attain a normal weight through wholesome foods and exercise.

Finally, you should be aware that one of the most important vitamins you should take when preparing for conception is folic acid. By taking just one milligram of folic acid per day in the first 6 weeks of pregnancy, you can dramatically decrease your baby's risk of neural tube defect, brain and spinal cord defects, and spina bifida. Since this vitamin has been shown to be so beneficial, you should begin taking it well before you even start trying to conceive, to be sure it is in your system from the day of fertilization.

THE THREE PRIMARY FERTILITY SIGNS

WAKING TEMPERATURE

Day	1	2	3	4	5	6	7	8	9	10	11	12	13	14	15	16	17	18	19	20	21	22	23	24	25	26	27	28	29	30	31

(Waking temperature chart showing a biphasic temperature pattern with a thermal shift after ovulation around Day 18.)

CERVICAL FLUID

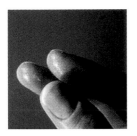 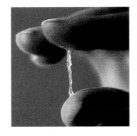 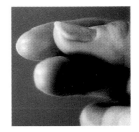

CERVICAL POSITION

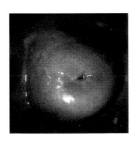 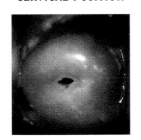 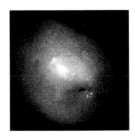

The chart and pictures above reflect the three primary fertility signs of one woman's cycle, which in this case was 30 days in length. These photos were taken on Days 12, 17, and 20. As she approaches ovulation around Day 17, increasing levels of estrogen cause her cervical fluid to become progressively wetter, developing into a pattern similar to the top photographs on the back of this page. In addition, her cervix becomes soft, high, and dramatically open. But quickly after ovulation, the strong effects of progesterone replace the influence of estrogen. Thus, her temperature shifts upward, her cervical fluid dries up, and her cervix reverts back to firm, low, and closed. (For the bottom pictures, her cervical fluid was removed so as not to obscure the opening. Also, note that the photos are unable to reflect the height of the cervix within the body, although they do reveal an obvious difference in its angle after ovulation.)

1

TYPES OF CERVICAL FLUID

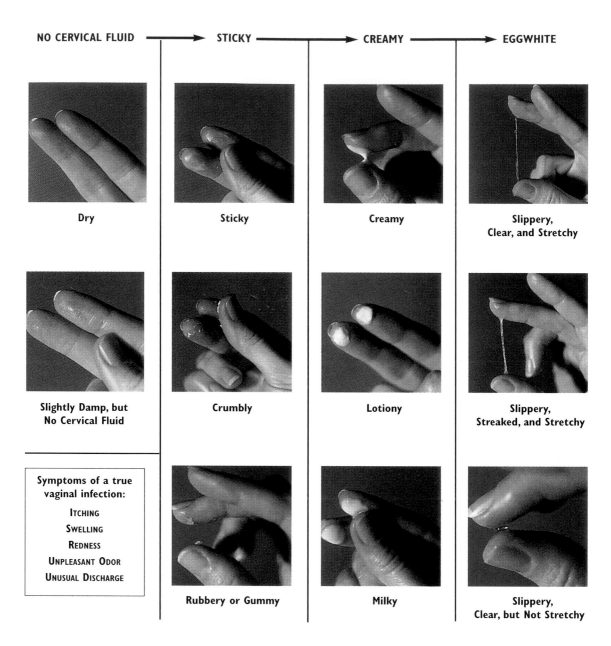

NO CERVICAL FLUID ——→ STICKY ——→ CREAMY ——→ EGGWHITE

Dry

Sticky

Creamy

Slippery, Clear, and Stretchy

Slightly Damp, but No Cervical Fluid

Crumbly

Lotiony

Slippery, Streaked, and Stretchy

Symptoms of a true vaginal infection:

ITCHING
SWELLING
REDNESS
UNPLEASANT ODOR
UNUSUAL DISCHARGE

Rubbery or Gummy

Milky

Slippery, Clear, but Not Stretchy

Most women tend to be dry for a few days after menstruation, but as they approach ovulation their cervical fluid becomes increasingly wetter. The above photographs show healthy variations in what women may experience. Symptoms of a true vaginal infection are shown in the box to the bottom left. A woman's Peak Day of fertility is the last day of a slippery, lubricative-quality cervical fluid or vaginal sensation.

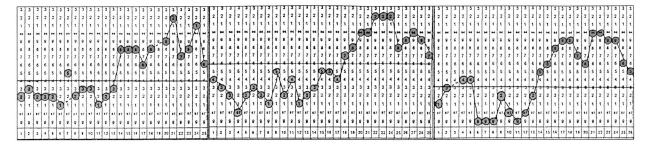

Seeing the Forest Through the Trees

Note the obvious pattern of thermal shifts indicating ovulation in three of the author's charts, placed side by side. Even though there are a few temperatures that appear out-of-line or even missing, you can clearly see a pattern of lows before ovulation (blue) and highs after ovulation (pink).

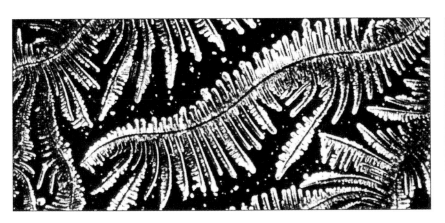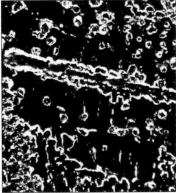

The Ferning of Fertile Cervical Fluid

When viewed under a microscope, the stretchy-type cervical fluid in the pictures on the opposite page look like a beautiful ferning pattern conducive to sperm motility (*left*). The drier, sticky types of cervical fluid do not have such a magical appearance (*right*).

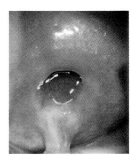

The Most Fertile-Quality Cervical Fluid

Fertile eggwhite-type cervical fluid exudes from this woman's open cervix right before ovulation.

THE BEAUTY OF REPRODUCTIVE BIOLOGY

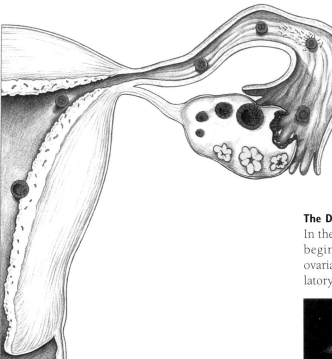

The Life of an Ovum
In the illustration above, a tiny egg within the ovary slowly develops its own follicle (red). After completely maturing, it bursts out of the follicle and through the ovarian wall, in the most significant event of the menstrual cycle: ovulation. In most cases, the just-released egg (blue) will continue on its journey, moving forward through the waiting fallopian tube.

The follicular material left behind in the ovary will soon form the corpus luteum (yellow), which emits progesterone. If fertilization does not occur, it will die within 12 to 16 days, causing progesterone levels to plummet and menstruation to follow.

If intercourse occurs in the short fertile phase surrounding ovulation, the sperm can meet the newly released egg within the tube, where fertilization takes place. The fertilized egg then continues the journey, implanting in the lining of the uterus about a week later.

The Drama of Ovulation
In the top photograph, the egg is just beginning to burrow through the ovarian wall. By the bottom the ovulatory process is almost complete.

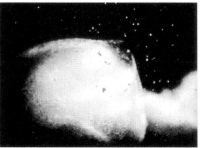

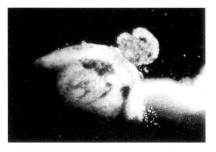

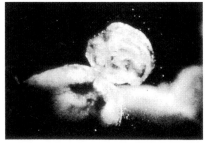

4

YOUR BODY, YOUR CYCLE: OVULATION IN PERSPECTIVE

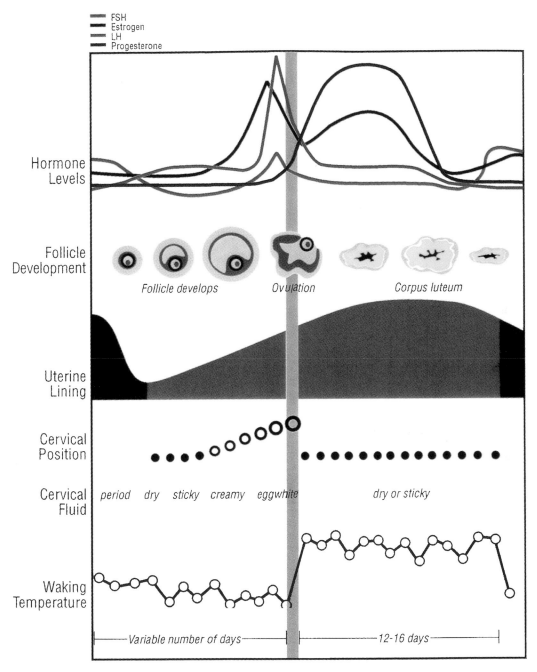

Note that the length of the phase before ovulation can vary widely, but the phase after ovulation is almost always 12 to 16 days. Within *individual* women, the postovulatory phase is remarkably consistent, usually not varying more than a day or so.

The Journey Continues

The newly released egg begins its voyage down the fallopian tube. Fertilization must occur within the egg's short life-span, which may be up to 24 hours, though 6 to 12 hours is more likely for any given egg. It is for this reason that the vast majority of conceptions are assumed to result from *pre-ovulatory* intercourse. Unlike the egg, sperm can survive several days, but only if fertile-quality cervical fluid is initially present to serve as a medium.

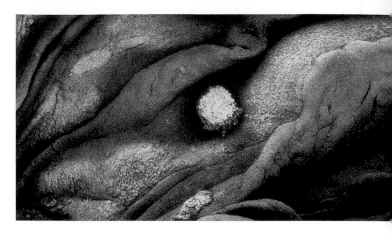

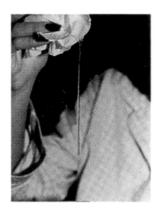

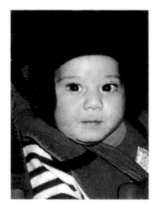

Stretching the Concept of Perfect Timing

To see how the cervical fluid (*far left*) led to the conception of this little guy, see page 17.

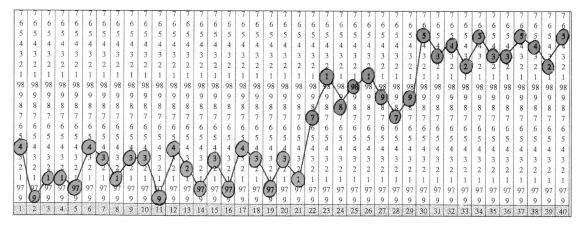

A Triphasic Pregnancy Chart

When a woman becomes pregnant, her temperature pattern often evolves into three levels, as can be seen by the three colors above. The second level is the result of the progesterone released after ovulation, while the third level is thought to be the result of the pregnancy hormone HCG, which circulates after implantation. Note that this woman ovulated about Day 21, not Day 14, as seen by the fact that her thermal shift didn't occur until Day 22.

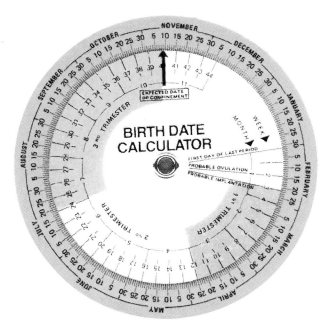

A Typical Pregnancy Wheel
The calculating device to the left is considered indispensable in determining a woman's due date. However, it is often inaccurate since it assumes that all women ovulate on Day 14, regardless of when they really do. This wheel is set for a woman whose first cycle day was February 1st, and thus ovulation was assumed to have occurred on February 14th. In reality, she could have easily ovulated a week or more later, as seen on the chart on the opposite page. Also note how the due date is referred to as the "Expected Date of Confinement," one of the many curious terms discussed in Appendix J.

Color-Coding Rows for Recording Secondary Fertility Signs Such as PMS and Ovulatory Pain
Charting your cycle can be beneficial for reasons beyond merely identifying your fertility. In the chart to the right, the woman records when she exercises as well as various secondary signs such as cramps and headaches, using colors to make her chart more graphic. This woman is able to track pre-menstrual and menstrual cramps as well as pain during intercourse, two possible symptoms of endometriosis. Color-coding this way will help her doctor better diagnose her condition. Additionally, she circles BSE for the breast self-exam she does on Day 7 of every cycle. A master copy of this basic chart, as well as others, can be found at the end of the book.

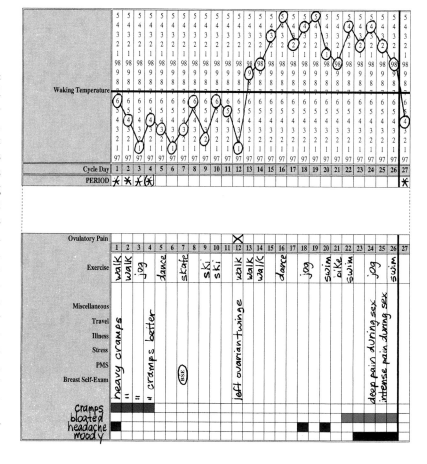

7

JANE RESPONSIBLE'S CHART

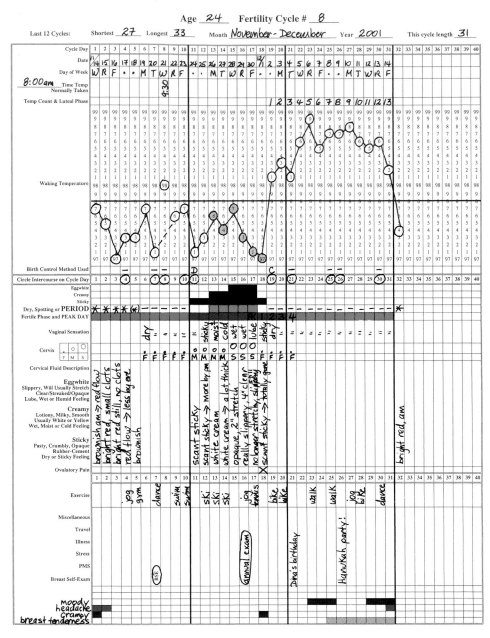

A blank master of this chart is printed on the second to the last page of this book. This particular chart is used for birth control, with the key below reflecting its fertile and infertile phases. Of course, cycles vary, which is why charting consistently is so vital.

■ Fertile phase   ■ Infertile phase   ■ Most fertile days

❧ CAFFEINE, NICOTINE, DRUGS, AND ALCOHOL

If you have unexplainable infertility, you and your partner should both seriously consider reducing or even eliminating caffeine, nicotine, drugs, and alcohol from your diet. In women, tobacco may decrease fertility, and caffeine seems to affect the ability to both conceive and nurture an embryo. Marijuana has been shown to disrupt a woman's ovulatory cycle. And as seen in Appendix I, antihistamines can dry up cervical fluid and thus interfere with sperm survival. Finally, alcohol is notorious for potentially causing Fetal Alcohol Syndrome in the offspring of mothers who drink while pregnant.

In men, the following products may suppress sperm production: marijuana, tobacco, alcohol, antimalarial drugs, steroids, and ulcer medications.

❧ DOUCHES, VAGINAL SPRAYS, AND SCENTED TAMPONS

As you've read in previous pages, douching alters the normal acidity of the vagina and is not necessary for most women. It adversely changes the normal Ph balance and can ironically lead to vaginal infections and PID (pelvic inflammatory disease). It can also alter the vaginal environment to such an extent that sperm can't survive. It may cause inflammations or allergic reactions that can kill sperm or impair sperm survival. And finally, it may wash away the very cervical fluid that sperm need to get through the cervix to the egg. Other than that, douching's no problem!

Vaginal sprays and scented tampons can also cause a Ph imbalance as well as an allergic reaction to the chemicals used in the products. As you would expect, the resulting imbalance can impede sperm survival.

❧ ANTIBIOTICS AND YEAST INFECTIONS

If you've ever had to take antibiotics for an extended period of time, you may have the unpleasant memory of battling yeast infections that might have resulted from the regimen. This is because antibiotics are notorious for killing the good bacteria along with the bad, often producing an overgrowth of candida, a type of yeast that renders the vaginal environment inhospitable to sperm. One of the ways to counter the effects of antibiotics is to eat yogurt with acidophilus or ingest acidophilus tablets, because this replaces the good bacteria killed by the antibiotics. Many clinicians also believe that inserting plain yogurt directly into the vagina is the most effective way to fight this type of infection, but women who are trying to get pregnant should never vaginally insert anything that may potentially introduce bacteria.

❧ FOR MEN: HOT TUBS, SAUNAS, BICYCLES, AND TIGHT CLOTHING

As you know, sperm are very sensitive to heat. While it's not clear how much is too much, it is wise if you're having problems conceiving to avoid anything that may expose the testes to excess heat. Hot tubs and saunas can be enjoyable, but from the sperm's perspective, it's basically saying "life's a fish and then you fry."

Bicycling is another activity that may affect sperm counts. The constant bumping of the testes, combined with the added heat generated from sweating in the scrotal area may contribute to diminished sperm counts. If the man's sperm analysis is fine, then by all means, enjoy the daily bike rides. But if the sperm count is marginal, it's one more practical thing you might consider changing.

Even hot work environments may have a harmful effect on sperm production. It should come as no surprise that standing in front of a pizza oven 8 hours a day may not be the most efficient way to build up a sperm count. And finally, as far as the common folk wisdom to avoid tight underwear and pants—it certainly can't hurt. Obviously, if you find bikini briefs sexier and your partner wants to wear them occasionally to seduce you, more power to him! But he would be wise not to wear them everyday.

The bottom line is that until you achieve the pregnancy you desire, you may want to avoid anything that causes the sperm to get too hot. And remember that it may take as long as 2 to 3 months after reducing such exposure for a new generation of healthy sperm to mature.

❧ CONDITIONS THAT MAY BE AMENABLE TO NONINVASIVE REMEDIES

There are a number of remedies you may want to try for fertility problems you detect through the Fertility Awareness Method. While there is considerable discussion today regarding the value of herbs, vitamins, and various alternative therapies such as acupuncture and chiropractics, I have generally chosen not to list these possible therapies unless I am aware of serious relevant studies within the medical literature. Although there is much here that should be able to help, I would still encourage you to consult with a qualified herbalist, nutritionist, or practitioner of alternative medicine if you feel this would lead to better results.

Limited Fertile-Quality Cervical Fluid

My professional experience is that one of the most commonly overlooked causes of subfertility is the lack of lubricative, slippery cervical fluid produced during a woman's cycle. Of course, the more days you produce it the more likely you'll be able to get pregnant. Women coming off the Pill or approaching menopause are particularly susceptible to this problem, as are women who have had cone biopsies performed on their cervix. If charting has confirmed that your cervical fluid doesn't seem wet enough, or isn't wet for at least two days, it may be a reflection of other reproductive problems. Still there may be a simple solution available. Before resorting to more involved medical therapies, you might want to try any of the following remedies:

- Avoid drugs that may dry up cervical fluid, such as antihistamines, atropine, belladonna, cough mixtures containing antihistamines, dicyclomine, progesterone, propantheline, or tamoxifen. If you must take Clomid, combining it with oral oestrogen may compensate for its drying effects. But oestrogen should never be taken without fertility drugs, because it may actually inhibit ovulation.

- Consider trying any of the relevant drugs listed in Appendix I but be aware that most of them should only be used with a doctor's prescription and for very specific conditions.

- Try taking an expectorant found in cough syrups such as Robitussin, or long-acting tablets of Humabid LA, both of which have the active ingredient *guaifenesin*. Along with helping to liquefy mucus in the lungs, it also has the added benefit of making your cervical fluid wetter. So if you only produce sticky or creamy cervical fluid, you could try this dosage: 2 teaspoons, 3 times a day, starting several days before your anticipated ovulation through to the 1st day of your temperature shift. (Caution! Be sure to use *plain* Robitussin, since other types can actually dry up your cervical fluid.)

- Take 5,000 to 8,000 IU of vitamin A daily. The Couple to Couple League in Great Britain (an NFP organization) has found that some women develop wetter and more fertile fluid with such a regimen. However, you should definitely consult with a qualified nutritionist before taking the vitamins, since an excessive amount is considered toxic. (Side effects may include such conditions as nausea, skin irritations, and, ironically, lack of menses.)

- Consider the use of real eggwhites as a lubricant if you don't produce much fertile-quality cervical fluid. While no studies have yet shown that you can actually use it as a *substitute,* several articles suggest it is compatible with sperm viability. This is because both sperm and real eggwhites are made of protein. Of course, you shouldn't try this if you're allergic to eggs, and you should be aware that there may be a slight risk of salmonella (as mentioned on page 169).

If these don't work, your doctor may prescribe oestrogen supplements to increase the amount and quality of the cervical fluid that you have.

Short Luteal Phases

If you discover that you have short luteal phases (defined as less than 10 post-ovulatory days without any bleeding), there are a few steps you may want to take before relying on the traditional medical remedy of Clomid, HCG injections, and progesterone suppositories, including the use of natural progesterone creams, available on prescription. You could therefore try using them as soon as you ovulate each cycle.*

Chapter 18 on PMS offers general dietary guidelines that have been shown to be helpful in treating both short luteal phases as well as the symptoms of PMS. Marilyn Shannon suggests that 200 to 600 milligrams a day of vitamin B6 may also help, but again, I encourage you to consult with a qualified nutritionist first.

Anovulation Caused by Being Underweight

As mentioned earlier, women who are considered underweight by general nutritional guidelines may not be producing the oestrogen required to trigger ovulation. These women may be able to end their anovulatory (and infertile) condition, whether it is caused by excessive exercise or simple undereating. The most fundamental advice is that they gradually gain weight by a combination of healthful diet and moderate exercise.

Irregular Menstrual Cycles

There are many alternative health practitioners who believe that certain cycle irregularities are easily resolved through the use of herbs. You should consult with a qualified nutritionist or health care provider who has expertise in herbs and their impact on various bodily functions.

---

* The most thorough treatment I have seen on the subject of progesterone cream is Dr. John R. Lee's *What Your Doctor May Not Tell You About Premenopause.*

In any case, and as you've already read, there are several underlying conditions that you can hopefully treat yourself, including excessively low or high body weight and intense stress. On the other hand, if you have no obvious causes for this problem, I would encourage you to be examined for PCOS, a serious medical condition for which irregular cycles are one of the primary warning signs (see page 204).

Long Infertile Cycles (Hypothyroidism)

If you are one of those women who suffer from unusually long cycles in which you have extended periods of fertile-quality cervical fluid, you should also observe whether you have low basal body temperatures. This is because the combination of these three symptoms often indicate low thyroid function (hypothyroidism), a condition that you may be able to treat by simple nutritional supplements. Marilyn Shannon suggests adding iodized salt to your diet, as well as lots of ocean fish, which is an excellent source of the iodine needed to treat the thyroid. She also recommends supplements of vitamins A, B, C, and E, in addition to zinc and selenium. Again, I would encourage you to see a qualified nutritionist before relying on these supplements.

Repeat Miscarriages

Miscarriages occur at a surprisingly high rate of about one in three pregnancies. If you discover that what you thought was an inability to conceive is in fact a problem of repeated miscarriages, there may be certain steps you can take at home before consulting a physician. To start, you should immediately eliminate smoking, alcohol, and drug consumption, including caffeine. Ideally all of that should be achieved a few months before a planned conception, as should the attainment of your ideal body weight. If charting reveals that you have short luteal phases (10 days or less), you may consider the general dietary guidelines discussed in the chapter on PMS (see page 255).

While miscarriage problems may be remedied by dietary changes, I do not mean to minimize the importance of seeking a physician's diagnosis, especially if it occurs more than once. In learning to chart and recognize the miscarriages when they occur, you have already gone far in helping the doctor guide you to a healthy pregnancy. (See page 212 for more on miscarriages.)

⒜ FOR MEN

Low Sperm Count

Unless clearly dealing with a case of blockage only treatable by surgery, there are several noninvasive treatments that men with subfertile sperm counts may want to consider before moving on to more serious medical procedures. Just remember that most everything a man tries on his own will probably not be detected in the ejaculate for two to three months. This is because it takes that long for newly created sperm to reach maturity.

Mild cases of zinc deficiency have been implicated in some low sperm counts. This is because the highest concentrations of zinc in the body are found in sperm and the prostate gland. Studies also suggest that a deficiency in vitamin A or B, and even selenium, can similarly affect male fertility. Almost half of the man's supply of selenium is located in the testicles and seminal ducts next to the prostate. For recommendations on dosages, consult a nutritionist.

Arginine is considered a nonessential amino acid, yet it seems to help a number of men with this problem. Specifically, studies have shown that taking an oral dose of 4 grams a day of pure powdered arginine dissolved in water can markedly increase sperm count and motility in some men.

Finally, low sperm count may be remedied by making some simple changes. As mentioned earlier, Jacuzzis, tight clothes, or anything else that may cause excess testicular heat should be avoided as much as possible. And perhaps the most obvious but overlooked change is simply to make sure that ejaculations are kept to a maximum frequency of once every 48 hours. For men with marginal counts, this may be all that is necessary to bring it up to normal.

Sperm Agglutination

One of the most dramatic results of a fertility study involved men with a condition called sperm agglutination (or clumping of sperm.) Twenty-seven men who had this problem were divided into two groups. One group of twenty men each received 1,000 mg a day of a vitamin C pill containing calcium, magnesium, and manganese. Every single man in that group got their wives pregnant during the study! By contrast, not one of the men in the control group was able to impregnate his spouse. Although the study was small, the results were striking. So if your partner is diagnosed with sperm agglutination, you'll certainly want to discuss this potential remedy with his doctor.

✌ OTHER FACTORS TO CONSIDER

Age

One of the most important reasons for the prevalence of subfertility is the relatively late age at which many people today attempt to start having children. The unfortunate biological reality is that as women reach their mid-30s, their infertility risk increases dramatically.

There are several reasons why couples in their 30s face a greater possibility of lower fertility. Some factors are easily remedied through simple education, while others are a regrettable function of biology. One of the most fundamental and easily rectified reasons for impaired fertility is that as couples age together, they tend to have intercourse less frequently, thus decreasing their odds of conception. While the average pair in their mid-20s may have sex up to three times a week, it's believed that typical couples in their mid-30s have intercourse twice weekly or less. Of course, charting would help them time their lovemaking to fully compensate for their possible decline in sexual frequency. Two acts of intercourse on perfectly timed days easily beats a dozen randomly performed acts throughout the entire cycle.

There are physiological changes that also affect overall fertility rates. As women age, the quantity and quality of fertile cervical fluid tends to decline. I've noticed that women in their 20s will generally have 2 to 4 days of eggwhite, while women approaching their late 30s will often have a day or less. This decline can lead to impaired fertility if intercourse is not timed properly. In addition, as women enter their late 30s, they tend to have more anovulatory cycles, and often those in which the egg is released have shorter luteal phases.

Unfortunately, what may be the most important age factor is not the ability of older women to conceive, but rather the odds of the fertilized egg surviving implantation. Research now shows that as women grow older, the percent of conceptions that end in miscarriage rises dramatically. This is certainly true for those pregnancies of which the woman is aware. But perhaps more significantly, there is strong evidence that as women approach 35, extremely early miscarriages occur more and more frequently. By her 40s, the average woman may face a 50% miscarriage rate, most of which are not detected.

What is not clear is the exact cause of this increase in miscarriages as women get older. There is some speculation that the mother's ability to nurture the egg is compromised as she ages. What appears more likely is that the older eggs themselves become increasingly less able to survive after fertilization. There is also the possibility that as men age, their sperm contribute to the increased risk of fetal loss. Whatever the precise reason, couples who delay having children until their 30s will unfortunately face a progressively greater risk of reproductive difficulties. And while both FAM and various high-tech strategies may help shift the odds back in your favor, you should know that it's definitely easier to conceive a child and carry it to term in your 20s than it is in your mid-30s or later.

Stress

It is frequently said that stress leads to infertility. While there is no doubt that stress is associated with diminished fertility, the opposite appears to be more accurate—that is, infertility leads to stress. So the old adage "just relax and you'll get pregnant" is well meaning but often misguided.

There are several ways, though, in which stress can indirectly influence fertility. One is simply that leading a busy life and all the stress that entails may leave little time or energy for a couple to actually have intercourse frequently enough to achieve pregnancy. (Of course, as you now know, intercourse doesn't need to be frequent as long as it is well timed.)

A second way is that stress itself may affect when ovulation occurs. In fact, one of the most common causes of delayed ovulation is both physiological and psychological stress. This is because stress can dramatically affect the functioning of the hypothalamus, that gland in the brain responsible for so much of the reproductive system. It is the hypothalamus that is responsible for the regulation of appetite, temperature, and most important, emotions. It also regulates the pituitary gland, which in turn is responsible for the release of FSH and LH. When stress affects the hypothalamus, the end result can be delayed emission of these reproductive hormones, which are necessary for the release of a mature ovum. (It is not known what triggers an early ovulation, but stress does not appear to play a role.)

As you know, the timing of ovulation will determine the length of the cycle—the later it occurs, the longer the cycle will be. Occasionally, if stress is severe, it can actually prevent ovulation from occurring altogether. If stress were to affect your cycle, then, one of two things would probably happen:

> **1.** You would have a longer-than-average cycle, with ovulation occurring later than usual and menstruation following 12 to 16 days afterward, if pregnancy did not occur. (See Chart 12.1, page 180.)

2. You would have a long cycle, but wouldn't release an egg (an anovulatory cycle). If this were the case, the cycle could theoretically extend for months. Or you would have a long cycle followed by anovulatory bleeding, which is the result of a drop in oestrogen (as opposed to progesterone). Remember that in an ovulatory cycle, the corpus luteum dies, and the sudden drop in progesterone causes the uterine lining to shed. But with anovulatory cycles, it is the drop in oestrogen that usually causes the bleeding. (See Chart 12.2 on the next page.)

While it is true that stress can prevent ovulation, it is my professional experience that it more commonly delays it. For this reason, it is especially important to learn to focus on the signs that indicate *approaching* ovulation. That way, if stress is causing delayed ovulation, you can at least take control by identifying when you are about to ovulate, and thus take advantage of the most fertile time. Of course, the sign that indicates impending ovulation is the wet cervical fluid (especially eggwhite quality) that develops just before you release an egg.

One of the ironies of how stress and the desire to get pregnant can interact is that couples may inadvertently prevent pregnancy by focusing on the mythical Day 14. For example, in women who usually have average-length cycles, a vicious circle can develop in which the stress of continually not achieving pregnancy may only delay ovulation. This in itself wouldn't be a problem, if the couple were taught how to identify when the woman was about to ovulate.

In women who typically have longer cycles, stress may not be delaying ovulation at all. However, if the couple is unaware of when the woman does ovulate, they may be having intercourse too early for conception to occur, thus subjecting themselves to the needless anxiety of misperceived infertility. With both examples, the most constructive advice is not a well-meaning admonition to "just relax." Rather, it would be to tell them to chart their cycles, and then time their lovemaking accordingly. (See Chart 12.3, page 181.)

Stress is also notorious for causing cervical fluid to either disappear altogether or to form patches of wetness interspersed with dryer days. It's as if the body keeps making attempts to ovulate, but the stress continues to delay it. If this should happen, remember that the temperature will ultimately indicate when you have finally ovulated. So if you observe patches of slippery- or eggwhite-quality cervical fluid, take advantage of those days until you see the confirmation that ovulation has indeed taken place by a rise in temperature.

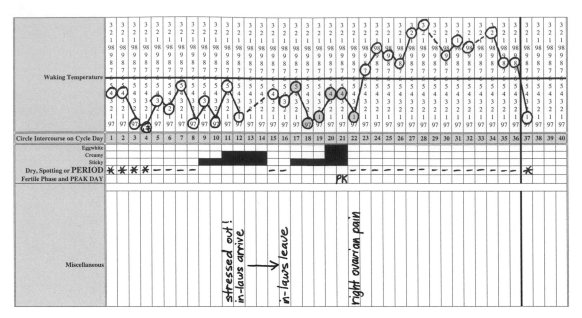

Chart 12.1. A long cycle due to stress. With her in-laws arriving for a week, is it any wonder that Shelly had a delayed ovulation leading to a long cycle? Note that she started to prepare to ovulate about the time they arrived, but didn't actually do so until after they left, about Day 22.

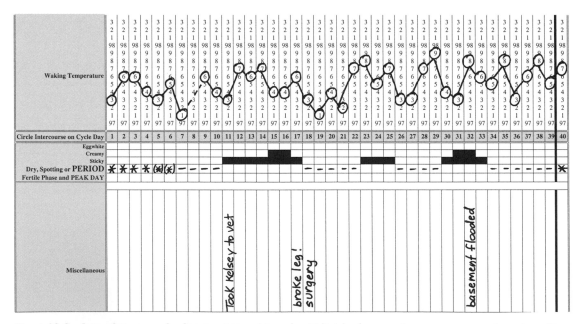

Chart 12.2. Anovulatory cycle due to stress. Note that Talia's body started to prepare to ovulate about Day 15, but then she broke her leg skiing. A couple of weeks later, as she was finally starting to recover and prepare again to ovulate, her basement flooded. At this point, her body decided to throw in the towel and not release an egg at all. On Day 40, she had anovulatory bleeding rather than a true menstrual period.

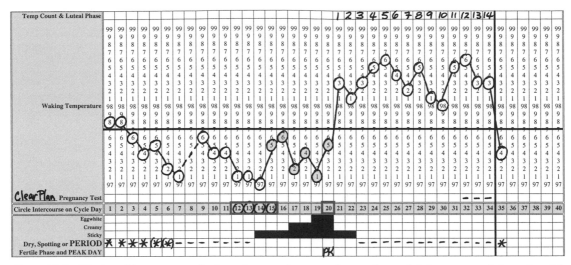

Chart I2.3. Mistimed intercourse during a long cycle. Note that ovulation didn't occur until about Day 20. Whether caused by stress or just typical of this woman's cycles, the end result is that intercourse the week before could not result in the conception they sought.

You should also understand that stress may not necessarily affect a cycle at all, and that it will affect individual women differently. In addition, continual stress may tend to normalize over time, so that the woman's body eventually stops perceiving it as stress, and thus cycles may revert back to the way they were before.*

Synthetic Hormones

Certain synthetic hormones have left a disastrous legacy of reproductive abnormalities on both the women who took them and their offspring. The most notorious of the group is DES, which was taken by pregnant women from the 1940s to 1970s to prevent miscarriages. Many of the daughters of these women have suffered a range of reproductive problems, from malformed uteri to a rare form of vaginal cancer. The sons of these women often have lowered sperm counts and other anomalies. If you are having trouble conceiving and suspect that your mother may have taken DES while pregnant with you, you should consult a doctor who is experienced with the treatment of DES offspring.

---

* Alice Domar of Harvard University, a pioneer in the study of the complex relationship between stress, depression, and perceived infertility, has shown that women who are helped to reduce stress or depression in their lives do tend to increase their odds of conception. However, her studies have not examined the precise issue of how stress or depression affect women's cycles, and how knowledge of that effect could, in fact, play a pivotal role in the successful timing of intercourse for pregnancy.

Even the Pill occasionally has been implicated in infertility for the simple reason that ovulation may be delayed for months or even years following its use. Charting your cycle will help you determine when your fertility is finally starting to resume again.

The Jewish Practice of Niddah

As you already know if you are a Jew who observes Niddah, this custom forbids you from having intercourse for seven days following the last day of your period. If you are an observant Jew who practices Niddah and meets any of the following three conditions, it may be affecting your ability to conceive:

- your cycles tend to be fairly short (i.e., less than 25 days or so)
- your cycles are average length but you bleed for at least seven days
- you have midcycle spotting

The reason the practice may be impeding your ability to get pregnant is that it forbids you from having intercourse during what may be your most fertile phase. For example, if you have cycles of about 24 days, you are probably ovulating about Day 10, but not allowed to resume intercourse again until about Day 13. And even if you have average-length cycles but your periods last 7 days or more, you would again find yourself abstaining until about Day 14 or so, possibly a bit too late for your particular ovulation. Finally, if you happen to be a woman who has occasional midcycle spotting, the Niddah would again require you to abstain at the time that you are most likely ovulating.

Needless to say, if you practice Niddah and you would like to conceive, I would highly recommend charting to determine whether this may be the reason you aren't getting pregnant. Then discuss it with your rabbi to see what modifications are acceptable according to Jewish law.

CHAPTER 13

Lovemaking Versus Babymaking

Just at the time when you are probably feeling the need for greater closeness with your spouse, the demands of trying to conceive interfere with the pleasure of your physical relationship. The intimacy and enjoyment of sex could help you escape the strain of infertility, but sex serves only as a reminder of the pain. It becomes a revolving door: you end up feeling anxious and frustrated, which is how you felt when you started.

—LINDA P. SALZER
from *Infertility: How Couples Can Cope*

Does this sound familiar? If you've been trying to get pregnant for a while, it's very likely you have experienced some of the emotions Linda Salzer communicates above. But so much of the anxiety associated with trying to achieve a pregnancy every cycle could be eliminated if couples were taught exactly when the woman can and cannot get pregnant. Knowing that women can only get pregnant a few days per cycle can actually be a liberating feeling for many couples, in that it leaves the rest of the cycle free for either:

- pure lovemaking, without the pressure of feeling that the entire cycle must be utilized to avoid missing an opportunity to conceive

or

- choosing not to make love and take a break from the routine of "babymaking"

Sexual problems often arise between couples touched by infertility because sex has taken on one main function: a means of reproduction. What is often lost is the emotional expression of lovemaking—the tenderness, passion, and joy. Charting the woman's cycle can free you once again to be spontaneous and tender for most of the cycle, knowing that you are in control.

Of course, some couple's fertility problems will require high-tech treatment, but ironically, these procedures may actually free them to enjoy lovemaking for what it is—and *not* as a means of conceiving. In essence, the frustration of trying to conceive is no longer theirs to endure, in much the same way that FAM relieves couples of this burden for most of the cycle.

Although a person's sexuality is separate from his or her fertility, society often equates them, leaving many people dealing with infertility to feel that they are somehow less sexual. This is extremely unfortunate since the two are quite different. When couples have sexual problems as a result of their quest to get pregnant, they may experience emotions ranging from unresolved anger and fear to anxiety or guilt. Even worse, communication between them often deteriorates.

🐚 MAINTAINING A SENSE OF HUMOR

It may reassure a couple to know that what they are experiencing is absolutely normal. Many endure similar feelings. Having a sense of humor about the stresses on your love life can help pull you through the rough times, as the following illustrates:

> *Diana had very irregular cycles, only having ovulated about eight times in the prior 4 years. Because she had excessively high levels of prolactin (the hormone that is normally present in breastfeeding women), she was prescribed Parlodel and Clomid to regulate her cycles. Along with the drugs and FSH shots, she had several ultrasounds taken. In addition, she would put her legs up on the wall for about an hour after intercourse. After about six months of trying, nothing worked. On the advice of her gynecologist, Diana and Steve tried using fresh eggwhites to simulate fertile-quality cervical fluid.*
>
> *Before making love, they removed an egg from the refrigerator, separated it, and inserted the eggwhite into a pastry decorating bag. After Diana comfortably positioned herself, Steve blew the ice-cold eggwhite into her vagina through the pastry bag nozzle. Diana laughed so hard she "farted" from her vagina and all the eggwhite squirted out in one fell swoop. So much for that cycle.*

During the next cycle they decided to try things a little differently. Having learned their lesson from the first time, they let the egg sit at room temperature first. Then they used an applicator (the type typically used for vaginal cream) to insert the eggwhite. They conceived that day—Mother's Day. Today they have a precious daughter, Tessa.

Admittedly, it can be hard to maintain a sense of humor amid the pain of infertility. But so many who have survived such frustration often say that it was their sense of humor that pulled them through.

℘ SEXUAL PROBLEMS THAT MAY ARISE DURING ATTEMPTS TO CONCEIVE

When I had my baby, I screamed and screamed. And that was just during conception.

—JOAN RIVERS

The Woman

Probably the most common sexual problem women experience while struggling with infertility is a lack of lubrication, which can make intercourse very painful. Just as men may have problems with erections, women may not feel sexual when lovemaking becomes less an expression of affection than a means to attain a goal.

As discussed in the preceding chapter, it is imperative that couples not use artificial sexual lubricants or saliva, since these can actually kill sperm. If they need to, they should only use eggwhites for lubrication. But the ideal would be to make time to tenderly take care of each other with lingering foreplay, allowing your natural lubrication to flow.

The Man

The impact of a couple's sexual difficulties can strongly affect the man. After all, the pressure is usually on him to achieve an erection and ejaculate during intercourse if conception is to occur, and thus it is not surprising that impotence is the most common problem men face when dealing with infertility.

Impotence is often related to general stress and fatigue, and thus to the extent that infertility brings new stress to life, it is commonly exacerbated during attempts to get pregnant. Of course the importance of charting in this context is that once men realize that they don't need to perform throughout the cycle, it can take the pressure off during the few days their partner is fertile.

The Couple

It is ironic but well known that the biggest problem a couple dealing with infertility may have is simple lack of sexual desire. Needless to say, waning sexual interest can be especially problematic when trying to get pregnant. Unfortunately, it can result from the entire range of emotional and physical anxieties that often accompany fertility problems.

If sexual apathy becomes an issue, I would recommend seeing a therapist who can help work through the sexual facets of infertility. I would also highly encourage you to contact CHILD and ISSUE. They are excellent organizations devoted to meeting the needs of couples struggling with fertility issues. (See Appendix M for addresses.)

␪ RECAPTURING THE ESSENCE OF LOVEMAKING

Infertility doesn't have to damage a couple's sexual relationship. In fact, it can have a positive influence by drawing them closer through the intimate sharing of their frustrations. Couples often develop a profound respect for each other's strength during such a trying time. Therapists suggest that the first step to revitalize your sexual relationship is to determine when your sexual relationship *was* fulfilling.

Were you more aroused during vacations? Did you feel more attracted to your partner after an intimate talk? A sexy movie? A relaxing dinner? Did you find your sexual relationship more exciting in the beginning of your relationship when you made more conscious efforts to be sexy for your partner? The key to rekindling sexual desire for your spouse is to try to remember what sparked your passion initially, and purposefully seek to repeat those wonderful moments. One means of doing this is to communicate your desires and frustrations so that you can be sensitive to each other's needs—and move on toward renewing your former sexual relationship.

If you are like most couples struggling with getting pregnant, you may need to work at keeping your relationship alive and stimulating. Find exciting new places to make love. Work at making yourself sexually enticing for your partner. Notice and comment on your partner's attractiveness. And plan special times together—away from the stresses of everyday life.

Perhaps most important, you now have the knowledge to realize that the very notion of babymaking, with all its pressures and implications, need only concern you in the few select days leading up to ovulation. For the rest of the time, you should be able to forget your fertility-related concerns and return to the carefree lovemaking that was, and should always be, a healthy part of your relationship.

What Next?
Tests and Treatments
That *May* Be Necessary to
Achieve Pregnancy

The world is moving so fast these days that the man who says it can't be done is generally interrupted by someone doing it.

—ELBERT HUBBARD

The most important advice for a couple trying to get pregnant is to chart the woman's cycle as the *first* step. It's astounding how something so fundamental is routinely ignored. Of course, there will be individuals for whom FAM won't be enough to get pregnant. Even then, charting will help determine what testing or treatment is needed, often bypassing inappropriate or unnecessary interventions.

℮ FACTORS NECESSARY FOR ACHIEVING PREGNANCY WITHOUT USING HIGH-TECH AIDS

In order to discuss what medical procedures you may need to get pregnant, you should first understand what is required for pregnancy to occur through intercourse alone:

- a woman who is ovulating
- a man who has sufficient sperm production (number, motility, and shape)
- intercourse with ejaculation
- adequate sperm transport and fertilization
- efficient embryo transport and appropriate environment for implantation

Practically speaking, this means that if you have any obvious impediments such as chronic anovulation or blocked fallopian tubes, I'm afraid the Fertility Awareness Method will not be able to help you. But there are some fertility problems that are still amenable to natural treatments. Believers in holistic remedies would encourage you to consider seeking help through those channels if you feel more comfortable doing so.

When first beginning to chart, you should verify that there are no obstacles to pregnancy that you can clearly identify. This would include anovulation, lack of fertile-quality cervical fluid, and excessively short luteal phases, as well as recurrent miscarriages. If your charting reveals nothing wrong, but you are still unable to get pregnant after *optimally* timing intercourse for 4 to 6 cycles, your partner should get a semen analysis. If his sperm count is subfertile, try timing intercourse by the FAM guidelines discussed on page 162 for another few cycles. If, however, his count is normal, you yourself should be given a fairly comprehensive fertility workup to determine the problem.

❧ THE MAN'S FERTILITY WORKUP

As mentioned earlier, when people think of fertility problems, they tend to think of it as primarily a woman's issue. But, as you know by now, fertility problems affect men and women equally. The reason a man should be tested first is that his own workup is fairly simple, cheap, and hardly uncomfortable! The foundation is the semen analysis, which is easily obtained by having the man ejaculate into a cup.

Remember that even though the analysis is usually referred to as a "sperm count," the expression is somewhat misleading. The count is only one facet of the whole analysis. As discussed in Chapter 11, the key to judging a man's fertility is not so much to look at the total number of sperm per ejaculate, but rather the total number of those sperm released that are of normal shape and motility.

Based on that analysis, a physician will be able to tell you whether your partner's sperm count is considered normal or subfertile. You should be aware that if the analysis shows a subfertile count, he would be expected to have at least two more analyses performed with at least 2 to 4 weeks in between in order to verify the results.

One additional investigation that is often routinely done with the sperm sample is called the sperm penetration assay, or the hamster egg penetration test. It is the best test currently available to determine the fertilizing capabilities of a man's sperm. As the name implies, the sperm is placed immediately next to hamster eggs to see whether they can penetrate them, since such penetration generally correlates with how well sperm can penetrate human eggs. Like any test, though, it's not perfect; 5 to 10% of men whose sperm do not "pass the test" are still able to eventually impregnate their partners. And likewise, some men whose sperm do fine in the test are still unable to fertilize their partner's eggs. However, it is considered fairly standard in a fertility workup, and should be taken for what it's worth.

Depending on the results of the semen analysis, the physician may perform a variety of other procedures. These include a physical exam to look for varicoceles, prostate problems or testicular anomalies, and blood tests to ascertain hormone levels. In addition, the doctor may need to take semen cultures to determine the presence of sperm clumping (agglutination) or genital tract infections, as well as X rays of his sperm-producing tissues. Once the source of the problem is identified, there may be a variety of treatments possible (see page 196).

ஃ THE WOMAN'S FERTILITY WORKUP

You'll now see why it is much more logical for the man's fertility workup to be performed first. The woman's is a substantially more extensive undertaking, usually involving several stages.

1. Preliminary Fact-Finding
The clinician should take a comprehensive medical history and review any previous fertility tests before performing a standard pelvic exam. The exam is to rule out any obvious physical problems of the uterus, ovaries, or cervix, such as fibroids, cysts, or infections.

2. Diagnostic Analyses
There are a number of fairly noninvasive means of determining potential problems. In women, the four general areas of concern in the reproductive system are:

- uterine and fallopian tube abnormalities
- cervical problems
- dysfunctional ovulatory cycles
- endometriosis

The tests and procedures discussed below are used to detect problems in any of the above areas. They are listed in order of least invasiveness.

Waking (Basal Body) Temperature Charting

As you know, this is the sign that is easiest to ascertain and puts control in your hands. Taking your waking temperature will help you determine whether:

- you are ovulating
- your luteal phase is long enough for implantation (at least 10 days)
- your progesterone levels are high enough in your luteal phase
- you may have a thyroid problem (either hypo- or hyperthyroid)
- you are still fertile in any given cycle as reflected by low temperatures
- you may have gotten pregnant, as reflected by more than 18 high temperatures
- you are in danger of having a miscarriage, as determined by a sudden drop in temperatures after an apparent conception
- you were pregnant before having what seemed to be just a "late period"

Hormone Blood Tests

Blood tests are one of the most fundamental means of determining if the woman is producing normal reproductive hormones or has a hormonal imbalance. They can determine levels of FSH, LH, oestrogen, and progesterone. They can help diagnose such vital facts as whether the woman is ovulating, has a normal luteal phase, or is possibly entering menopause. The chart on the next page summarizes the most commonly performed blood tests.

Cervical-Fluid Ferning Test

This is a test in which cervical fluid is removed from the woman's vagina and observed under a microscope to determine if it has the characteristic fertile ferning pattern. In order for the test to be valid, though, it is imperative that it be done *when the woman's cervical fluid exhibits its most fertile characteristics* (i.e., her wettest, most slippery days), and not necessarily on Day 14, as is commonly done. If the cervical fluid is indeed fertile, it will form a beautiful ferning pattern on the slide. (See photograph on page 3 of color insert.)

HORMONE BLOOD TESTS

In order of day of cycle it is usually drawn.
All test results vary depending on the laboratory used.

Hormone	Best Time to Take Test	Purpose of Hormone
Follicle Stimulating Hormone (FSH)	Day 3 and Day 10, if part of Clomid Challenge Test	Stimulates follicle development. If FSH levels are too high, it could indicate possible menopause or declining fertility.
Estradiol	Day 3 and possibly mid-luteal phase (7 to 10 days after your LH surge)	Stimulates egg maturation and endometrial maturation for the implantation of a fertilized egg. Responsible for the fertile quality of the cervical fluid around ovulation.
Luteinizing Hormone (LH)	Around ovulation	Triggers ovulation when it surges.
Pooled Progesterone	Days 20, 22, and 24	Evaluates adequacy of progesterone production and rules out a luteal phase problem. (Many physicians feel that BBT charts or a surge value is all that is needed.)
Progesterone	Mid-luteal phase (7 to 10 days after your LH surge)	Necessary for sustaining the uterine lining and maintaining early pregnancy. Causes the rise in basal body temperature and drying of cervical fluid in the post-ovulatory infertile phase.*
Prolactin	Any cycle day	Stimulates the production of breast milk and inhibits the ovarian production of estrogen. Occasionally present in excessive levels in non-breastfeeding women, potentially causing fertility problems.
Thyroid Stimulating Hormone (TSH)	Any cycle day	Stimulates the production of thyroxine in the thyroid gland, the endocrine gland that regulates hormones in the body. Excessively high or low levels may affect fertility.
Testosterone	Any cycle day	Necessary for the production of estrogen. When produced in high levels, may impact fertility.
Dehydroepian-drosterone sulfate (DHEAS)	Any cycle day	Produces the same effects as male hormones (androgens). When produced at high levels in both men and women, may cause fertility problems.

* If you are trying to conceive through traditional intercourse and the one progesterone blood test mid-luteal phase reflects low levels, it may be more accurate to get a series of five blood tests, one every other day starting about the 3rd day after your LH surge or the 2nd day of your thermal shift. Also, you may want to inquire about a newer test utilizing saliva instead of blood.

Postcoital Test

This test is done to determine whether the couple's sperm and cervical fluid are compatible. In other words, can the man's sperm survive inside the woman's cervical fluid? In order to determine this, a sample of cervical fluid is taken from the woman's vagina within two hours of intercourse. Again, for the test to be valid, it is imperative that it be done when the woman has fertile-quality cervical fluid, and not necessarily on Day 14, as it often is. If the two are compatible, the clinician will be able to observe live sperm swimming forward in the cervical fluid.

Ultrasound

The only way to determine definitively if ovulation has occurred is with ultrasound. This procedure offers a means of being able to actually observe if and when ovulation occurs. It's especially useful in detecting the condition LUFS (Luteinized Unruptured Follicle Syndrome), in which the woman's body produces all the signs of ovulation, including a thermal shift, but without actually releasing an egg. (See page 206.)

Ultrasound can also be helpful in detecting ectopic pregnancies—those which develop outside of the uterine lining. Its main disadvantage is that it is not very practical on a daily basis since it requires a doctor's appointment.

Endometrial Biopsy

The endometrial biopsy sounds ominous but is fairly simple. We tend to associate the word "biopsy" with cancer, but the test has nothing to do with that. Its purpose is to determine if the uterine lining (endometrium) is sufficiently developed during the luteal phase of the cycle. The lining must be mature enough to be able to sustain the implantation of a fertilized egg.

The test is usually done a couple of days before the woman's expected period. A tiny piece of the uterine lining is removed and biopsied. Unlike the tests listed above, it can be uncomfortable because it may cause cramping or a sharp pain from partially dilating the cervix. The timing of this test is critical, because if it's done too soon after the egg is released (especially in the case of delayed ovulations) it can deceptively appear as if the woman has an undeveloped endometrium. Likewise, if it's done too late after ovulation, the woman may start her period before the test has been completed. Charting is thus strongly recommended in order to time this test appropriately.

HSG (Hysterosalpingogram)

The purpose of an HSG is to determine if the woman's fallopian tubes are open. It involves shooting dye through the cervix and uterus to see whether it spills out the fallopian tubes into the pelvic cavity. Although the test can be quite useful, it does have its limitations. For one thing, the tubes occasionally spasm during the procedure, giving the appearance of being blocked, when in reality it may have been the test itself that caused the tubes to appear closed.

Another potential problem is that if the tubes are only scarred but not blocked, the HSG would not necessarily reveal that. The concern with scarring is that it could lead to a tubal pregnancy, in which the fertilized egg begins to burrow into the tube rather than the uterine lining.

3. Surgical Investigation

If the tests in section 2 above fail to identify a problem, there are several surgical diagnostic procedures that can be very helpful in pinpointing potential impediments to pregnancy. Among them are the following:

Laparoscopy

The best way to have a "window into the womb" is through a laparoscopy—exploratory surgery that is used to view the internal pelvic area, especially the ovaries and fallopian tubes. The procedure is most commonly used to detect endometriosis. It usually involves a tiny incision in the navel through which a lighted tube is inserted to view the pelvic region. Although the procedure is fairly routine, it is usually done with general anesthesia.

Hysteroscopy

This procedure is performed specifically to view the inside of the uterus. It is primarily done to determine if the woman has fibroids, or other conditions that may affect her ability to carry a pregnancy to term.

Falloscopy

This is a newly developed procedure that uses state-of-the-art devices to look directly inside the miniscule interior of the fallopian tubes. It is done primarily to diagnose any tubal abnormalities that could block the route of sperm migrating toward the egg or an embryo traveling back to the uterus.

THE WOMAN'S FERTILITY WORKUP:
COMMON DIAGNOSTIC TESTS AND EXPLORATORY SURGICAL PROCEDURES

(in alphabetical order)

Test	Best Time to Take Test	Purpose of Test
Basal body temperature charts	Throughout cycle	To determine whether you are ovulating and how long your post-ovulatory phase is.
Cervical fluid ferning slide	The few days leading up to ovulation, when your cervical fluid is slippery and wet	To determine if your cervical fluid forms the characteristic ferning pattern indicating that it is fertile enough for sperm to survive within it or if you are making adequate estrogen. Note, though, that the test is not quantitative and does not predict if the sperm can swim in it.
Clomid Challenge Test	Day 3—FSH and Estradiol Day 10—FSH	To evaluate ovarian reserve and chances for pregnancy before assisted reproductive technologies.
Endometrial biopsy	One or two days before expected period in order to assure validity	To determine if luteal phase is sufficient and uterine lining is suitable for the fertilized egg to implant (but its clinical validity is disputed).
Hormone blood tests (miscellaneous)	Various times throughout cycle (see table on page 192)	To determine critical factors about your cycle such as whether you produce enough FSH, estrogen, LH, and progesterone, all necessary for successful conception and implantation.
Hysterosalpingogram (HSG)	The week after your period ends	To determine if the fallopian tubes are clear and the uterine cavity is normal.
Hysteroscopy	Usually before ovulation	To determine if the uterine cavity is normal (not routinely performed).
Laparoscopy	Usually before ovulation	To diagnose and treat pelvic disease such as adhesions or endometriosis.
Postcoital Test (PCT)	Close to ovulation (ideally from intercourse during presence of your most fertile cervical fluid)	To determine whether the man's sperm can survive in the woman's cervical fluid. (There should be 5 to 10 sperm per high-power field.) (This test is rarely performed anymore by reproductive endocrinologists due to its disputed clinical validity, because the predictive value is poor and the results do not change the recommended therapy.)
Saline infusion sonography or sonohyterogram	Before ovulation	To determine if the uterine cavity is normal.
Ultrasound	Just before HCG injection and sometimes after	To evaluate follicle maturation, ovulation, and endometrial thickness and character. (Several ultrasounds may be done as ovulation approaches to determine follicle size and uterine maturity.)

4. Chromosome Analysis (if necessary)

Some people are born with congenital problems that aren't evident until they try to get pregnant. Chromosome analysis can reveal the nature of the problem, which may be related to sexually dysfunctional anatomy.

5. Genetic Counseling (if necessary)

Some families may carry a recessive gene for certain birth defects. If you or your partner has such a family history, you may wish to get genetic counseling to determine what your chances are of giving it to your offspring.

❧ WAYS OF RESOLVING INFERTILITY: AN OVERVIEW

Once you've identified a fertility problem, you can often resolve it through one of the following treatments:

1. Optimizing the chances of getting pregnant by using FAM to time intercourse when you are the most fertile
2. Correcting the basic underlying problem
3. Bypassing steps in reproduction through assisted reproductive technologies

The following is a brief synopsis of the fertility treatments listed above.

1. Optimize Chances of Getting Pregnant by Timing Intercourse at the Most Fertile Time

As discussed in detail in Chapter 11, the most fertile time in a woman's cycle is the *last day* of the most fertile-quality cervical fluid or vaginal sensation. If a man's sperm count is normal, the couple should have intercourse every day that the woman has wet cervical fluid through to the first morning of the rise in temperature. If a man's sperm count is low, the couple should have intercourse every *other* day of wet cervical fluid through to the first morning of the rise in temperature.

2A. Correct the Man's Basic Underlying Problem

As with women, the man's fertility may be improved simply by changing diet and eliminating caffeine, nicotine, recreational drugs, and alcohol. Some people believe that homeopathic and naturopathic treatments as well as nutritional supplements may also be useful. Still, men facing infertility problems usually have a variety of overlapping symptoms that require medical intervention. While fertility specialists generally view male infertility as easier to detect but more difficult to cure than the female counterpart, it is also true that some of the more prevalent problems can be successfully treated. Male infertility may be due to problems relating to any combination of the following:

- low sperm count
- varicoceles
- damaged sperm ducts
- hormonal deficiency
- testicular failure
- sperm antibodies

A. Low Sperm Count

The most common cause of male subfertility is low sperm count, believed to be due to a variety of causes. Among these are hormonal deficiency, bacterial infections, and varicoceles, all of which may be treated by standard medical procedures discussed below. Success rates vary depending on the cause. Unfortunately, low sperm counts often have no detectable source, though abnormal testicular maturation dating back to embryonic development is suspected.

Regardless, it's possible that sperm production can be increased through the use of various fertility drugs such as Clomid, Pergonal, and HCG (all of which are more commonly associated with women's fertility procedures). In addition, low sperm counts can be treated with a variety of high-tech procedures to take advantage of the sperm that exist, and indeed, even men with zero sperm counts have an exciting new option available (see Testicular Failure, next page).

B. Varicoceles

The most likely cause of diminished sperm counts are varicoceles in the scrotal sac. About 30 to 40% of all infertile men have them, though often they have no impact on fertility. They almost always occur in the left testicle, since the spermatic vein enters the renal vein at a right angle on that side, allowing pressure to build. The most plausible reason why this would affect sperm is that the pooled venous blood overheats the sperm production centers of the testicles. And, as you know, heat can kill sperm.

Either general or local anesthesia can be used to operate on them. The effective sperm count improves in about 80% of infertile men after surgery, but only half of these men typically go on to impregnate their partners. This would suggest that male infertility is often caused by a series of overlapping problems.

C. Damaged Sperm Ducts

Blocked sperm ducts may account for about 10 to 15% of all male infertility. Scarring in the vas deferens may prevent the sperm from reaching the cervical fluid as it flows through the urethra. This is often caused by an infection that is the result of an STD. The vas deferens may also be blocked by a varicocele that is pressing against it. Some of these cases can be corrected without surgery, but most would require a minor operation to eliminate the blockage or scarring. Microsurgery is generally extremely effective in restoring fertility to men whose only problem is obstruction of sperm outflow.

Amazingly, it is now possible to avoid the invasiveness of the tubal surgery above by removing sperm directly from the man's epididymis. This is done through two newly developed procedures called microsurgical epididymal sperm aspiration (MESA) and percutaneous epididymal sperm aspiration (PESA), the latter of which uses an ultrathin needle to retrieve the sperm. Both procedures are done in conjunction with one of the assisted reproductive technologies discussed on page 206.

D. Hormonal Deficiency

The next most common cause of male subfertility is hormonal deficiency. It is usually due to an insufficient or erratic release of FSH and LH, the sex hormones necessary for sperm production (these hormones, discussed extensively throughout this book, are also produced by the male reproductive system). If hormonal deficiency is causing low sperm count, it may be possible to treat the problem with gonadotropins. Male hormonal problems are generally complex and difficult to cure, though the chances of success are much greater when the problem results in marginal sperm count, as opposed to the complete cessation of sperm production.

E. Testicular Failure

Another fairly common problem is testicular failure, in which the amount of reproductive hormones being released from the pituitary is sufficient, but the testes fail to respond appropriately and therefore do not produce sperm. The causes for this condition range from illnesses such as mumps and various STDs to physical traumas caused by surgery, tumors, and drugs. It may even be caused by a sports injury, in which a sudden blow to the testes may lead to reduction in the flow of oxygen to the spermatogenia, thus causing the cells to die. Unfortunately, there appears to be no effective treatment that will improve sperm production in cases where no sperm are present.

However, if there are some sperm, fertility drugs may be able to increase the numbers. And as mentioned earlier, it is now possible to retrieve sperm directly from the testicles even if the man's count is zero! In a new and remarkable procedure called testicular sperm extraction (TESE), special high-powered microscopes and delicate microsurgical instruments take sperm directly from the testicles. Even more remarkably, the latest related breakthrough as of this writing is a procedure that allows for the harvesting and successful fertilization of "spermatids," or sperm buds, for those men who have no fully functioning sperm within them.

F. Sperm Antibodies

In some men, the problem is caused by production of antibodies to their own sperm, so that the immune system effectively destroys the sperm as soon as they are produced. This occurs in about 10% of infertile men, though the numbers may be higher among those who underwent a vasectomy and then reversed it. If a man has developed antibodies against his own sperm, he may be prescribed steroids, which are potent drugs that suppress the immune system (clearly such treatment has its disadvantages). There is also some evidence that adrenal hormones may restore fertility in certain cases.

Another option is to have the sperm washed. This is a procedure in which the semen is mixed with culture media in a test tube and then rapidly spun. Although it doesn't dislodge antibodies, it does permit separation of the best swimmers, allowing for artificial insemination high in the woman's reproductive tract. In fact, intrauterine insemination (IUI) is the most common treatment for sperm antibodies. If IUI is unsuccessful, then the couple can try one of the assisted reproductive technologies such as IVF or GIFT.*

---

* It is also possible that the *woman* may develop antibodies against her partner's sperm. If this happens, there are a number of treatments that can be used. If her cervical fluid is incompatible with his sperm, hormones can be prescribed to change its composition, or she can use normally unnecessary douches to change its acidity. If she has antibodies in her cervical fluid, she may be prescribed steroid treatments (such as prednisone) or, interestingly enough, condom therapy. Condom therapy to get pregnant? Actually, the principle is that the couple should use condoms during intercourse for a period of six months in hopes of weakening the antibodies in the woman's immune system that attack her partner's sperm. When the couple does resume unprotected intercourse, it needs to be timed precisely for conception, lest she once again start building antibodies against his sperm.

Many of the above-mentioned conditions as well as some less common fertility-related problems can now be clearly treated. And as the revolution in reproductive medicine continues, it now looks like there is even hope for those men who produce no sperm at all. Of course, these new technologies can be expensive and are not guaranteed to work for all men, but even in those cases, such couples could use a donor for artificial insemination.

2B. Correct the Woman's Basic Underlying Problem

A. Change in Diet or Nutritional Status

As discussed in Chapter 12, being either too thin or too heavy can compromise a woman's fertility. If a woman is too thin, she may cease ovulating altogether. And if she is too heavy, her extra fat can excrete excess oestrogen that paradoxically suppresses the normal hormonal feedback system.

Additionally, some women are more sensitive than others to unbalanced diets or those that are lacking in necessary vitamins and nutrients. Because the discussion of appropriate nutrients for optimal fertility is a book in itself, I would recommend *Fertility, Cycles, and Nutrition* by Marilyn Shannon.

B. Naturopathic and Homeopathic Treatments

Naturopathy is a system of medicine that treats health conditions by utilizing the body's inherent ability to heal. Homeopathy is a system of medicine in which minute amounts of natural substances from plants, minerals, and animals are used to treat chronic conditions that fail to respond to standard Western medicine. Both systems have devoted adherents, including those who believe various infertility problems may be successfully treated through their practice.

For those determined to exhaust all natural possibilities before moving on to more conventional approaches, I have recommended a couple of books that deal with these and other forms of alternative medicine, including herbal treatments and acupuncture (see Appendix N).

C. Drug Therapy

The chart on the next page lists the most commonly prescribed fertility drugs, for use both alone and with Assisted Reproductive Technologies (ART). Whenever any drug is prescribed, you should always verify with your physician precisely what the drug is for and what the potential side effects are.

FERTILITY DRUGS

The drugs listed below are often used for more than one function, and often in combination. Each woman's protocol may differ.

How drug is given: C (Cream)   G (Gel)   I (Injection)   NS (Nasal Spray)   O (Oral)   P (Pump)   VS (Vaginal Suppository)

Brand		What It Is	Generic Name	What It Does
STIMULATES OVULATION				
Clomid Serophene	O O	Selective estrogen receptor modulator (SERM) Synthetic anti-estrogen which indirectly stimulates FSH and LH, as well as higher levels of progesterone	Clomiphene Citrate	• Induces ovulation • Regulates cycles • Increases egg production • Corrects luteal-phase deficiency
Pergonal Humegon Repronex	I I I	FSH and LH made from the urine of postmenopausal women Synthetic FSH and LH	hMG Human Menopausal Gonadotropin	• Induces ovulation • Increases production of eggs in ART* • Increases levels of progesterone
Metrodin Fertinex Follistim Gonal-F	I I I I	FSH made from urine of post-menopausal women 100% pure, human recombinant FSH	FSH Follicle Stimulating Hormone	• Induces ovulation • Increases production of eggs in ART* • Increases levels of progesterone
Factrel Lutrepulse	I P	GnRH	GnRH Gonadotropin-Releasing Hormone	• Indirectly stimulates the ovary of women whose hypothalamus fails to produce enough GnRH (used only if other drugs have failed)
Profasi Pregnyl APL Novarel Ovidrel	I I I I I	Placental hormone made from urine of pregnant women, mimics LH A recombinant pure form of HCG	HCG Human Chorionic Gonadotropin	• Triggers ovulation • Supports corpus luteum following ovulation • Enhances the quality of the uterine lining • Improves progesterone production
BLOCKS PRODUCTION OF HORMONES				
Lupron Synarel Zoladex	I NS I	Gonadotropin-Releasing Hormone Agonist †	GnRH agonist	• Inhibits premature LH surge • Prevents premature release of eggs in ART* (in short-acting form) • Will stop FSH production and therefore estradiol, creating a pseudo-menopause (in long-acting form)
Parlodel Dostinex	O O	Dopamine Agonist †	Bromocriptine	• Suppresses the overproduction of prolactin, a condition which can disrupt ovulation and impact the quality of the luteal phase • May diminish the rate of miscarriages
Antagon	I	Gonadotropin-Releasing Hormone Antagonist (GnRH antagonist)	GnRH antagonist	• Inhibits premature surge of LH in ART*
FACILITATES CONCEPTION AND SUPPORTS PREGNANCY				
Progesterone Crinone Progesterone Prometrium	VS G I O C	Natural or synthetic progesterone	Progesterone	• Matures and sustains the uterine lining following ovulation. Its use to prevent miscarriage, though, is disputed.
Estrace Premarin	O O	Micronized estradiol Conjugated estrogen	Estrogen	• May encourage the production of fertile-quality cervical fluid, but only when prescribed along with other fertility drugs

* ART refers to Assisted Reproductive Technologies such as IVF, GIFT, and ZIFT.
† Agonists are synthetic versions of natural hormones, but are longer lasting and considerably more potent than the hormones they mimic.

1.) Drugs to Stimulate Ovulation

Two of the most commonly prescribed drugs to induce ovulation are Clomid and Pergonal. Clomid is considered the least invasive of the two and, in principle, is prescribed when a woman is either not ovulating at all or only sporadically. It is also used when she has a short luteal phase. In reality, Clomid is often prescribed as a matter of routine even when the woman's fertility problem is not known. Pergonal, on the other hand, is one of an extremely potent class of drugs that is usually prescribed only when Clomid doesn't work. Pergonal is usually used for the assisted technologies of IVF, GIFT, and ZIFT.

Your doctor may also prescribe any number of other drugs to induce ovulation, all of which stimulate the maturation of your egg follicles. Included among these are Humegon and Repronex (which may have the added advantage of actually enhancing the production of cervical fluid), Fertinex and Metrodin (often prescribed to women over 40 who have an imbalance of FSH and LH), and finally Follistim and Gonal-F (which are among the newest fertility drugs that use modern DNA technologies). Regardless of the particular ovulatory drug chosen, you should definitely be aware that some studies continue to suggest that there may be an increased risk of ovarian cancer if such drugs are used for an extended period of time.

2.) Drugs to Block Production of Hormones

Occasionally, it is necessary to suppress ovulation in order to abate conditions such as endometriosis. Women are typically prescribed anovulatory drugs for about six months or longer, after which they are then instructed to try to get pregnant. These drugs are also used in conjunction with high-tech treatments.

It is also worth noting that some women have an excessively high level of hormones that may disrupt their normal ovulatory cycle. For example, Parlodel is used to reduce prolactin, the hormone that normally circulates in women who are breastfeeding.

3.) Drugs to Further Facilitate Conception and Support Pregnancy

Oestrogen is critical for the development of fertile cervical fluid. Often, when women are prescribed Clomid to induce ovulation, it has the unfortunate side effect of drying up the necessary cervical fluid. In these cases, oestrogen can be prescribed along with Clomid to counteract its drying effects.

Progesterone is usually given to support a short or insufficient luteal phase. It's typically given either by injections, vaginal suppositories, or oral tablets. It acts to prevent a newly pregnant woman from menstruating before the egg has had a chance to implant, thus decreasing the odds of a miscarriage.

D. Surgery

Nowadays, surgery means not only traditional cutting with a scalpel, but perhaps just using a simple laser beam. It may be performed to correct obstructions such as tubal scarring and cervical polyps. In addition, surgery can remove adhesions such as those caused by endometriosis and scarring from pelvic inflammatory disease. Finally, it can be used to remove growths such as fibroids in the uterus. While the prospect of undergoing an operation is admittedly not pleasant, advances in technology do mean that many procedures can now be done on an outpatient basis.

A Special Note on Four Distinct Fertility Problems

Before discussing possible high-tech treatments, there are four conditions of which you should be aware. The first, endometriosis, is one of the most widely diagnosed fertility problems. The second, Polycystic Ovarian Syndrome, has recently come to be seen as one of the most common hormonal disorders for women. The third, Luteinized Unruptured Follicle Syndrome, is rarely detected but has recently emerged as a prime suspect in inexplicable infertility cases. Finally, Premature Ovarian Failure is perhaps the most unsettling, but fortunately, it is also fairly rare.

• Endometriosis

One of the most peculiar causes of infertility is endometriosis, a surprisingly prevalent disorder in which normal endometrial tissue, which is supposed to line the uterus, begins to grow elsewhere in the body. The misplaced tissue may develop anywhere within the abdominal cavity, growing in small superficial patches, in thicker, penetrating nodules, or within cysts in the ovary. The condition is highly unpredictable in that it may remain in a few very small areas or spread invasively throughout the pelvis. One of the most puzzling aspects of endometriosis is that the degree of pain it causes is not a valid indicator of the severity of the condition. It may cause absolutely no symptoms even though it has spread extensively, or cause excruciating pain even though there is minimal spreading.

A paradox of endometriosis is that pregnancy is one of the few natural conditions that seems to cause the disease to regress temporarily. Yet it is the condition itself that often causes infertility. There are basically two types of treatment: hormones or surgery.

The goal of hormonal treatment is to simulate pregnancy or menopause, the two natural conditions known to inhibit the disease. Women are prescribed either birth control pills, synthetic progesterones called progestins, Danazol, or analogs of GnRH such as Lupron, Synarel, or Zoladex. These drugs are typically taken for at least six months in order to be most effective. While less invasive than surgery, hormonal therapy has its limitations. It only works in mild cases, has many side effects, and requires much more time to diminish the disease.

Surgery, on the other hand, can remove adhesions, implants, or blood-filled cysts. Laparoscopy can often be used to drain fluid and remove small patches through laser or electrical current. But not all cases can be treated through the laparoscope. Occasionally, more extensive surgery is necessary when scar tissue is thick or involves delicate structures.

Finally, some patients need a combination of both medical and surgical therapy. Regardless, women are encouraged to try to achieve pregnancy within six months of completing treatment, because it often recurs as severe as it was before. But if a woman doesn't respond to any of the above, she still may be able to achieve pregnancy through one of the assisted technologies such as IVF.

• Polycystic Ovarian Syndrome (PCOS)

Over the last few years, the medical community has come to realize that PCOS may be the most prevalent hormonal disorder that women have, and that along with endometriosis, it is one of the most common causes of infertility. What essentially happens with this condition is that the developing follicles that are normally ovulated each cycle actually remain trapped inside the ovary. After a while, they swell with fluid and turn into cysts that develop on the internal ovarian wall. If not treated, a hard shell may also form around the outside of the ovary, which of course will make a successful ovulation even less likely in the future.

As mentioned, PCOS is a hormonal problem, specifically caused by the fact that the ovaries begin to produce a troubling excess of the male hormone testosterone, which is normally only produced in very tiny amounts. In addition, excessive quantities of LH and FSH are also produced. The cause of these hormonal imbalances is still not totally understood, although increasing evidence now strongly points to the interaction of high blood insulin levels and insulin-sensitive ovaries.

Aside from the obvious infertility that results from an inability to ovulate, several symptoms are associated with PCOS. As one might expect, menstrual cycles may be extremely irregular or even nonexistent. In addition, PCOS can cause excessive facial and body hair, male-pattern hair loss, acne, and even obesity. It may also lead to higher risks of endometrial cancer (since nonovulating women do not regularly shed their uterine lining), and it is associated with diabetes. If your doctor suspects PCOS, there are a number of ways to verify that you have it, including an ultrasound of your ovaries to observe the size and presence of cysts, as well as various blood tests to measure the level of such hormones as LH, FSH, and testosterone.

Women with this condition often have a paradoxical fertility sign of appearing to be extremely fertile, when in reality they are less so than the average woman. This is because they produce excessive amounts of FSH and LH, leading to exceedingly high levels of oestrogen, which in turn causes them to produce slippery-quality cervical fluid seemingly all the time. But rather than signaling impending ovulation, they often discover that their temperatures remain monophasic, instead of showing the classic biphasic pattern following ovulation. This is because they are, in fact, not ovulating.

Although there is no known cure for PCOS, there have fortunately been great strides made in its treatment. Traditionally, the most common strategies were either surgery or drugs that stopped the production of sex hormones. For women who wanted to get pregnant, these treatments were often combined with ovulatory drugs such as Clomid and, if thought necessary, laparoscopic surgery followed by some type of IVF procedure.

More recently however, the emphasis has been on drugs designed to regulate the body's production of insulin, including Metformin, which is often used by diabetics to help control their own insulin levels. There have also been promising results with a nutritional supplement called D-chiro-inositol, which also lowers insulin levels and allows for a natural ovulation.

- **Luteinized Unruptured Follicle Syndrome (LUFS)**

You should be aware that even if you have all the classic signs of ovulation, including fertile cervical fluid and clear biphasic temperature patterns, it is still possible that you may not actually be ovulating. This is because some women experience on rare occasions a condition called LUFS. In such a case, the luteal phase is typically so short that it's obviously not a fertile cycle. The woman often has no physical symptoms other than infertility itself, but ultrasound reveals that the ovum remains stuck within the luteinized follicle, unable to pass through the ovarian wall to a possible conception.

It is now estimated that up to 30% of unexplained infertility is due to this condition. If ultrasound did reveal that you have LUFS, it's still possible that one of the assisted reproductive technologies could help you conceive.

- **Premature Ovarian Failure (POF)**

Women with Premature Ovarian Failure have a condition in which their ovaries stop producing eggs a decade or more before normal menopause. It may emerge suddenly, or more gradually over several years, with the appearance of irregular cycles along with classic premenopausal symptoms such as hot flashes, vaginal dryness, and eventually the disappearance of periods altogether.

The standard way to determine if you have entered premature menopause is an FSH and oestrogen blood test drawn on Day 3 of your cycle. If it is elevated over several repeat blood draws, it usually indicates that you are starting to experience POF. Unfortunately, such a condition makes it difficult to stimulate a woman's ovaries into releasing an egg, since they rarely respond to drugs.

3. Bypass Steps in Reproduction Through Assisted Reproductive Technologies

The procedures that follow are listed in approximate order of invasiveness, from least to most. AI, IUI, and FAST all involve placing the sperm inside the woman, either outside the cervix, within the uterus, or directly into the fallopian tubes. IVF, GIFT, and ZIFT all involve artificially removing the eggs from the woman's ovaries. The differences here are a function of where fertilization occurs (in or out of the body) and where the egg and sperm are returned to the body (uterus or fallopian tubes).

These technologies usually involve "sperm washing," a process that dramatically increases the motility of the sperm by mixing it with a culture media and then placing it in a centrifuge. It is considered much more effective if the woman's ovulation is artificially stimulated through ovulatory drugs such as Pergonal.

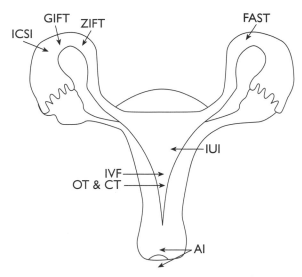

Site of Reproductive Technologies. High-tech procedures involving removal and reinsertion of the egg are on the left in red. Low-tech procedures involving insertion of *sperm only* are on the right in black. Arrows indicate the site of insertion.

A. Artificial Insemination (AI) and Intrauterine Insemination (IUI)

These are the simplest and least technologically complex of the assisted reproductive technologies. AI typically involves using a catheter to gently insert the man's sperm just outside or within the cervix, whereas IUI involves placing the sperm directly into the uterus (thus the expression intrauterine insemination). For both, the sperm may be that of your partner or a donor. Nowadays, IUI is the preferred choice because it more effectively bypasses numerous potential fertility problems, including low sperm count or poor sperm motility, antisperm antibodies, infertile-quality cervical fluid, irregular cycles, endometriosis, and unexplained infertility.

In any case, with both AI and natural intercourse, conception is most likely to occur if the sperm is deposited at the cervical opening on the woman's Peak Day, which as you know, is the last day of wet-quality cervical fluid or lubricative vaginal sensation. With IUI, however, the best time to deposit the sperm is in the hours immediately before and following ovulation, which can usually be determined by a combination of charting, ovulation predictor kits, and ultrasound. This is often accomplished by performing two procedures 24 hours apart.

B. Fallopian Sperm Transfer System (FAST)

This is one of the newest and most promising artificial insemination technologies. It usually involves placing washed sperm directly into each of your fallopian tubes in the hours following drug-induced ovulation, as close to the egg as possible. By doing this, it is believed that fertilization is likely to occur more quickly and easily, and as of this writing, the first small but significant studies seem to suggest that this is the case.

C. In Vitro Fertilization (IVF)

IVF is a procedure that is most commonly done on women whose fallopian tubes are blocked, although it is also useful in those situations where there is unexplained or male factor infertility as well as ovulatory problems and advanced maternal age. It involves removing several eggs from the woman's ovaries and fertilizing them with her partner's sperm in a petri dish outside her body, then placing the 2-day-old embryo in her *uterus*. The challenge with IVF is not fertilization, but implantation, since the embryo must be transferred from the petri dish and implanted in the uterus earlier than would naturally occur.

D. Gamete Intra-Fallopian Transfer (GIFT)

This procedure solves the implantation problem of IVF, but requires that the woman's fallopian tubes be open. As with IVF, the eggs are removed, but the sperm and eggs are inserted into the *fallopian tube* and left to fertilize on their own. GIFT is generally considered more effective than IVF because the placement of the sperm and egg into the tubes (rather than the uterus) re-creates the natural conditions necessary for a successful implantation.

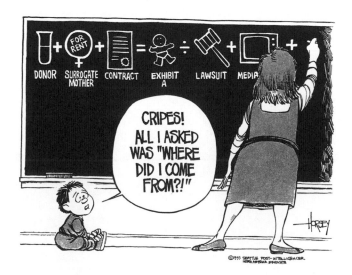

E. Zygote Intra-Fallopian Transfer (ZIFT)

This procedure is a logical answer to the situation where the man's sperm quality is marginal, but the woman's tubes are still open. With ZIFT, the egg is first fertilized in a petri dish, and the resulting zygote is returned to the *fallopian tube,* after which it continues to naturally travel down to implant in the uterus.

F. Intracytoplasmic Sperm Injection (ICSI)

This is one of the most promising techniques developed for those conditions in which the man's sperm count is low or the sperm he does have has been unable to fertilize an egg in previous IVF attempts. In addition, it is usually done when the woman has such conditions as tubal scarring or mild endometriosis, and thus it often is used to bypass the reproductive impediments that are found in both partners. It is a procedure in which a single sperm is inserted directly into the ova through the assistance of high-tech instruments. After fertilization is achieved, the newly created embryo is placed in an incubator for about 2 to 3 days before it is deposited in the woman's uterus.

G. Ovum Transfer (OT) and Cytoplasm Transfer (CT)

One of the most dramatic advances in fertility technology allows a postmenopausal woman to carry and deliver a child. Using a petri dish, her partner's sperm are used to fertilize the eggs from a younger donor. The embryo is then transplanted into the uterus of the woman desiring pregnancy. Of course, the embryo is related to the man, but not biologically related to her.

There are also situations in which women still produce good follicles and many eggs, but cannot conceive because the surrounding cytoplasm, a gel-like fluid that lines the shell of the egg, is compromised. Now however, an exciting option has recently emerged that would allow them to be biologically related to the embryo. In a procedure called cytoplasm transfer, the cytoplasm of a donor's egg can be used to encase the egg of the biological mother.

It should also be noted that until recently the option to freeze a woman's own eggs was never possible because they were simply too fragile to withstand the procedure. But it now appears that with emerging technology, women will soon be able to do this when they are still young, allowing them the possibility of carrying their own babies to term when they are older and ready to become parents.

THE DIFFERENCE BETWEEN IVF, GIFT, AND ZIFT

	IVF	GIFT	ZIFT
Fallopian tubes need to be open	No	Yes	Yes
Where fertilization takes place	Petri dish outside the uterus	Fallopian tube	Petri dish outside the uterus
Where egg and sperm (or the fertilized egg) are returned to	Uterus	Fallopian tube	Fallopian tube
Good option for poor sperm quality	Yes, if tubes closed	No	Yes, if tubes open
Surgery and hospitalization required	No	Yes	Yes

The table above summarizes the three most common high-tech procedures. I have specifically chosen not to list an estimated success rate per cycle because the data available in the medical literature and from the infertility clinics is extremely inconsistent and confusing. One reason for this is because there are so many variables that affect the rates, including such things as maternal age, the cause of infertility and the numerous variations within the procedures used. It's also worth noting that a straight pregnancy rate is often claimed (whether a miscarriage results or not), when it is the "take home baby rate" that is obviously more relevant for intelligently analyzing your options. The bottom line is that the technology continues to improve, but success is never assured. And even for those who eventually succeed, it often takes at least several cycles before a healthy pregnancy results.

What is generally accepted is that GIFT and ZIFT have greater success rates than IVF. Still, many couples choose to try IVF because it is a simpler and less costly procedure that can be performed on an outpatient basis. And obviously in certain cases, such as when the woman's fallopian tubes are blocked, GIFT and ZIFT are not even options. It should also be noted that IVF allows clinicians to verify that fertilization has indeed occurred (this is not possible with GIFT). This is especially helpful for couples where the man's sperm quality is poor and it's uncertain whether his sperm can fertilize her eggs.

The Steps Necessary for IVF, GIFT, or ZIFT

Before you seriously consider any of these technologies, you should be aware that they all involve a series of procedures that can be both physically and emotionally uncomfortable. As of this writing, IVF, GIFT, and ZIFT remain the most widely used high-tech options, and all three involve variations of the following:

1. The woman is prescribed a series of hormones throughout her cycle (usually in the form of injections) which typically include a combination of drugs such as the following:

   - **Pergonal** (a purified preparation of FSH)*
   - **Lupron** (a drug that prevents a premature LH surge)
   - **HCG** (Human Chorionic Gonadotropin, a hormone that acts like luteinizing hormone when injected)
   - **Progesterone** (the hormone you normally make in the latter phase of your cycle, but which may cease being released as an effect of Pergonal)

2. The man's sperm are "washed" to improve their quality, maximizing the chances of success.

3. In the final step, a dozen or so of the woman's matured eggs are aspirated from her artificially stimulated ovaries with a vaginal, ultrasonically guided needle. Then, depending on the procedure chosen, fertilization will be attempted in either a petri dish (ZIFT or IVF) or her fallopian tubes (GIFT). If the eggs are fertilized in the petri dish, several will be returned to either her tubes (ZIFT) or her uterus (IVF).

---

* If you've heard some outlandish story about how Pergonal has been harvested from the urine of postmenopausal nuns in Italy—for once, 'tis true! One of the paradoxical effects of menopause on a woman's body is to produce massive quantities of FSH as a way of trying to trigger the ovaries to continue to ovulate. Since FSH is needed to induce ovulation in clinically stimulated cycles such as those prepared for artificial insemination, IVF, GIFT, and ZIFT, isn't it logical to use nun's urine? You're probably thinking "Why didn't I think of that? Nuns' urine. It's so obvious." (For an even more bizarre hormonal source, see page 267.)

℘ DEALING WITH MISCARRIAGES

Unfortunately, all the high-tech procedures discussed above will probably not help if you are experiencing repeated miscarriages. For unlike any other infertility issue, this is not a problem in achieving pregnancy, but rather in keeping the embryo viable after conception has occurred. It is also unfortunate, but true, that as women age into their 30s, miscarriages become the most prevalent cause of infertility, with undetected ones probably composing the vast majority of fetal loss.

While the assisted reproductive technologies have little role to play in the miscarriage problem, there are hopeful medical advances being made. Of course, before you can begin seeking treatment, you must first be aware that you have the problem. As you have already learned, charting can play a critical role in this area. FAM can usually identify miscarriages as they occur (as seen by at least 18 temps followed by sharply dropping temps and eventual bleeding), or identify the abnormally short luteal phases that would make a successful implantation highly improbable.

If you do discover that you are in fact getting pregnant but losing the embryo, you should at least know that the majority of women in your situation will still be able to go on and have healthy babies. In fact, most women should be able to start trying to conceive again within a cycle or two. But keep in mind that each woman and situation is unique, so the length of time you may want to wait will depend on numerous factors, including how early in the pregnancy the miscarriage occurred, what actually caused it, whether or not you are still bleeding, and, of course, whether you are emotionally prepared to try again.

Aside from the obvious steps you should take to make sure you are in the healthiest condition possible, I urge you to consult a qualified fertility specialist. Better yet, you should bring the doctor your Fertility Awareness charts. By doing so, you will not only feel more in control, but you may very well be expediting the process that leads to a healthy baby.

Deborah and Burt used FAM to get pregnant, but the pregnancy sadly ended in a miscarriage due to a blighted ovum (a strange phenomenon in which a sac develops, but an embryo never does). Because they had no problem initially getting pregnant, they decided not to resume charting when they were ready to try again.

Deborah had one normal cycle following her miscarriage, but the cycle after that was extremely long and confusing to them. When she had spotting on Day 54, she didn't know whether it was ovulatory spotting, implantation bleeding due to pregnancy, or the signs of a possible miscarriage. She only realized then how frustrating it was to not have charted that cycle, because it left her completely in the dark. She got a pregnancy test, which came back negative. Of course, she still wasn't sure if the test was accurate, because she might have ovulated so late that the test could have indicated a false negative if her body had not yet had a chance to produce enough HCG to be detected.

As it turned out, Deborah was not pregnant. Either she didn't ovulate that cycle, or had an extremely delayed ovulation. In any event, their confusion could have been eliminated had they simply charted. Needless to say, they learned from this experience how valuable charting is, even for those who seemingly have no problem getting pregnant. After waiting a few cycles, they tried again. This time they charted, and were thrilled to discover they were pregnant through temperatures that remained above the coverline beyond 18 days. Sure enough, Deborah later gave birth to a darling baby boy.

Causes of Miscarriages

Infections

One of the surprising things about the role of infections in miscarriages is that the more common ones are not considered responsible. So having a bad cold, the flu, or a fever during pregnancy is *not* likely to harm your fetus. But there are certain infections that may, including mycoplasma, toxoplasmosis, chlamydia, listeria, malaria, and monilia (this last one only when an IUD is in place at the time of accidental conception).

In addition, there are infections associated with certain procedures that may cause a miscarriage, including those from a cervical stitch used to tighten a weak cervix, an IUD, an organism called campylobacter, and prostaglandins in semen during intercourse itself (which is only of concern to women who have previously miscarried). If a cervical or semen sample reveals an infection, you and your partner will most likely be prescribed an antibiotic such as erythomycin. In fact, many fertility specialists now routinely prescribe this drug in particular because it is considered safe for both the mother and baby. More important, it has proven to be one of the most beneficial treatments in preventing miscarriages in general, especially those of unknown causes.

Finally, certain viruses are dangerous during pregnancy, including the most notorious, German measles (rubella), and herpes (if the initial viral attack occurred during the first 20 weeks of pregnancy). Others that may also cause miscarriages include mumps, measles, hepatitis A and B, and parvovirus.

Endocrine Problems (Hormonal)

One of the most common hormonal problems leading to early miscarriages is that of an abnormal luteal phase. As you've read, in order for a fertilized egg to have a chance to implant and mature, the corpus luteum must maintain the latter phase of the cycle for at least ten days. In addition, once pregnancy occurs, it must continue to live long enough for the developing placenta to take over the function of providing nutrition for the embryo. The corpus luteum should live about 10 weeks beyond conception, so if you had a miscarriage before then that was within the first few weeks of pregnancy, one of the first things the doctor would suspect is a possible corpus luteum deficiency.

Of course, you yourself should suspect a potential problem if your basal temperatures reflect a luteal phase of 10 days or less.* If it does, your doctor will most likely perform a blood test and endometrial biopsy to confirm this. If you do indeed have a problem with progesterone production in the latter phase of your cycle, your doctor will likely recommend a natural form of progesterone, to be taken as soon as you ovulate each cycle. (Once pregnancy is confirmed, it should probably be taken through to the 3rd trimester.) Many doctors will also prescribe Clomid in the first phase of the cycle, in the hope that it will promote an optimal ovulation and a healthy progesterone level afterward.

Uterine Abnormalities

One of the most common causes of miscarriages in the second trimester is what is unfortunately referred to as an "incompetent cervix." As the name implies, it is a weak cervix that tends to dilate before the fetus has reached full term. Some women are born with congenital abnormalities of the uterus which are shaped in such a way that the baby can't grow big enough before it runs out of room and causes the cervix to dilate. Uterine anomalies are often the result of a woman's mother having taken DES while pregnant with her.

If your physician suspects that recurring miscarriages may be due to structural problems of your uterus, she will probably perform a hysterogram. This procedure is basically an X ray that uses injected dye to determine its shape. Two other diagnostic procedures often used to view the uterus are a laparoscopy, in which a narrow tube is inserted through the naval, and a hysteroscopy, in which a similar device is inserted through the vagina and cervix.

---

* While most of the medical literature suggests that a 10-day luteal phase should be sufficient for implantation, it's also true that 10- or even 11-day luteal phases could be a potential problem in certain cases.

One of the least invasive treatments, especially in the case of a weak cervix, is to place a suture in it to prevent it from dilating prematurely. But if the uterus is malformed or has uterine adhesions, it can usually be successfully treated only through surgery.

Finally, if you have fibroids (or benign tumors) in or on your uterus, you are not alone. By age 40, about 40% of women have them. They generally don't require any treatment unless they grow exceedingly fast or cause severe bleeding or pelvic pressure. Your physician will often recommend doing nothing, in the hope that the fibroids themselves will not interfere with the pregnancy, since their removal is often more invasive than necessary.

Genetics (Chromosomes)

A large percentage of early and first miscarriages are believed to be due to chromosomal damage. Fortunately, chromosomal miscarriages are not considered a recurring problem, and thus the chance of another one due to similar reasons is small.

Antibodies (Immune System)

One of the most peculiar types of problems now thought to lead to a significant percentage of miscarriages is that of the mother producing antibodies that, in essence, reject her own fetus. Through blood tests, tissue typing, or an endometrial biopsy, the doctor can determine if you are producing such antibodies and, after a precise diagnosis is made, treat you accordingly with any of the following:

- Baby aspirin throughout your pregnancy to prevent blood clots, which if left untreated can act to cut off the embryo's supply of nutrients.
- Prescription anti-inflammatory and anticlotting drugs to treat inflammatory health problems such as rheumatoid arthritis or lupus, which if not resolved can lead to the production of antibodies that can attack the uterus and the embryo's placenta.
- Injections of your partner's white blood cells to trigger the necessary production of the blocking antibodies that embryos need to protect themselves during pregnancy.
- Immunoglobulins, which act to absorb excess "killer" cells.
- A new drug called Enbrel (not available in the UK) to treat certain destructive immune system cells, including macrophages and natural killer and mast cells.

Medical Disorders

Finally, miscarriages tend to occur more frequently in women who have medical conditions such as uncontrolled diabetes, thyroid disease, high blood pressure, or heart disease. If your physician diagnoses any of these, they will probably refer you to an internist for treatment before you attempt to get pregnant again.

The Dilemma of Advanced Maternal Age

There is an unfortunate biological reality that all women wishing to be mothers should internalize as soon as they become adults. The fact is that women in their late 30s and older are at much greater risk of miscarriage, for the simple reason that as they age, the eggs within their ovaries continue to age with them. It is not completely understood why older ova lose their ability to sustain a healthy pregnancy after they are fertilized, but it's clearly symptomatic of the same biological phenomenon causing the increased risk of birth defects in the babies of older women.

While medical advances continue to be made, solving the problem of miscarriage among women in their 40s continues to be one of the greatest reproductive challenges. I urge you to keep up to date, and of course if at all possible, try to have the children you want before the issue ever arises.

Types of Pregnancy Loss Beyond Vaginal Miscarriages

In addition to regular miscarriages in which the fetus is expelled through the vagina, there are a few other types of failed pregnancies of which you should be aware.

Ectopic Pregnancy: A condition in which a fertilized ovum attaches itself *outside* of the uterus (usually in the fallopian tube) and begins to grow.

Missed Abortion: A most unfortunate term to describe a fetus that has miscarried, or died, but has not been expelled naturally.

Blighted Ovum: A pregnancy in which no fetus ever developed in the pregnancy sac.

Molar Pregnancy: A rare condition in which a normal pregnancy goes awry, becoming a benign tumor at about 10 weeks.

> ## WARNING SIGNS OF MISCARRIAGES
>
> - temps continuously falling after at least 18 days above coverline
> - brown spotting (well beyond the postovulatory implantation spotting that is common 7 to 10 days after conception)
> - red bleeding of any intensity
> - cramping
> - dizziness
> - burning headache
> - joint swelling
> - excessive nausea or vomiting
> - fever
> - extreme or sudden fatigue
> - fainting
> - severe or sudden backache
> - sudden loss of pregnancy symptoms
> - pelvic pain

🙠 FAM, INFERTILITY, AND MODERN MEDICINE

Reproductive medicine continues to make headline-capturing advances. While I believe that a low-tech option such as FAM is the preferred solution to infertility problems whenever possible, you should be aware of FAM's limits. Just as important, you should now know that even if you can't have a baby by completely natural means, charting will certainly help you identify the problem and exploit the various solutions that the miracles of modern medicine increasingly offer.

PART FIVE

BEYOND FERTILITY: PRACTICAL BENEFITS OF CHARTING YOUR CYCLE

CHAPTER 15

Maintaining Your Gynecological Health

Sex is a pleasurable exercise in plumbing, but be careful or you'll get yeast in your drain tap.

—RITA MAE BROWN

Have you ever thought about how odd it is that intimate details about your body are filed in a medical office across town? Why shouldn't you have access to such records in your own home? Once women learn to chart, they take control of all facets of their health care—from annual exam results to the symptoms that may prompt them to seek medical help.

The first form in the master charts section at the back of the book can be used as a master sheet for your annual exams. Enlarge it by 125% and then copy it onto the back of the chart of the cycle in which you get your yearly physical, taking it with you when you go. You'll find it a practical way to keep track of your weight, blood pressure, and general gynecological health, including such things as breast exam, mammogram, Pap test, vaginal culture, or any possible STDs. You can use the back of the regular charts to record anything else worth remembering.

Most women have fairly common conditions that are considered medically normal, but may appear problematic simply because they are not taught about the healthy female body. In addition, as mentioned earlier, there are true gynecological conditions that can be more easily identified through charting, including:

- vaginal infections
- abnormal bleeding
- nabothian (cervical) cysts
- endometriosis
- premenstrual syndrome
- breast lumps

221

By now, this list should be familiar to you. But I think it's important to repeat why charting is so beneficial for your gynecological health. One of the points I made in the beginning of this book is that charting enables a woman to understand her body in a practical way. As you'll recall, I said that a woman who charts every day is so aware of what is normal for her that she can help her clinician determine irregularities based on *her* symptoms rather than the average woman's symptoms. Charting her menstrual cycle allows a woman to actively contribute to her gynecological well-being by working with her health care provider. This concept cannot be stressed enough. The remainder of this chapter will discuss both normal and abnormal gynecological conditions and how FAM can be used to distinguish the two.

❧ NORMAL, HEALTHY CERVICAL FLUID VERSUS REAL VAGINAL INFECTIONS

Healthy Cervical Fluid

From a health perspective, the obvious benefit of learning about your own pattern of cervical fluid is to be able to determine if and when you have a true vaginal infection.

> *Marsha is an American FAM instructor teaching in Israel. While getting her master's degree in public health in the States, she had an annual Pap test. Since she was charting her cycles, and planned her appointment for midcycle, she happened to have a lot of slippery, stretchy cervical fluid. As the physician removed the speculum, he exclaimed. "My dear, you have an infection," to which she replied. "Excuse me? I feel fine and don't have any symptoms." He replied "Look at this discharge!" showing her the Pap stick with the obvious cervical fluid on it. "Well, I know I'm in my fertile phase and these are just my fertile secretions." The nurse stood behind him, winking and nodding in agreement with her. He curtly and abruptly responded: "Well, we can't know for sure. I'm going to prepare these slides for STDs, including gonorrhea, syphilis, and chlamydia" and then proceeded to prescribe a week's antibiotics to take until the results came back.*
>
> *Needless to say, she didn't take the drugs. Nor did the results test positive for any infections. As she cynically sighed, "I knew this was normal for me. But what about the average woman who doesn't know FAM? What kind of message does this send her?"*

Is it any wonder that women grow up believing they are dirty all the time and need to douche and spray away the "discharge"? The continual advertising of douches and feminine sprays only acts to reinforce the confusion between healthy cervical fluid and what is in fact a true infection. Millions of dollars a year is spent promoting vaginal douches alone.

If you think this is harmless, consider a well-known talk show whose topic one day dealt with gynecology. No sooner had the two OB/GYNs finished explaining why douches and sprays were unnecessary and potentially infection-producing, when the show cut to a commercial. And what was the commercial about? You guessed it—vaginal sprays! Only a minute earlier, one of the gynecologists cynically commented that the income he generated treating women who had developed infections from using these products was enough to send all his children to college. And nowadays, with over-the-counter products readily available for yeast infections, how many women buy them every month to try to eliminate the supposed infection that keeps recurring?

Realistically, though, there are going to be times when you really *do* have a vaginal infection. Obviously, knowing your own pattern will enable you to detect the onset of infection almost immediately, treating it before you become uncomfortable. One of the reasons women are often misdiagnosed, as was the instructor above, is that a "symptom" during one time in a woman's cycle may be nothing more than a fertility sign in another. So, for example, wet secretions midcycle is absolutely normal, but may be an indication of infection if it occurs in the latter phase. (One exception to this is explained on page 326.) Of course, the sooner you detect a potential infection, the sooner you can treat and eliminate it.

Symptoms of Vaginal Infections That Can Be Distinguished from Normal Cervical Fluid

Fortunately, once you know your own cervical-fluid pattern, you'll be able to clearly see that true infections almost always appear with any number of unpleasant symptoms that distinguish them. Vaginal infections can range from STDs such as chlamydia and herpes to various forms of vaginitis and, of course, the generic yeast infection. While it is beyond the scope of this book to identify the individual symptoms and treatments for all these conditions, the following symptoms are definitely not part of healthy cervical fluid secretions, and should therefore be seen by a qualified clinician:*

---

* For a comprehensive discussion of various gynecological infections and conditions, I would encourage you to get a good general women's health book such as *Our Bodies, Ourselves for the New Century: A Book by and for Women* by the Boston Women's Health Book Collective.

- abnormal discharge
- itching, stinging, swelling, and redness
- unpleasant odor
- blisters, warts, and chancre sores

Avoiding Infections

There are certain precautions you should take to avoid contracting infections in the first place. Aside from the obvious consequences of douching, you should be aware that wearing clothing that is either damp or too tight may create an unhealthy vaginal environment. Also be sure to always wear cotton underwear and lingerie that allows your body to breath.

🐚 NORMAL VERSUS ABNORMAL BLEEDING

Normal Bleeding

A normal menstrual period typically lasts about five days and usually follows a variation of these two patterns:

Light → heavy → medium → light → very light
Heavy → heavy → medium → medium → light

In addition, women may have spotting or bleeding at other times in their cycle besides menstruation. In fact, one of the most misunderstood facets of the woman's cycle is that of normal spotting or occasional bleeding (spotting is usually brownish because the blood is exposed to more oxygen as it trickles out of the body). A common mistake many women make is to assume that all bleeding episodes are periods. In reality, true menstruation is the bleeding that occurs about 12 to 16 days following the release of an egg. Any other type of bleeding is either anovulatory bleeding, normal spotting, or symptomatic of a problem.

Ovulatory Spotting

Simply stated, some women have a day or two of light bleeding right around ovulation. Not only is this spotting normal, but it's another fertility sign that can help identify where they are in their cycle. It's usually the result of the sudden drop of oestrogen just before ovulation and tends to occur more often in long cycles.

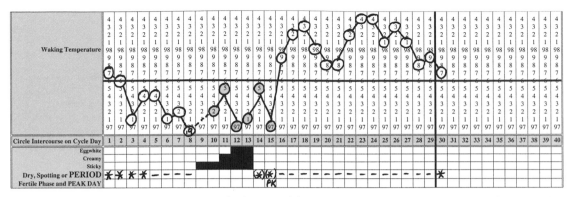

Chart 15.1. Ovulatory spotting. It is perfectly normal for women to have spotting around ovulation, in this case on Days 14 and 15. (Ovulation is clearly seen to have occurred by the thermal shift on Day 16.) Had the spotting occurred several days away from ovulation, it could have been a sign of abnormal bleeding.

Another FAM instructor describes her experience using a diaphragm before she learned a natural method of birth control. Every now and then, when she would remove it after making love, there would be a little blood and slippery cervical fluid mixed in with the spermicide. She would find it very confusing and wonder whether her partner had injured her cervix during intercourse. It wasn't until years later that she realized that the blood she had seen periodically was merely ovulatory spotting collected in the diaphragm.

Anovulatory Bleeding and Spotting

Occasionally women don't release an egg, for several reasons. One is that oestrogen doesn't reach the threshold necessary for the egg to be released. When this happens, the drop in oestrogen is enough to cause a slight shedding of the lining of the uterus. At other times, oestrogen may continue to stimulate the growth of the uterine lining to such an extent that it can't support itself sufficiently, and breakthrough bleeding occurs. In women over 40, the cause of anovulatory bleeding is often the result of a decreased sensitivity to the hormones FSH and LH. The result is that the woman may not ovulate, and without progesterone to sustain the lining, spotting or bleeding may occur. In all these cases, though, the bleeding is not technically menstruation.

The way to determine if a woman did indeed ovulate is through charting the temperature. Remember, ovulatory cycles reflect a classic temperature pattern of low before ovulation, followed by high after.

Implantation Spotting

Likewise, if a woman was trying to get pregnant and noticed spotting rather than bleeding anytime from about a week after her thermal shift, she should consider taking a pregnancy test because it may be "implantation spotting" rather than a period. When the egg burrows into the endometrial lining of the uterus, a little spotting may occur. She can also confirm if she is pregnant by noting if her temperatures continue to remain high beyond 18 days. This would indicate that the corpus luteum was staying alive to support a pregnancy.

Breastfeeding Spotting

Women who have just delivered a child may find that after the initial lochia has stopped, they have an episode of spotting at about 6 weeks postpartum. It's usually due to the withdrawal of hormones that had been circulating at high levels when the woman was pregnant. In addition, while breastfeeding, hormone levels can fluctuate due to the varying needs of the baby. Because of this temporary hormonal imbalance, breastfeeding women may experience a number of anovulatory spottings. (See Appendixes B and C on how to use FAM while breastfeeding.)

Spotting After Office Procedures

Women will often spot after office procedures such as Pap tests, cervical biopsies, cryosurgery, cautery, laser surgery, pelvic exams, IUD insertions, and abortions. This is normal.

Spotting with Birth Control Pills and Oestrogen Replacement Therapy

In addition, women will usually experience withdrawal bleeding during the week in which they are not taking either the Pill or postmenopausal hormone replacement therapy.

Clotting During Menstruation

Blood clots during menstruation are common and usually not considered a problem. However, if you find them annoying and would prefer to treat them, you may want to discuss several options with your doctor, including the use of anti-inflammatory drugs or, ironically, even birth control pills.

Abnormal Bleeding

Your periods should typically follow a pattern of increasing and decreasing in flow or just decreasing from a heavy flow on Day 1. In either case, the patterns should be somewhat similar to one of the two mentioned on page 224. If they don't, or if you have what is referred to as postmenstrual, brown bleeding, defined as two or more days of brown or even black bleeding at the tail-end of your period, it is probably caused by an irregular shedding of the endometrium and small fragments of endometrial tissue. It is almost always thought to be a result of sub-optimal luteal function in the prior cycle. It is usually treated by focusing on supporting your luteal phase in much the same way that you would if you had premenstrual spotting, as discussed on page 295.

In addition, if you are trying to conceive and you experience several days of brown spotting either before your period or from Day 6 onward, it could be an indication of a problem with your luteal phase. In order for implantation to occur, the uterine lining must be sufficient for the egg to burrow into it before it is shed during menstruation. So one of these patterns of spotting around your period should probably be discussed with your physician.

As you now see, spotting can be absolutely normal. But it can also be an indication of a potential problem. If you note unexplainable bleeding on your chart, you should consider seeking medical care. Fortunately, most cases of abnormal bleeding are also accompanied by other symptoms.

Finally, you should be particularly alert to such signs as cramping or abdominal pain, abnormal vaginal discharge, fevers and chills, or any kind of pain during urination or intercourse. Such symptoms, when accompanied by abnormal bleeding, could be characteristic of a variety of conditions, from pelvic infections to various STDs. And even without other symptoms, erratic heavy bleeding could be due to fibroids, excess oestrogen, or other more serious conditions, all of which require medical attention.

❧ NORMAL NABOTHIAN CYSTS ON THE CERVIX VERSUS ABNORMAL CERVICAL POLYPS

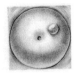

Normal Nabothian Cysts on the Cervix

These cysts are a fairly common female condition. They are little bumps that appear on the surface on the cervix and are caused by cervical cysts which may become temporarily blocked. Women who haven't been taught about these cysts may panic the first time they feel one, not realizing they are completely harmless. Women often feel them the first time while checking their cervix or inserting a diaphragm or cervical cap. They usually disappear on their own, but if they don't, you should probably have them checked by a clinician the first time you feel one to rule out anything else. Then simply draw them on your chart in the miscellaneous section and keep track of them. You can chart them as in the example on page 330.

Abnormal Cervical Polyps

Polyps are small, tubular or tear-shaped growths that protrude from the mucus membranes of the cervical canal. Unlike nabothian cysts, which are quite firm, these tend to be somewhat spongy. And even though they are considered abnormal, they're almost always benign. You may not even be aware you have one unless you experienced one of their symptoms—unusual bleeding. This is due to their vulnerable position in the vagina, making them susceptible to being tapped, especially during intercourse. They are typically not painful, but may cause excess cervical fluid due to irritation of the mucus glands. If you think you may have one, you should consult a physician.

✺ NORMAL CYCLE-RELATED PAIN VERSUS ABNORMAL PAIN

Normal Cycle-Related Pain

Unfortunately, female pain can be a little tricky. Certain pains during a woman's cycle can be absolutely normal. For example, midcycle pain, which is often referred to as *mittelschmerz,* is thought to be caused by a number of factors:

- the follicles swelling within the ovaries
- the egg passing through the ovarian wall
- a small amount of blood being released at ovulation, irritating the pelvic wall
- contraction of the fallopian tubes

This is all considered normal, and even a secondary fertility sign. When you feel *mittelschmerz,* you can be pretty certain that ovulation is about to take place or just occurred.

Another example of cyclical pain is headaches, which tend to occur in the postovulatory (luteal) phase. If a woman weren't charting, she might not realize that they are related to her cycle instead of being a potential problem. If she finds a pattern of headaches on her chart at only certain points in her cycle, she can be more confident that these headaches are probably hormonally based.

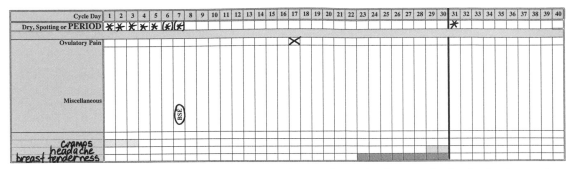

Chart 15.2. Various pains throughout the cycle. Colors can be used to keep track of cyclical pains or other symptoms. Note that you should fill in the specific symptoms you want to track in the far left column of the chart.

Abnormal Pain

On the other hand, if you notice pelvic pain that is intense or occurs at other times in the cycle, it could be an indication of any number of conditions, including endometriosis. This is where the uterine lining (the endometrium) begins to grow outside of the uterus, often attaching to other parts of the internal reproductive system. It can result in adhesions and scarring, and potentially impede fertility. One of the classic symptoms of endometriosis is pelvic pain before and during menstruation, as well as during intercourse (see page 203).

By accurately tracking your symptoms on your chart, you can help your doctor determine if you need further testing to diagnose the cause of the pain. For this reason, women should learn to recognize what is considered normal, cyclical pain, as opposed to that which is more intense or occurs at unexpected times of the cycle. This is obviously because the latter cases are more likely to indicate a potential health problem. A simple but graphic way to keep track of symptoms during your cycle is through the use of colors, as shown on page 7 of the color insert.

❧ NORMAL CYSTIC BREASTS VERSUS CANCEROUS BREAST LUMPS

Normal Cystic Breasts

Charting your cycle can help you differentiate between normal cyclic breast changes and abnormal breast lumps. The texture of breasts in women with fibrocystic breasts tends to be fairly lumpy, becoming more so in the postovulatory phase of their cycle. By knowing when they have begun that phase, they can determine if their lumps are normal and cyclical, and make the necessary lifestyle adjustments to try to lessen the discomfort of fibrocystic breasts. (Dr. John R. Lee, in his excellent book *What Your Doctor May Not Tell You About Premenopause,* recommends a variety of treatments, including the application of 15–20 mg. a day of progesterone cream during your luteal phase.) But if the lump(s) remain throughout the cycle, charting can be extremely beneficial in tracking whether further examination should be made by a health practitioner.

Charting is an excellent way to remind you to do a monthly breast self-exam on Day 7 of your cycle. (Note the BSE symbol in the Miscellaneous row at the bottom of the master chart.) The reason that you should perform the exam on that day is because it is the hormonally optimal time since your breasts are least susceptible to lumps or tenderness caused by progesterone. After completing your self-exam, circle the notation on the chart.

In addition, the American Cancer Society recommends that women who are not considered at high risk should start having annual mammograms starting at age 40. As with your breast self-exam, you should ideally have it done in your preovulatory phase.

Cancerous Breast Lumps

The prospect of breast cancer is extremely frightening to all women. However, you should know that most lumps are benign and that cancers of the reproductive system are curable if detected and treated early. You, yourself, can directly affect your chances of finding cancer early if you maintain a healthy lifestyle, get annual pelvic exams and Pap tests, do monthly breast self-exams, and make a point to promptly attend to suspicious symptoms.

Cycle Day	1	2	3	4	5	6	7	8	9	10	11	12	13	14	15	16	17	18	19	20	21	22	23	24	25	26	27	28	29	30	31	32	33	34	35	36	37	38	39	40
Miscellaneous																																								
Breast Self-Exam							BSE																																	

Chart 15.3. Charting breast self-exam.

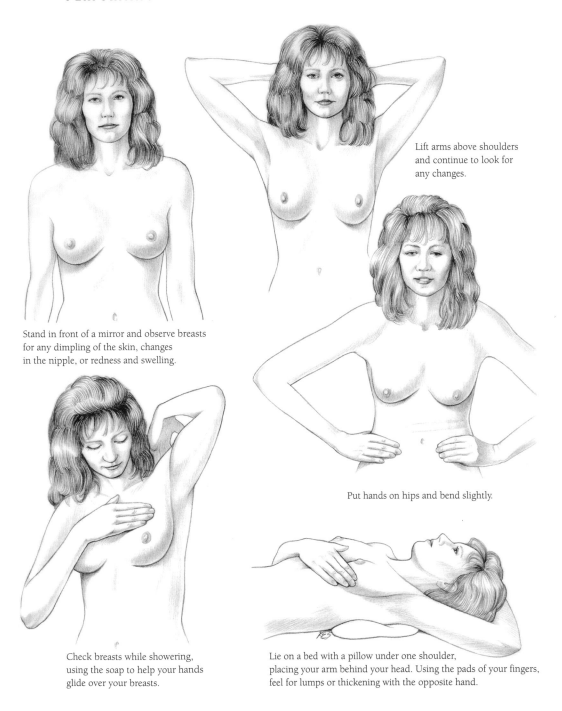

Lift arms above shoulders and continue to look for any changes.

Stand in front of a mirror and observe breasts for any dimpling of the skin, changes in the nipple, or redness and swelling.

Put hands on hips and bend slightly.

Check breasts while showering, using the soap to help your hands glide over your breasts.

Lie on a bed with a pillow under one shoulder, placing your arm behind your head. Using the pads of your fingers, feel for lumps or thickening with the opposite hand.

The following are warning signs to look for in your breasts. The important point is to notice whether they remain indefinitely, or disappear with the new cycle. Obviously, anything that persists should be examined by a clinician.

- breast lump or thickening (firm, nonmovable lumps are important to watch for, especially because they are usually painless.)
- lump in underarm or above collarbone
- swelling under the arm
- puckering or dimpling in one area of the breast
- persistent skin irritation, flaking, redness, or tenderness of breast
- sudden change in nipple position (such as nipple inversion)
- bloody nipple discharge

🔖 SCHEDULING THE BEST TIME FOR PHYSICAL EXAMS, CONTRACEPTIVE FITTINGS, VACCINATIONS, AND SURGERY

Another benefit of charting is that it can help you identify the most effective time in your cycle to have physical exams, contraceptive fittings, vaccinations, and surgery. The best time to schedule a Pap test is about midcycle, when the cervix is naturally dilated. In the case of fitting for diaphragms or cervical caps, having it done at the wrong time can mean the difference between complete contraceptive protection and an unplanned pregnancy! Since the cervix clearly changes around ovulation, it only makes sense to get fitted at the time when the method *is most likely to fail.* Remember that when a woman is fertile, her cervix becomes soft, high, and open. That is the best time to do it.

As mentioned earlier, you should do your breast self-exam on Day 7 of your cycle. For the same reason, you should schedule your routine mammogram around the same time, ideally about Day 7 or 8. This is because your breast tissue is less radiographically dense in the preovulatory phase. Regardless, if you're going to have two steel metal plates squish your breasts, it might as well be done when there is as little discomfort as possible!

A practical piece of advice would be to have a rubella vaccination performed just after your period. This would assure that you aren't pregnant at the time. This is critical for this particular vaccine, since the effects of the rubella virus on the fetus of pregnant women is potentially disastrous.

WOMAN HAVING BIMANUAL PELVIC EXAM AND PAP SMEAR

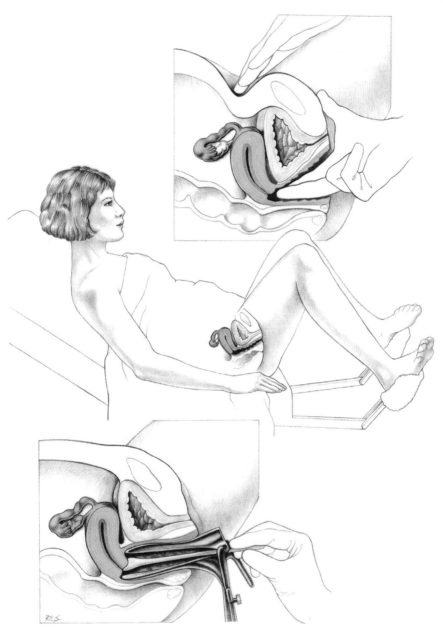

A pelvic exam typically includes a bimanual and a Pap test. The clinician inserts a finger into the vagina to be able to stabilize the uterus from the inside while gently pressing down on the abdomen to palpate the uterus and ovaries from the outside. The Pap test is done primarily to detect the presence of pre-cancerous cells of the cervix. You should ask your doctor about a new form of the test called the Thin Prep System, which is considered to be more accurate.

Of less significance but certainly interesting are the results of a couple of small studies that found that postoperative nausea and vomiting is increased in women undergoing laparoscopic tubal sterilization during the first 8 days of their cycle. Of course, this is not overwhelming evidence, but it is worth noting that surgeries may be affected by when they're performed.

Some recent studies have suggested that having breast cancer surgery after ovulation may increase your chances of living longer without a recurrence of the disease. One theory for the difference in outcome is that oestrogen in the first part of the cycle could stimulate the growth of cancer cells. You should be aware, however, that these findings do not yet reflect a general consensus.

Since further research may prove that timing surgeries to a particular phase of your cycle increases the odds of a positive outcome, you should ask your physician about it. If the surgery is not serious, it may not be so important. But if it involves something as profound as your survival, I would encourage you to do your homework, and research the latest studies with a discriminating eye.*

🙋 STAYING HEALTHY AND KEEPING INFORMED

The information in this chapter has been written to help you distinguish between what is normal and what may require medical attention. Ideally, you should also get an annual exam. The example on the opposite page can serve as a useful record of your overall health in much the same way your fertility charts track your cycles. A master copy of the form is included with the master fertility charts at the back of the book. Enlarge it about 125%, then copy it onto the back of the chart of the cycle in which you get an annual exam.

---

* The breast cancer studies found in the medical literature may have shown less than convincing results because all of them divided the survival rates of the women into groups based on what cycle day surgery was performed, and not whether they were truly in their pre- or postovulatory phase. Indeed, one particularly interesting study I read in *The Lancet* (June 18, 1994, p. 1545) subdivided 1,775 patients into two groups, with those having allegedly undergone surgery in the postovulatory luteal phase composing Days 15 to 36. Of course, any women who eventually had a cycle of 30 days or longer were almost certainly placed in the wrong group, since as you now know, such women most likely ovulated on Days 16 through 22, and not on Day 14, as was assumed.

None of the studies since the publication of this book's first edition have addressed this problem of the study design, which would require researchers to *truly* divide the women into pre- and postovulatory status. This is not surprising given the logistical hurdles involved in doing so. But if research along these lines could be done (working with women who do chart their temperatures), there is a greater chance of finding a definitive answer to this question.

Annual Physical Examination
Health Practitioner
Dr. Mary Compassionate

Cholesterol _190_ Ratio _3.1_ HDL _65_ LDL _120_   Day of cycle _16_ Date _29.11.01_

Blood (CBC) _OK_   Age at time of examination _30_

Urine test _OK_   Height _5'6"_ Weight _10st_

Cervical smear _OK_   Pulse _76_

Chlamydia test (optional) _not done_   Blood pressure _120 / 80_

Other Tests _—_   Shots/Boosters/Vaccines
Tetanus

	Status	Comments
Breast examination		Dr. Compassionate agreed that the soft lump that I found during my breast self-exam is probably nothing to worry about, but she scheduled a mammogram just to rule out anything.
Mammogram	OK!	The lump on my right upper breast was just a milk duct. Watch it to confirm that it disappears on its own.
Cervix	OK	She pulled out a great 4" clear stretchy thin string! Looked at my cervix in mirror — os was open!
Uterus	OK	
Ovaries		The doctor found a tiny ovarian cyst on the left side. Should subside on its own.
Heart	OK	
Lungs	OK	
mole on my back		She said it looks fine, but referred me to a dermatologist to have it checked.

Prescriptions _—_

Recommendations _Suggested I consume a lot of calcium-rich foods to build my bones and prevent osteoporosis later in life._

Referrals _Dr. Rea Sure_

CHAPTER 16

Appreciating Your Sexuality and Nurturing Your Relationship

"How is your sex life? How often do you have sex?" asked their respective therapists. Alvy Singer reflected. "Hardly ever, maybe three times a week," he whined. "Constantly . . . I'd say three times a week!" Annie Hall complained. He felt deprived. She felt exhausted.
—Scene from Woody Allen's *Annie Hall*, 1977

*D*oes that sound familiar? A woman's sexuality doesn't have to be the mystery so many people think it is. In reality, there are a number of reasons why women and men differ sexually.

Most women tend to view lovemaking as an emotional and intimate experience, not just a physical act. So women tend to get aroused if they feel trust and affection in the hours and even days leading up to intercourse. Men, on the other hand, tend to place more importance on the visual and other stimuli at the actual time of sexual interaction.

In addition, a woman's physical experience of sex is quite different from a man's simply because her clitoris is located outside of her vagina. This one fact can dramatically affect every aspect of her emotional and physical sexuality. Men need to realize this.

Finally, a woman's sexuality is often closely tied to her cycle. Many women themselves don't understand this. Is it any wonder, then, that men often find women somewhat confusing? But men who help their partners chart often maintain they finally understand female sexuality in a way that often eluded them before. They describe the newfound wisdom that they've acquired in understanding an aspect of women that is so frequently misunderstood. These next few pages will hopefully clarify the puzzle and make you appreciate the secret of your sexuality.

236

Why Orgasms During Intercourse May Be Hard for You to Attain

In the case of some women, orgasms take quite a bit of time. Before signing on with such a partner, make sure you are willing to lay aside, say, the month of June . . .

——BRUCE JAY FRIEDMAN

As you probably know, the most sensitive part of the man's body is near the tip of the penis. On the woman, it is the clitoris. The problem is that because the clitoris is situated outside the vagina, intercourse is often not as intense for women as it is for men. In fact, studies indicate that a large majority of women are unable to achieve orgasm through intercourse alone.* Internalizing this one physiological fact and really understanding how it can impact a woman's sexuality is critical for men to develop a truly loving, sexual relationship with their partner.

Because a lot of people don't fully understand basic human anatomy, misunderstandings result. For example, women often fake orgasms because they don't want to hurt their partner's feelings or they don't think it's worth the longer time and effort it would take to have one. This type of deception can poison an intimate relationship, which is unfortunate because it could so easily be resolved if both people understood the difference between male and female physiology. Needless to say, communication between the partners is the key to developing a fulfilling and warm sexual relationship.

It's a good thing we don't live in the 1870s. John Davenport would have us believe women shouldn't have orgasms at all. As he described it in *Curiositates Eroticae Physiolgiae* (1875), the result of orgasm in women was that:

> She burns and as it were, dries up the semen received by her from the male, and if by chance a child *is* conceived, it is ill-formed and does not remain nine months in the mother's womb.

Indeed. In any case, it's over a century later, and we certainly don't believe that female orgasms are harmful anymore. But the length of time it takes for a

---

* This is pretty amazing in light of the brainwashing bestowed upon a whole generation of women by Sigmund Freud. His theory of female sexuality was rooted in the delusional belief that women who weren't able to attain a "vaginal orgasm" through intercourse alone were immature and in need of psychotherapy.

woman to climax can be frustrating if people don't understand how normal it is for women to take longer than men. Even if communication between a couple is completely open and healthy, women usually require more stimulation to reach an orgasm.

Many men assume that as soon as the woman has become lubricated, she is ready to be penetrated. For most women, this is not true. Vaginal lubrication is one of the *first* signs of arousal. It only signals that she is gradually becoming more interested in further love play. Most women still need considerable time and *sensual* (rather than sexual) touching to become fully aroused. In fact, one of the most common complaints women make about men as lovers is that they rush through the motions and are too narrowly focused on the genitals, rather than the whole body. You've probably heard it before, but in this context it's worth repeating the adage: "Women make love in order to touch, men touch in order to make love."

What You Can Do to Increase Vaginal Feelings During Intercourse

For some women, being asked if she has had an orgasm during intercourse is a sign that her partner doesn't really understand what excites her. In his excellent book, *Sexual Solutions,* Michael Castleman asks men to develop a different sexual perspective:

> Imagine your own feelings if a woman climaxed courtesy of your oral-clitoral stimulation, then asked you: "Did you come?" Many men would resent the question: "How can you even ask if I've come? I've been stimulating you. You haven't touched me where it counts! Women feel the same way.

Still, many women can increase their chances of having an orgasm during intercourse by learning what positions best stimulate their clitoris. Many women who can climax this way say the optimal position is straddling on top of their partner, with one of them directly stimulating her clitoris. Most women agree that intercourse in the missionary position is simply not enough to lead to orgasm.*

---

* One of the most failproof ways for women to achieve an orgasm is through using a vibrator. Many couples include it as part of their lovemaking. If a woman has never had an orgasm, she may want to try using a vibrator by herself to learn what level of intensity works for her. The best type of vibrators are those that can easily stimulate the clitoris and *not* those that are shaped like a penis.

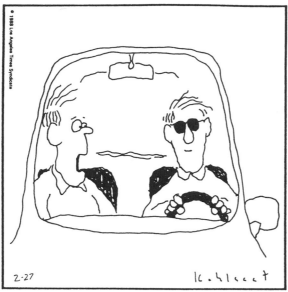

"It's a little disorienting when Louise tells me that I can always be replaced by a pulsating shower."

In addition, many people don't realize that the vagina is a muscle that can be strengthened just like any other. Both men and women find that sex can be more fulfilling when the woman has control over her vaginal muscle. The way to strengthen it is through Kegels or vaginal contractions. By simply tightening and releasing the vagina every day, you can increase sexual satisfaction for both of you. You can do any combination of Kegels that's comfortable. A key advantage of these exercises is that they can be done any time, anywhere, without others being aware of it. So, for example, you can do Kegels while talking to your grocer or giving a presentation at a corporate meeting. The point is to do them as often as necessary to maintain a healthy, strong vagina that promotes sexual gratification for you and your partner (see page 88).

Why You May Tend to Feel Sexier Midcycle

Juicy, luscious, delectable, succulent, and delicious . . . no, I'm not talking about a pineapple. I'm referring to fertile cervical fluid as described by the renowned childbirth educator Sheila Kitzinger. As you know, women often develop abundant amounts of slippery, wet cervical fluid as they approach ovulation. Since it feels wet and lubricative, women are conditioned to associate it with sexual excitement. Of course arousal fluid tends to dissipate in a few seconds when waved in the air. True fertile cervical fluid will remain on your finger.

Besides the similarity between fertile cervical fluid and sexual lubrication, something else is responsible for women often feeling more sexual midcycle. The high levels of oestrogen around ovulation act to heighten sexuality in many women. They may also notice that their vaginal lips feel fuller and tend to blossom open. Again, this is related to the increased hormones before ovulation. These physical changes can make women feel especially sexual at this time.

This increased sexuality can admittedly be somewhat untimely for women who use FAM for natural birth control. They often feel that their fertile phase is the time they especially want to have intercourse. But many FAM users view the fertile phase as a time to be especially creative with other forms of lovemaking, knowing that in a few days they can resume intercourse again (of course, barriers can also be used).

Why Intercourse Can Be Uncomfortable During Certain Phases of the Cycle

You may occasionally feel a deep pain during intercourse. Or perhaps you notice discomfort during certain sexual positions, especially if you straddle atop your partner. Remember that when your oestrogen levels are low and you're outside your fertile phase, particularly after ovulation, your cervix tends to be low in your vagina. During these times, it is possible that your partner's penis can actually tap your cervix during intercourse.

The reason you may feel the discomfort only when you straddle him is that the cervix tends to drop lower in that position. This makes sense when you consider that the best way to check the cervix is by squatting, since this is the position that pushes the cervix to its lowest point. This doesn't mean that you can't ever enjoy sex in that position, but you should be aware of the fact that when you're not fertile, your cervix may be too low to be comfortable.

How Birth Control Can Affect Your Sexuality

It should come as no surprise to you that birth control can be a source of tension between many couples. Because no method is perfect, there may be drawbacks that undermine a couple's intimacy by tending to place the burden on the woman. For example, if a woman feels resentful that she has to endure urinary tract infections from the diaphragm, or vaginal dryness from the Pill, she may not be as receptive to intercourse as the man would be.

But if her partner participates in her charting, she will probably be much more sexually responsive. In essence, through his actions he can show her how respectful he is of her body and comfort, and how much he wants to share in the responsibility of contraception. The fact is that birth control doesn't have to be a devisive issue in the bedroom.

Among my first clients was a charming couple, Erin and Nick. As we were reviewing her charts, I realized the writing was barely legible. It said something about her menstrual cramps that day, but I couldn't decipher it. When I asked her what it said, she held it up to her eyes, squinted, then turned to Nick and said, "Honey, what did you write here? I can't read it either." As it turned out, the entire chart was in his writing, down to the most intimate details of her menstrual cycle.

How Your Partner Can Participate in Your Charting— and Why He Should

> *Men fear women.*
> *Men fear women period.*
> *Men fear women's periods.*
> *Men fear women not getting their periods.* *

Men are often criticized for not taking a bigger role in birth control and even pregnancy achievement. But the truth is that many men are very caring and loving and would be happy to be more actively involved if only there was a way they could. As you've seen, with the Fertility Awareness Method, there is. The beauty of charting is that a man can be as involved as his partner—taking her temps, jotting down her fertility signs, determining when her fertile phase has begun and ended. And rather than perceiving it as work, most people agree that the minute or two a day is so enlightening that it can be fun rather than a chore. Men who help their partners chart find that they discover a lot about them in the process. Ultimately, FAM can draw couples together.

The reality is that aside from the condom, withdrawal, or a vasectomy, the Fertility Awareness Method is the contraceptive most conducive to male involvement. Remember that the FAM rules were designed for the combined fertility of the man and woman together. Men are fertile every single day, whereas women are only fertile a few days per cycle. The first part of the woman's fertile phase is a reflection of the man's fertility (that is, the potential for sperm to survive 5 days in fertile cervical fluid). The second part is a reflection of the woman's fertility (that is, the potential for an egg to survive one day, with an additional day added for a possible double ovulation).

---

* Adapted from *Beyond Putting the Toilet Seat Down* by Jack York and Brian Krueger.

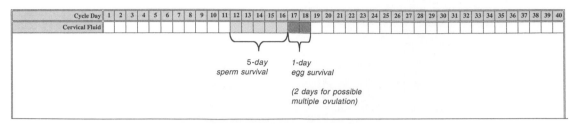

Chart 16.1. The woman's fertile phase is determined by egg *and* sperm viability.

More succinctly stated, then, a woman's fertile phase is a function of the respective fertility of both partners. Indeed, as Dr. Suzanne Poppema of Seattle so eloquently mentioned in an NPR interview, "I've taught our sons to know that they are responsible for each and every sperm that leaves their bodies until they know the sperm are either dead or have been used to help create a pregnancy."

Many men who learn about the menstrual cycle are struck with the idea that the length of their partner's fertility is primarily determined by their own continuous fertility, and thus feel equally responsible for contraception. By being so aware of their partner's cycle, they are more understanding and cooperative because they can no longer feign ignorance. It's worth remembering that many accidental pregnancies result from a lack of communication between the two partners. FAM is a wonderful way to involve both individuals equally in such an important aspect of a couple's life.

The Fertility Awareness Method encourages couples to communicate, simply because it is more effective if both partners understand it together. As you've seen, men often choose to do the actual charting. In order to record the woman's fertility signs, he may ask her about all facets of her cycle—from what kind of cervical fluid she had to whether she had breast tenderness or felt depressed during the day. In other words, the man can become intimately in tune with his partner's biology and emotions by simply recording her chart. The potential for furthering intimacy is obvious. "If you can talk about cervical fluid," one of my male clients once joked, "you can talk about anything!"

CHAPTER 17

Choosing the Sex of Your Baby

> For those of you who just skipped ahead to this chapter, it is critical
> that you fully understand the information discussed in Chapters 5, 6,
> and 11 before attempting to follow the guidelines presented here.

*T*rying to choose the sex of the baby you conceive may strike many
as unethical or just plain bizarre, but others find it exciting and
even fun. Over the years, several theories have been posited to
help people increase the chances of conceiving a boy or girl, yet they've contra-
dicted each other, leading many to discount the possibility altogether. Indeed,
such theories have been hypothesized since the Middle Ages, though one wonders how seriously they were taken at the time. The noted Italian physician Tro-
tula wrote in 1059:

> If they wish to have a male child let the man take the womb and vulva of a
> hare and have it dried and pulverized; blend it with wine and let him drink
> it. Let the woman do the same with the testicles of the hare and let her be
> with her husband at the end of her menstrual period and she will conceive
> a male.

Fortunately, the gender selection technique discussed in this chapter has
eliminated the hare.

Since the 1970s, Dr. Landrum Shettles, M.D., Ph.D., has developed a scientifically based, fairly simple way in which to increase your chances of having a
boy or girl. He has written an informative book called *How to Choose the Sex of
Your Baby* (Doubleday, 1997); also see www.sexselection.co.uk. This chapter
adapts many of the critical points in his book but emphasizes Fertility Awareness
principles to help improve your odds. You may wish to read Dr. Shettles's own
work for more thorough coverage of the topic.

While various studies have shown the Shettles method to be quite successful, I must emphasize here that its overall effectiveness is still widely disputed in the medical community. I do not profess to be an expert on this subject, but I discuss it in this book because once you know the fundamental principles of Fertility Awareness, this method of gender selection is relatively easy to apply. In addition, it seems that of all the natural theories proposed, Shettles's method is the best supported by scientific studies.

Of course, even the method's most ardent supporters do not suggest it is anywhere near foolproof. Dr. Shettles himself claims that it is about 80 to 90% effective for choosing boys, and 75 to 80% effective for choosing girls, when the method rules are followed correctly. The reason for the lower rates for girls is that it is more difficult to appropriately time intercourse when trying for a female.

The most fundamental principle on which the Shettles method is based is that sperm determine what sex a baby will be. The male sperm (Y chromosomes) are smaller, lighter, faster, and more fragile than the female sperm (X chromosomes).* The female sperm are generally bigger, heavier, slower, and heartier, and thus tend to live longer than the male sperm. All of this means that if you desire a boy, you should time intercourse as close to ovulation as possible so that the fast, light, male sperm reach their prize first. Likewise, if you prefer a girl, you should time intercourse as far from ovulation as you can while still allowing conception to occur.

The primary evidence on which Shettles bases his method is that male sperm generally beat female sperm when put through a racecourse of alkaline, fertile-quality cervical fluid in laboratory containers. Sperm retrieved from the woman's reproductive tract also confirm that male sperm are faster, but that female sperm are more resilient.

Evidence that Indirectly or Partially Supports the Shettles Method Can Be Divided by Gender Outcome

Male

- Artificial insemination (AI) results in a preponderance of male offspring, which makes sense, given that AI is always done as close to ovulation as possible. The closer to ovulation, the more likely the male sperm will race up to the egg before the slower, heavier female sperm.

---

* For simplicity's sake, for the remainder of this chapter, I will refer to sperm carrying the male Y chromosome as "male sperm," and sperm carrying the female X chromosome as "female sperm."

- Younger men and women tend to have more male conceptions than older individuals. It's hypothesized that the reason for this is that younger men generally have higher sperm counts and younger women tend to have more copious, alkaline-quality cervical fluid—both of which favor male conceptions.

Female

- More girls tend to be born to couples who use in vitro fertilization for achieving their desired pregnancies. Researchers speculate that more female sperm are capable of surviving the stresses imposed on them through the rigorous laboratory procedure.
- Men with low sperm counts tend to have more female sperm. (Shettles theorizes it may be because the same factors that would cause a low sperm count are likely to kill many of the more fragile male sperm, such as heat, certain drugs, and toxic substances.)
- Some studies show that undersea divers in Australia and high-performance military aircraft pilots elsewhere have predominantly fathered daughters. Researchers theorize the reason may be due to the fact that both are subject to unusual environmental stresses including shifting atmospheric pressures, varying oxygen tension, possible radiation, and excessive scrotal heat from tight-fitting wet suits and flight suits. It makes sense that the sperm that would survive such abuse are the hardier female sperm.
- Anesthesiologists tend to father more girls than boys. It's also known that they are exposed to many toxic substances in the course of their career, so it's understandable that the female sperm are the ones that are more likely to survive in greater numbers.
- A study of men with non-Hodgkin's lymphoma revealed that 154 out of 190 children born were girls, again revealing the resilient nature of female sperm.

Both

- Fraternal twins (from two different eggs) are usually the same sex, which would support the idea that timing of intercourse is of critical importance in determining the sex of the baby. Since fraternal twins are conceived within 24 hours of each other, the conditions within the mother's reproductive tract are presumably the same for each conception.

Although the debate continues, it is true that many carefully controlled studies from Japan to Nigeria seem to clearly show what Shettles has now proposed for over 20 years: *The critical variable in terms of gender selection is the timing of intercourse in relation to ovulation.*

FERTILITY AWARENESS AND GENDER SELECTION

Before seeing how Fertility Awareness specifically fits in with the Shettles method, you should chart at least three cycles before attempting gender selection in order to really know your own cycle well. If just starting to chart, it is best to either abstain or use condoms so as not to mask cervical fluid. This will help you to accurately identify its pattern while preventing a pregnancy that wasn't well-timed for the gender you want.

Timing Intercourse for a Boy

> You should have intercourse on your Peak Day, as well as the following day.

If you desire, you can initially have intercourse in the first part of the cycle, but only on dry days. Once you start to have any cervical fluid, you should abstain in order to minimize the risk of conceiving a girl. *Then, have intercourse on what you perceive will be your Peak Day as well as the day after.* (In order to determine your Peak Day, review page 91.)

Remember that, ideally, you are trying to time sex as close to ovulation as possible. Dr. Shettles says that you should try to time intercourse for the day of ovulation itself, but, in reality, it makes more sense to time for the Peak Day, which is often the day before. This is because by the time ovulation occurs, the cervical fluid will have frequently dried up already, thus dramatically reducing the possibility of conception for any gender. In any case, without the use of ultrasound, there is no practical way to truly know which precise day you are ovulating.

One of the reasons to chart a few cycles first is to *determine how many days of fertile cervical fluid you usually have.* Generally speaking, most women tend to have a fairly consistent number of eggwhite days each cycle. (Those who don't produce eggwhite will usually produce creamy, wet cervical fluid.) You can clearly see that the better you know your cervical fluid pattern, the more likely you will time sex accurately, and thus conceive the baby boy you both desire.

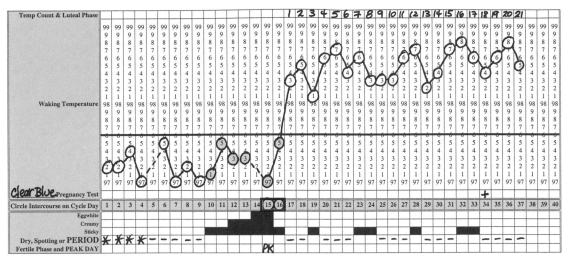

Chart 17.1. Timing intercourse for a boy. Note that when timing for a boy, the couple should try to have intercourse on the Peak Day, as well as the following day. Here, the Peak Day was on Day 15, and thus intercourse was timed accurately.

A Note on Basal Body Temperatures

For most women, temperature charting has little strategic value in gender selection. For predictive purposes, the only women to benefit from charting their temperatures in this situation are those few that show a dip before the thermal shift. In those women, the dip usually does coincide with the day of ovulation, and thus it could be useful in timing for a boy. For all other women, temperatures are still practical, but only for identifying when ovulation occurred in retrospect, and thus for seeing how accurately you timed intercourse for either gender.

Using Ovulation Predictor Kits for Choosing a Boy

I believe that cervical fluid is the most appropriate way to time intercourse for gender selection purposes. However, if you do decide to use ovulation predictor kits, Shettles recommends you choose one that will allow you to test your urine any time of day, not just the morning's first urine. This is because a woman is most likely to detect an LH surge that indicates impending ovulation when she tests between 11 A.M. and 3 P.M. You should test again after 5 P.M. The two tests should be spaced about ten hours apart, with noon and 10 P.M. considered ideal. Wait about twelve hours after you first detect the LH surge to have intercourse, since sex immediately after detection may increase the chance of conceiving a girl.

Finally, you should be aware that women with irregular or long cycles should not start testing until they notice their cervical fluid start to get wet. This will ensure that the kits are at least being used at the most appropriate time, as ovulation approaches.

Timing Intercourse for a Girl

> You should have intercourse several days before your Peak Day, but preferably not closer than 2 days before.

It may take a little more patience and perseverance to conceive a girl, because the timing is trickier. You'll want to have intercourse far enough away from ovulation to assure that mostly female sperm remain, but close enough to still allow a conception to occur. As with tying for a boy, the better you know your cervical fluid pattern, the more likely you'll be able to time sex correctly.

The key is to time intercourse from *4 to 2 days before your Peak Day*. (In order to determine when that is, review page 91.) What this means, practically speaking, is that you should first try four days before you anticipate the Peak Day. However, if that fourth day is no wetter than sticky, you should initially try the third day before. If that doesn't work, try a day closer the following cycle. But for the first few cycles, do not have sex any closer than 2 days before you expect your Peak Day.

If you have gone several cycles without conceiving, you may decide to try intercourse on what you estimate to be only one day before your Peak Day. The fact is that doing this greatly increases the odds of conceiving, but the risk of having a boy also goes up. I personally suspect that a girl is still more likely because it appears that ovulation most often takes place the day after the Peak Day, or a full 2 days after you would have had intercourse. However, it's also true that ovulation may occur on the Peak Day itself, in which case the Shettles method would predict a male conception. You now see why it's harder to time for a girl! *Remember, the point is to try to have intercourse as far from ovulation as you can and still have conception occur.* After the cutoff date, you should abstain from intercourse or use barriers until you are outside your fertile phase. If you continued to have sex right up through ovulation, you would dramatically increase the risk of conceiving a boy.*

---

* Obviously, if you have any problems with infertility, it is probably not worth following the guidelines for having a girl.

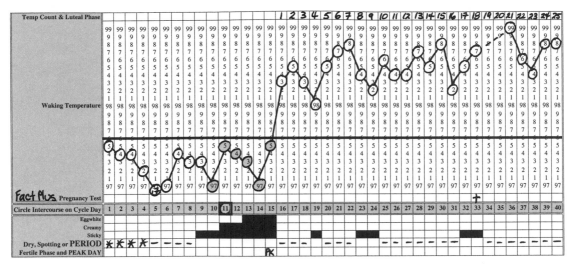

Chart 17.2. Timing intercourse for a girl. Note that when timing for a girl, this couple has sex on Day 11, which they estimate to be 4 days before their Peak Day. If they fail to conceive, they may try in later cycles just 2 or 3 days before the estimated Peak Day (the equivalent of Days 13 and 14 in the sample above).

Why Basal Body Temperatures and Ovulation Predictor Kits Are Essentially Useless for Choosing a Girl

Because gender timing for a girl involves having sex as far in advance of ovulation as possible while still allowing for conception, neither temperature charting nor ovulation kits are helpful. As you know, the temperature shift will generally only tell you that you've already ovulated, not that ovulation is approaching. Since you are trying to conceive several days before this shift will occur, the bottom line is that it has no strategic value.

Likewise, ovulation kits are almost as useless for timing intercourse to conceive a girl, since they only detect the LH surge, which itself only occurs a day or so before ovulation. If intercourse for a girl is truly well timed, it will have almost certainly occurred before either the temperature or kit could tell you where you are in your cycle.

ᨘ A BRIEF WORD ON SOME HIGH-TECH ALTERNATIVES

Although the Shettles method of gender selection is the one that most logically complements the principles you have learned from FAM, you might want to explore other techniques that have emerged in the past several years. Among the most promising are the Microsort and Ericsson methods of sperm selection. With both of these, the male and female sperm are separated by sophisticated devices before artificial conception takes place through any number of assisted reproductive technologies. Finally, a somewhat controversial option is Embryo Selection, a type of IVF in which only those embryos of the gender desired are implanted back in the woman's uterus.

ᨘ CONCLUDING REMARKS ON GENDER SELECTION

The guidelines presented in this chapter may greatly increase your odds of conceiving the gender of your choice. However, I should emphasize again that even Shettles's most ardent supporters do not claim that they are foolproof. Thus, if you are someone who would be greatly disappointed by the birth of your *second* choice, you should strongly reflect on the potential risk before trying to conceive. If you do choose to make the attempt, good luck!

GUIDELINES FOR MAXIMIZING THE ODDS OF SUCCESSFUL GENDER SELECTION (SHETTLES METHOD)

	Boy	**Girl**
Ideal Timing of Intercourse	Day of ovulation, or the day before.	4 to 2 days before ovulation.
Timing Sex with Cervical Fluid	Have sex on your Peak Day (the *last* day of eggwhite cervical fluid or lubricative vaginal sensation), as well as the following day.	Have sex several days *before* your Peak Day (the last day of egg-white cervical fluid or lubricative vaginal sensation), but not closer than 2 days before. Note that 1 day before increases the odds of conception, but also the odds of of conceiving a boy.
Timing Sex with Ovulation Predictor Kits	Test 2 times a day. Have sex 12 to 24 hours *after* LH surge.	Not useful for girl gender selection.
When to Stop Having Intercourse Before the Target Day	Can have intercourse every preovulatory *dry* day, but then abstain until the target day.	Can have intercourse every day right up to the last target day.

CHAPTER 18

Premenstrual Syndrome: It's Not All in My Head?

*A*h, yes. Premenstrual syndrome. The common condition whose cause eludes researchers and doctors alike. At times, it seems as if there are as many theories about PMS as there are symptoms. "It's a progesterone deficiency." "No, it's due to a vitamin deficiency." "Actually, it's related to prostaglandins." "Wrong. It's obviously due to a neuroendocrine imbalance."

The only thing that researchers and clinicians can agree on is the validity of the condition itself, and the fact that it can be debilitating for many women. So what is PMS? Basically, it is a recurring condition that can cause a variety of unpleasant physical and emotional symptoms in the luteal (postovulatory) phase of the woman's cycle. Although most women tend to experience it in the week or so leading up to menstruation, it can happen anytime from ovulation on. It primarily affects women over 25 and tends to worsen with age. The timing of the symptoms is often consistent within each woman, and thus charting may give you the opportunity to deal with it constructively.

✺ THOSE DELIGHTFUL SYMPTOMS

It's been estimated that as many as nine out of ten women experience at least some form of PMS during their reproductive years. Since it is unclear what causes it, there are different theories as to how best to treat it. There are numerous excellent books on the subject. If you are adversely affected by PMS, I would encourage you to explore your options, since there are practical ways in which you can alleviate many of your symptoms.

Even the way symptoms are categorized varies among clinicians. Still many classify them into some variation of what Dr. Elizabeth Vliet refers to as "the seven PMS clusters," which are shown in the box below.

TYPES OF PMS SYMPTOMS*

Affective	Depression, irritability, anxiety, anger, tearfulness, panicky feelings
Behavioral	Impulsive actions, compulsions, agitation, lethargy, decreased motivation
Autonomic	Palpitations, nausea, constipation, dizziness, sweating, tremors, blurred vision, hot flashes
Fluid/Electrolyte	Bloating, water-weight gain, breast fullness, hand and foot swelling
Dermatological	Acne, oily hair, hives and rashes, herpes, and allergy outbreaks
Cognitive (Brain)	Decreased concentration, memory changes, word-retrieval problems, fuzzy thinking, foggy-brain feelings
Pain	Migraines, tension headaches, back pain, muscle and joint aches, breast pain, and neck stiffness

---

* This chart is adapted from Dr. Vliet's comprehensive book, *Screaming to Be Heard: Hormone Connections Women Suspect and Doctors Still Ignore* (2001).

৯ DIAGNOSING AND CHARTING PMS

The most important point in diagnosing PMS is that you determine whether the symptoms are *cyclical* in nature. If you experience them occasionally throughout your cycle, they would not be considered PMS. Of course, what makes it cyclical is the hormonal changes that occur in an ovulatory cycle. This means that technically women who don't ovulate shouldn't experience classic PMS. That would include preadolescent girls as well as those who are pregnant or post-menopausal. One would also expect women on the Pill to not experience PMS symptoms since they don't ovulate either, but for inexplicable reasons, they often have heightened symptoms.

When trying to determine if you even have PMS, the first step is to chart your symptoms along with your fertility signs. By recording both, you can verify their cyclical nature and what factors may trigger them. Most women with PMS tend to notice the same symptoms from cycle to cycle. The best way to monitor the various symptoms is to write them to the left of the narrow columns at the bottom of your master chart, as in the example of Chart 18.1 below. Most women find that color-coding is an excellent way to immediately visualize when they occur in the cycle. Use colors that you associate with various conditions. For example:

Irritable	Fluorescent green (or some other irritating color)
Headache	Red
Depressed	Blue
Chocolate cravings	Brown

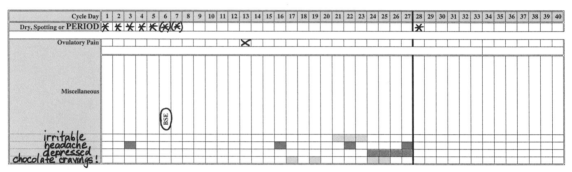

Chart 18.1. Charting PMS signs. Dana records various PMS signs using different colors near the bottom of the chart. This allows her to quickly determine whether her symptoms are cyclical or indicative of a problem requiring medical attention.

✍ TREATING PMS

Once you have determined the cyclical nature of your PMS symptoms, you can then decide on the appropriate steps to take. Many women find that just being able to anticipate when they will occur can help alleviate them. When you realize that your depression, irritability, or headache is only a sign that your period is a few days away, you should have less cause for concern. Often the symptoms themselves create needless anxiety as women wonder if they are "going crazy" or suffering from a serious illness. The knowledge and control that comes with charting can be the first step in managing PMS.

There are many self-help therapies that seem to work well for women, but if you suffer severe symptoms, I would encourage you to get medically evaluated before attempting to treat yourself through change in diet, vitamins, or minerals.

Severe PMS (such as depression or panic attacks) can be an indication that you have underlying problems that may require hormone therapy.

Treatments range from alternative health care to traditional medical therapy, with self-help approaches somewhere in the middle. Your goal should be to discover the best solution for your particular situation. I have listed self-help treatments first, since they tend to be the easiest and most accessible for most women.

Self-Help Approaches

Self-help therapy is geared toward preventing PMS altogether, rather than just treating the symptoms. Of course, you may not always be able to do so, in which case you may want to take one of the nonprescription drugs discussed on the next page. If you are charting your cycle, be on the lookout for when your temperature rises, so that you can be especially attentive to the following suggestions.

Dietary Considerations

The fact is there is probably no better way to control PMS symptoms than proper diet. The nutritional guidelines that almost all experts recommend emphasize a well-balanced diet of whole grains, fruits, and vegetables, including legumes. And as expected, PMS symptoms can be greatly alleviated by dramatically cutting back on everything that you no doubt love, including all foods that are high in sugar, salt, and fat. Drugs such as alcohol, nicotine, and caffeine—and, yes, even chocolate—should be avoided. You should increase your intake of complex carbohydrates while decreasing your intake of protein, as well as eat more frequent, smaller-portioned meals. Finally, you should know that many nutritionists believe that a variety of vitamins, minerals, and herbs can go a long way in alleviating various PMS symptoms.

Exercise and Yoga

You just can't seem to get away from advice to exercise, can you? Whether your concern is weight loss, lowering cholesterol levels, maintaining cardiovascular fitness, or PMS, the bottom line is that exercise is an excellent therapy for numerous ailments. One reason is that it activates the production of endorphins, a naturally occurring stimulant in your body. This explains why people usually feel so good after exercising. The trick to using exercise to benefit you the most is to maintain a regular exercise program of at least three to five times a week, about 30 minutes each session.

In addition to vigorous exercise, yoga is an excellent source of relief for many PMS sufferers. Traditionally, the goal of yoga has been to promote balance and harmony. Adherents of yoga will tell you there's nothing better for promoting health on all levels—physical, mental, emotional, and spiritual.

Rest

Of course, once you've exercised, you have to rest sufficiently to maintain optimal health. The common wisdom is that people should get at least 7 to 8 hours of sleep per night. Some need more. Ultimately, your body will tell you what feels best. Some women find that something as simple as going to bed earlier helps lessen PMS symptoms.

Stress Reduction

Who today doesn't experience stress at least occasionally? Of course, some stress is inevitable. Still, do whatever you can to eliminate at least some of it from your life, whether it be through massage, yoga, meditation, dancing, or going to a movie. Whatever you do, at least be aware that stress in the postovulatory phase is going to exaggerate your PMS symptoms.

Coping with Emotions

For many women, one of the most distressing aspects of PMS is the sense of feeling emotionally out of control every cycle. It's as if their emotions are exaggerated ten-fold. It can be especially distressing to women who are used to thinking of themselves as caring and warm people. They often feel as if their anger, anxiety, or depression are out of character for them. But remember, women in our society are socialized to always be nice, always be the caretaker, always be giving, and never show dissatisfaction. Perhaps a better way to perceive your premenstrual emotions is to recognize that it is a time when you finally allow yourself to express the frustrations society expects you to suppress.

Of course, if you feel that the intensity of your emotions during this time is incapacitating or harmful to your relationships, you may benefit from the help of a therapist in addition to a clinician. Because therapists are more objective, they can often help clarify your seemingly complex emotional state, even if the problem is hormonally based. Remember, PMS doesn't cause emotions, but it will exaggerate what is already there.

Nonprescription Drugs

There are currently a variety of over-the-counter drugs that are designed to deal with specific PMS symptoms. These drugs, which include various analgesics, antihistamines and diuretics, have proven effective against such symptoms as uterine cramps, headaches, and breast tenderness. Again, I suggest that you read the relevant sections of a more comprehensive PMS book or, at a minimum, talk to an informed pharmacist. Finally, it should be clear that while drugs such as Tylenol and Advil will certainly relieve many discomforts, a concerted regimen of healthy diet and vigorous exercise would do more by minimizing such symptoms in the first place.

Alternative Health Care

Homeopathic and naturopathic treatments seem to be helpful for some women, but you need to consult a qualified practitioner who is trained to diagnose you as a whole, and not just examine your symptoms. Some find relief through either acupuncture or acupressure, both of which perceive PMS as the result of imbalance or blockage of vital energy, or *chi*. Osteopathy, reflexology, and aromatherapy may be helpful as well. Of course, in all these cases, you need to consult a professional to determine if these might work for you. Many of the more specialized PMS books discuss the theory and practice of alternative treatments in more detail.

Using Drugs and Alternative Therapies Together

You may prefer to try to eliminate PMS through the natural alternatives just discussed. However, your symptoms may be so severe that you might want the quick relief drugs can provide. The good news is that natural and medical therapies aren't mutually exclusive. You can use medication for severe symptoms while simultaneously changing your lifestyle to try to prevent PMS symptoms in the future. Eventually, then, you could go off drugs altogether and rely strictly on natural means to control your symptoms.

Traditional Medical Treatments

There are a number of standard medical therapies that you may want to try. But before consulting with your physician, it will help to have charted your symptoms for several cycles so that they can efficiently arrive at the most accurate diagnosis.

Diuretics

Many doctors prescribe diuretics for women whose PMS causes weight gain, bloating, and breast tenderness due to fluid retention; however, some clinicians believe the first treatment should be to balance hormones and improve diet, allowing the symptoms to diminish on their own.

Hormone Therapy

Unfortunately, because there are conflicting theories regarding the primary cause of PMS, the proposed hormonal treatments also vary. Those who think that it is due to low oestrogen levels in the luteal phase believe than an oral contraceptive with the least amount of progestins may provide substantial relief for those with *severe* PMS. But those who think it is due to a progesterone deficiency believe that natural progesterone creams rather than artificial progestins utilized during the latter two weeks of the cycle can be very effective in diminishing symptoms.

If you prefer to use the more natural approach, you should try to consult with a doctor who is familiar with the use of the newest progesterone creams. Although there may be some risk to certain women, they are generally easy to use and have few side effects. And because they are derived from wild yams and soybeans, they are considered a natural substance. Progesterone therapy has now gained wide acceptance as a treatment with potentially great benefits for many women.*

Tranquilizers, Antidepressants, and Mood Stabilizers

If you suffer serious postovulatory anxiety, mood swings, or depression, your doctor may prescribe any number of tranquilizers or antidepressants. Some work by elevating levels of neurotransmitters like serotonin and norepinephrine—chemicals in the brain that regulate personality, mood, sleep, and appetite.

Antiprostaglandin Medication

Probably the most painful symptom of both PMS and menstruation is uterine cramps. We now know that they are caused by imbalances in prostaglandins—chemicals produced in the uterine lining that increase prior to menstruation. Luckily, there are effective drugs such as Motrin that eliminate the cramping.

PMS, Conventional Medicine, and Long-Term Solutions

You should keep in mind that there are always potential side effects whenever you take any drugs. Remember that while medications can be extremely useful in eliminating PMS symptoms, they will only be effective as long as you are taking them. Since PMS is known to get worse with age (lucky us!), that could mean years on drugs or hormone therapy for women who are severely affected. While the dietary suggestions and other natural alternatives can involve considerable sacrifice, you should at least know that you have a number of choices that offer relief.

---

* For a thorough discussion of the use of progesterone creams, see Dr. John R. Lee's *What Your Doctor May* Not *Tell You About Premenopause: Balance Your Hormones and Your Life from Thirty to Fifty* (1999).

☙ KEEPING SANE ALL CYCLE LONG

The reality of womanhood is that PMS is an unfortunate fact of life for most, and even a fairly debilitating experience for some. Like menstruation, it is hardly an experience that most women would choose to have. But treatments do exist, and you do have some influence in restricting its severity, if not achieving its complete prevention. Perhaps as important, you may have the ability through charting to pinpoint your own PMS pattern, allowing you to take preventative action in the days immediately prior to its usual arrival.

No small advantage of such warning may also be to educate your partner, who could be sensitized to the cyclical basis for your physical and emotional changes. By being attuned to your cycle, your partner can understand why, for example, you may be feeling depressed or premenstrually unresponsive, sexually or otherwise. Such knowledge on their part won't make PMS go away, but with both of you sensitive to your cycle, it can help minimize its impact.

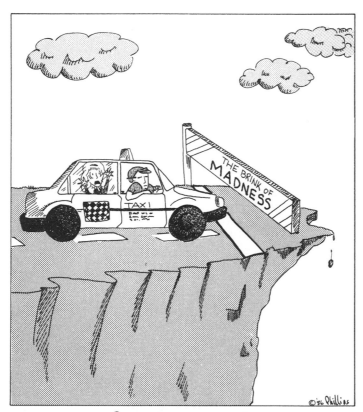

Peggy is driven to
the brink of
Madness

Demystifying Menopause

Perhaps with education and proper perspective, we can look forward to the day when people will stop viewing menopause as a crisis, or even as "the change," and see it more appropriately as "yet another change." For living is constant change. That is its essence and its promise.

—DR. KATHRYN MCGOLDRICK, former editor in chief of the
Journal of the American Medical Women's Association

Menopause. The word itself evokes countless emotions in women—everything from dread and fear to excited anticipation and relief. But it wasn't until fairly recently that the word was even uttered aloud. For some reason, it was a stage in a woman's life that was simply not discussed in polite company. Perhaps a lot of the stigma formerly associated with menopause related to a woman's primary role being defined as a mother, since it is true that menopause signals the end of the biological potential to reproduce.

Luckily, things have changed considerably. Women's roles have expanded dramatically, and society no longer defines a woman simply by her capacity to give birth. Today, many women are making the decision not to have children altogether, yet they still feel very feminine and fulfilled.

Needless to say, the topic of menopause is so huge that I couldn't do it justice in just one chapter. I would encourage you to read about it more thoroughly in any number of excellent books available today, many of which are listed in Appendix N. The simple fact that this topic and more specifically, the associated issue of hormone replacement therapy represent a continually evolving body of knowledge that will demand of you serious research if you are to make the most informed and best decisions for your own health.

℘ WHAT EXACTLY IS MENOPAUSE?

"I thought it was when women stopped having periods."
"Isn't it when women run out of eggs?"
"I think it's when women reach about fifty."
"It's when a woman can finally enjoy sex without having to worry about getting pregnant."

Actually, all of the above have kernels of truth, but I should clarify a few terms. "Menopause," in the strict biological sense, refers only to the final menstrual period. The "premenopause," or "climacteric," is the 10 to 15 years preceding the final period, during which the ovaries gradually stop maturing eggs and releasing large amounts of hormones. (Actually, there is disagreement as to whether post-menopausal women still have a few ova left that simply no longer respond to hormonal stimuli or in fact have completely run out of them.) "Perimenopause" usually refers to the few years on either side of your last period. Finally, the "change of life" is the somewhat euphemistic term used to include the emotional, intellectual, and obvious physical changes that a woman experiences during this transitional time.

In the end, menopause is a uniquely individual experience. Some women glide right through it, barely noticing any changes at all. Others have a harder time, often choosing medical help to cope with the challenges it presents. The only definitive statement that can be made is that menopause is when menstruation stops, which for the average woman is about age 51.

℘ CLASSIC SIGNS OF IMPENDING MENOPAUSE

The most obvious way to tell if you are nearing menopause is by noticing the three classic signs that most women experience to varying degrees:

- menstrual cycle irregularities
- hot flashes
- vaginal dryness

Medical professionals refer to the above as symptoms, but it makes more sense to refer to them as signs. After all, "symptoms" imply disease, and certainly menopause is nothing more than a natural passage of life. Many women have questioned the medicalization of menopause, just as they have insisted on natural approaches to birth control, pregnancy achievement, and childbirth. They want to perceive it as a healthful part of their lives—perhaps different, but with distinct advantages.

Gail Sheehy, author of the groundbreaking book *The Silent Passage: Menopause,* describes what it was like to educate people about this universal transition:

> *As I traveled around the United States giving lectures and appearing on TV and radio talk shows, the conversation about menopause had to be started up from scratch in each city. . . . Reactions from male talk show hosts were sometimes comical.*
>
> *"Menopause," gulped a Cleveland man on the midday news. "Is that like— impotence?"*
>
> *"Um, no," I murmured lamely. ". . . Baldness. Is that like Alzheimer's?"*

Menstrual Cycle Irregularities

One of the first signs of impending menopause is a change in your menstrual cycle. About 80% of women experience some kind of cyclic change, often as early as seven years before. Typically, women first find that their periods become heavier and more frequent as their cycles shorten. But eventually, their periods start to become lighter and less frequent as their cycles become longer, and ovulation becomes more sporadic. These latter changes are due to ever-decreasing levels of oestrogen.

If you do find that your periods are getting unusually heavy, there are some practical tips that you may want to reconsider. Try to avoid excessively hot showers and baths whenever you're bleeding. In addition, you should avoid alcohol and aspirin throughout the cycle, both of which inhibit blood clotting. But the best thing you can do is to maintain a lifestyle of steady and vigorous exercise, which will help adjust the hormonal imbalances that are causing the heavy bleeding in the first place.

Of course, irregular or heavy bleeding could be symptomatic of various medical conditions, including pelvic infections or even a uterine fibroid, which is a fairly common occurrence as women get older. Therefore, it's especially useful during this time to continue charting and report any conspicuous abnormality to your clinician.

A Word About Menopause and Ovulation Predictor Kits

A tempting way to detect if you are still ovulating is through one of the many ovulation predictor kits widely available. But you should be aware that these kits can be especially unreliable if you are indeed nearing menopause. The reason for this is that premenopausal women tend to have exceedingly high levels of LH that don't necessarily trigger ovulation.

In addition, using the kits to detect menopause is impractical since a woman may ovulate so sporadically during this time that it would be nearly impossible to pinpoint when to even use them. Because they only come in 5- or 9-day supplies and cost from £12 to £30 a kit, you would be spending a pretty penny to verify whether you're still ovulating. Charting is cheaper, easier, and simply more accurate.

Confusing Irregular Cycles with a Pregnancy

Keep in mind that unless you chart your cycles, menopause may make you think you are pregnant when you are not. The reason for this is that you may seem to skip periods (which, as you should know by now, are just very long cycles). In fact, "missed periods" may be normal during this transition, though it could also be a sign of pregnancy. If you are charting, there are two ways to tell the difference between the two:

- You are probably pregnant if you have more than 18 consecutive days of high temperatures, especially if you also experience tender breasts and nausea. (However, you'll need to confirm it with your doctor. Home pregnancy tests are unreliable during menopause due to fluctuating pituitary hormones.)
- You are probably *not* pregnant if your temperature pattern shows consistently low temperatures, or a delayed ovulation that indicates that you are merely having a long cycle. These extended cycles become increasingly likely if you are experiencing hot flashes and vaginal dryness.

Hot Flashes

You may be one of the lucky minority who manage to coast through menopause with no discomfort whatsoever. Unfortunately though, up to 85% of women experience hot flashes at one time or another during their menopausal years. They can start while your cycles are still regular and often continue through to about two years after your last menstrual period. In some women, they may persist several years longer. The unpleasant episodes may last anywhere from a few seconds to a few minutes. They may occur once a week or even once an hour! (Oh joy.)

You may experience hot flashes as nothing more than the feeling you get when you've just stuck your foot in your mouth at a dinner party—that familiar passing warmth on your face or upper body. But you may also experience them as a drenching sweat accompanied by chills. In rare cases of extreme intensity, they may even occur with heart palpitations and feelings of suffocation. Many women describe feeling an "aura" just before—a distinct sense that they are about to have a hot flash. Some even feel anxious, tense, dizzy, nauseous, or a tingling in the fingers a few seconds in advance.

Researchers believe hot flashes are caused by changes in the hypothalamus, the master gland in the brain that controls, among other things, the body temperature and cyclical fertility hormones. These changes are a result of declining levels of oestrogen, which essentially trigger the body to turn on a misguided hormonal cooler. In essence, then, hot flashes reflect an inappropriate lowering of the body's natural thermostat.

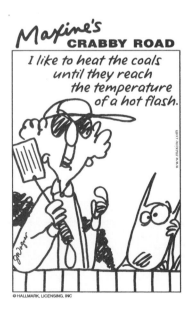

There are several practical things you can do that will make life easier while going through what may be a several-year transition. You should try to wear clothes made of cotton and other fibers that allow you to breathe, because the key is to literally stay cool. It's best to avoid hot weather, or at least have continual access to cold water.

As with everything else, get plenty of vigorous exercise and maintain a well-balanced diet, including lots of fresh fruits and vegetables. Many women find relief from including soy-based products in their diet. Soy is a naturally occurring plant compound that mimics oestrogen. You should, however, be wary of some of the hype surrounding it. It should only be consumed a few times a week because it can also block the absorption of needed nutrients. The ideal forms reduce that drawback and include tofu, tempeh, and miso. Of course, if you are like my colleague, you too may exclaim, "Tofu? Yuck! I'd rather have hot flashes!"

The most commonly prescribed medical treatment for hot flashes is hormone replacement therapy (HRT). By replacing the oestrogen that has plummeted to such a low level, HRT is nearly 100% effective in eliminating them. However, HRT is not without its side effects and potentially serious problems, as discussed on page 268.

Finally, many women who chart may find a pattern to their hot flashes. Recording them can help you feel more in control, by allowing you to be psychologically prepared for when they return.

Vaginal Dryness

One of the most commonly experienced and least discussed effects of menopause is the drying of vaginal tissue, again due to progressively dropping oestrogen levels. Women are typically too embarrassed to talk about it, feeling that it must be their unique problem. But in fact most women find that their vaginas take longer to become sexually lubricated as menopause approaches. Some may even feel irritated by the type of stimulation that they previously found pleasurable.

While menopause can definitely lead to vaginal dryness, there are practical things you can try to keep your vagina lubricated, including taking more time for foreplay and using water-based lubricants such as K-Y jelly. If you still find that you have vaginal dryness that makes intercourse uncomfortable or even painful, you may want to try oestrogen therapy in cream form. This should relieve dryness or soreness in the vagina, usually within a week or two. Creams are often recommended over pills because they don't pose as many side effects or health risks as oral medications do. However, be aware that many clinicians believe that any time you use oestrogen, you should balance it with progesterone.

♋ MENOPAUSE AND SEXUALITY

Menopause has a paradoxical effect on female sexuality. But just to set the record straight: It does not signal the end of a woman's sex life! While it's true that it tends to cause vaginal dryness, it finally frees women of the fear of pregnancy. The liberating feeling that results can be more than enough to compensate for the extra effort that it may take to become sexually lubricated. In fact, many women find their sex lives improve when they no longer have to worry about pregnancy or menstruation.

♋ HORMONE REPLACEMENT THERAPY

> *These days, it isn't raging hormonal imbalance that drives a post-menopausal women berserk. It's raging medical debate. Some 30 to 40 million American women want a definitive answer on oestrogen, and instead, they're getting the daily odds.*
>
> —ELLEN GOODMAN

Probably no other phrase in medical terminology evokes more confusion and contradictory reactions than hormone replacement therapy. Should menopausal women take artificial hormones or not? The debate is often extremely heated, and ultimately inconclusive. The bottom line is that there is no ideal answer. Each woman's situation is unique, and will have to be thoughtfully discussed with her own physician.

Part of the controversy over HRT stems from the fact that when it was first prescribed in the 1930s, not much was known about the potential long-term effects of the therapy. It wasn't until years later when it was discovered that the type of oestrogen therapy then being practiced would increase a woman's risk of uterine and breast cancer. In 1975, articles in the *New England Journal of Medicine* showed that women who took oestrogen were several times more likely to develop cancer of the endometrial lining than those who did not.

Pharmaceutical companies and many doctors stress that things are dramatically different today. They cite several reasons for prescribing the new models of HRT, including the fact that the modern therapies contain a lower dosage of oestrogen and are combined with progestins (a form of progesterone) to balance the negative effects of oestrogen. Nevertheless, the most recent and conclusive studies suggest that there still may be a slightly increased risk of breast cancer, strokes, and heart attacks.

Today, one of the most commonly prescribed oestrogens is Premarin. It's what is referred to as a conjugated oestrogen, and is considered the most natural oestrogen available. And where is it extracted from? The urine of pregnant horses, of course!*

Deciding What's Right for You

While most women let the severity of their menopausal signs play the dominant role in deciding whether to take HRT, you should also be sensitive to more subtle factors that could tip the scales in your own particular case. Indeed, the development of bone loss, glucose intolerance, or even higher cholesterol should be discussed with an informed physician, as should other factors such as your family medical history. Regardless, if you do ultimately choose to take HRT, you should remember that every woman's body and medical situation is different, and that the amount and type of hormones you take should be a function of your own specific health needs.

What Hormone Replacement Therapy Cannot Treat

It's often tempting for menopausal women to look to HRT as the magic pill that's going to resolve all sorts of problems. The fact is that there are a number of things that HRT will specifically *not* prevent, including depression, wrinkled skin, and weight gain (unfortunately, your metabolism slows down as you age). But it is true that HRT may make you feel better by treating the symptoms that cause your anxiety.

What Hormone Replacement Therapy Can Treat

There is no question that HRT can relieve hot flashes and vaginal dryness. It also helps maintain the acidity of the vagina, making it more resistant to infections. And far more significantly, most researchers agree that HRT can help prevent osteoporosis.

---

* In fact, that's how Premarin got its name:

| Pre | mar | in |
| (pregnant) | (mare's) | (urine) |

Regardless, the use of the words "natural" and "synthetic" can be counterintuitive. "Natural" substances like Premarin are hardly naturally occurring in the *human* body, whereas some "synthetic" hormones created in a laboratory, such as 17-beta estradiol, are bioidentical to what is found in people.

It should be made clear that HRT will only help these specific problems while you are taking the hormones. Once you discontinue, the problems will often return. This is particularly true with hot flashes. You should also remember that hormones will not restore bone density to their premenopausal level. It will simply prevent bone loss for as long as you remain on the therapy.

Risks of Hormone Replacement Therapy

If HRT is so beneficial, why don't all menopausal women take it? There are several reasons, including some serious medical concerns. The most recent and significant studies suggest that despite the addition of progestins to counter the adverse effects of oestrogen, HRT may lead to a slightly increased risk of both breast and uterine cancers, as well as strokes and heart attacks. This increased danger may be even greater for those who already have a higher risk of breast or uterine cancer, including women who have a family history of those conditions, are diabetic, or are substantially overweight.

Side Effects

In addition to the increased medical risks, there can be annoying side effects. Among the more common are nausea (if taking high-dose oestrogen), fluid retention, and fibroid enlargement. And of course you will continue to have cyclical vaginal bleeding, though it is usually shorter and lighter than typical menstruation.

HRT: Balancing the Data

The reality of HRT is that potentially serious problems need to be weighed against some very real and substantial benefits, with each individual woman judging how the pros and cons balance out when applied to her own personal situation. If you are considering HRT, you will definitely need to consult with a clinician experienced in Hormone Replacement Therapy. This is clearly an important and complicated subject, and one in which I urge you to keep current. There are many factors to consider, but ultimately you can make an intelligent decision, as long as you are informed.

℘ FERTILITY AWARENESS FOR BIRTH CONTROL DURING THE PREMENOPAUSAL YEARS

Some medical practitioners warn against using natural birth control when you begin to have menopausal signs because of the irregularity of cycles during this time, but this advice shows a misunderstanding of how the Fertility Awareness Method works. Yes, it is true that cycles tend to become more sporadic for women in their 40s. But the key to FAM is that each individual *day* is observed for possibly fertile conditions, and thus the cyclic consistency is almost irrelevant.

What *is* relevant is that many premenopausal women may have fertile cervical fluid patterns for increasingly longer periods of time (such as preovulatory sticky day after day). This is both the potential frustration and irony of FAM in the years approaching menopause, for while the method's conservatism may tell a woman she is fertile more days then ever, the fact is that as she ages, her potential fertility is diminishing rapidly.

The truth is that using FAM during the menopausal years can be confusing, but depending on your own particular cycles, it may also be easier than ever before. Indeed, you may go for months at a time with nothing but dry, infertile days. Regardless, using FAM will provide you with an amazing window into the workings of your body as it travels through "yet another change."

How to Determine Whether You Are Near Menopause

Using FAM during menopause may involve some modifications, but before using the special guidelines, you obviously need to determine how close to menopause you actually are. As discussed previously, you will generally have distinct symptoms to alert you, in addition to the fact that you will most likely be in your 40s as the transitional time arrives. As you know, the most distinct signs signaling the premenopausal transition period are menstrual cycle irregularities, hot flashes, and vaginal dryness.

℘ CHARTING YOUR FERTILITY SIGNS AS MENOPAUSE APPROACHES

If you decide that you want to chart your cycles for birth control, brace yourself for quite a ride. You can still use the method effectively, but this phase may be a challenge. Whatever your choice, charting will reflect your hormonal changes, giving you a sense of control over your seemingly unpredictable body.

When charting premenopausally, anticipate significant changes in your typical fertility pattern. Each of your fertility signs will reflect your new hormonal fluctuations as your body prepares for the cessation of ovulatory cycles.

Waking Temperatures

One of the most obvious reflections of your diminishing fertility will be your waking temperatures. Rather than seeing the usual thermal shifts every cycle, you will start seeing new variations. Initially, you may notice that your cycles become shorter and more frequent, and thus your thermal shifts occur sooner than usual. In addition, you may notice that the number of postovulatory temperatures decrease, reflecting shorter luteal phases than you normally have.

And finally, you'll notice more and more anovulatory cycles in which your temperature remains low throughout, indicating that you didn't release an egg that cycle. All of these variations in your temperature pattern are absolutely normal as you approach menopause, and should only serve to remind you of the benefits of charting to help you understand what is happening in your body.

Cervical Fluid

As the number of follicles in your ovaries begin to decrease, you will stop ovulating as often. You will also produce progressively less oestrogen, which in turn will decrease the amount of fertile-quality cervical fluid you produce. For example, if you used to observe about 3 days of eggwhite every cycle, you may now only have it one day, if at all. Yet without ovulation, progesterone won't be present to rapidly dry up what cervical fluid there is. All of this means that it may become harder to identify your Peak Day.

Your usual fertile pattern of cervical fluid will start to be replaced with more days of either dry, sticky, or even a watery secretion without any of the fertile characteristics such as slippery, stretchy, or lubricative. Your vaginal sensation may become a continuous, unchanging dry or sticky feeling. Or you may experience patches of cervical fluid, as your body makes noble attempts to ovulate in the face of impending menopause.

Cervix

Being able to observe your cervix during phases of anovulation can be especially helpful, since such cycles can be fairly confusing. You will probably notice that as menopause approaches, your cervix is more often firm, closed, and low, confirming longer phases of infertility and clarifying confusing cervical fluid or temperature patterns.

Secondary Fertility Signs

Along with the obvious changes you may notice in your three primary fertility signs, you will probably see changes in your secondary signs as well. You may even notice certain fertility signs for the first time as discussed below.

Midcycle Spotting
If you're someone who never used to have midcycle spotting around ovulation, you might be surprised to start experiencing it now. Its appearance is due to the fact that ovulatory spotting tends to be more common in long cycles, and one of the hallmarks of premenopausal cycles is their increasingly longer lengths.

Mittelschmerz
If you are used to having midcycle pain around ovulation, you may notice that you don't experience it as often as you stop ovulating as frequently.

Breast Tenderness
One of the nice benefits of anovulatory cycles is that you don't usually experience the postovulatory breast tenderness characteristic of normal cycles. This is because, when ovulation doesn't occur, there isn't any progesterone to cause the breast discomfort.

❧ THE CONTRACEPTIVE RULES AS MENOPAUSE APPROACHES

Once you have determined that you are indeed experiencing menopausal signs, the way you will use Fertility Awareness can be fairly straightforward: *You should follow all the standard rules of FAM for birth control discussed in Chapter 9, except that you should not rely on the First 5 Days Rule.*

What this means in practice is really quite simple. You should chart your cycles as you always have, but you should no longer assume that the first 5 days of the cycle are infertile. The reason for this is that your premenopausal cycles are subject to hormonal fluctuations which may cause a dramatically early ovulation.

Again, we are dealing with degrees of risk. Although there is little data to cite, it is likely that the first 3 days of a period are nearly as safe as the first 5 days were before you had that first hot flash. But to be most conservative, you should assume you're fertile until you can verify a *dry* day, which as you know, is essentially impossible as long as you're bleeding.

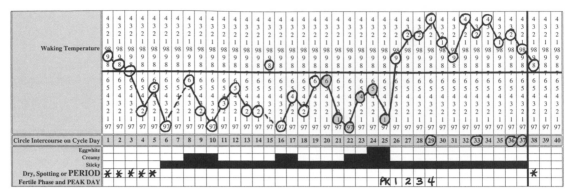

Chart 19.1. A challenging premenopausal Basic Infertile Pattern. Deborah has the misfortune of having a premenopausal BIP of sticky, day after day, interspersed with wet patches.

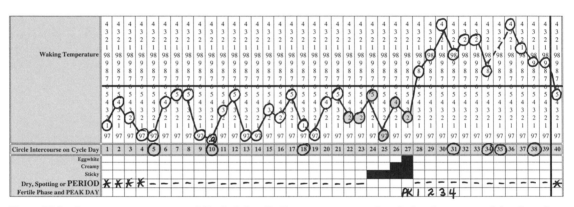

Chart 19.2. An easy premenopausal Basic Infertile Pattern. Later, Deborah develops a BIP of dry day after day. With charts like this one, FAM for birth control will be a breeze.

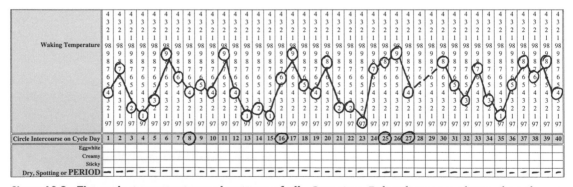

Chart 19.3. The easiest premenopausal pattern of all. Over time, Deborah stops ovulating altogether, as evidenced by continuous dry days with no thermal shift.

"Hard Cycles, Easy Cycles"

As menopause draws closer, you may find that you go for months without any dry days. Instead, you might have a continuous and extended preovulatory pattern of sticky days, perhaps interspersed with patches of wet cervical fluid. The occurrence of unchanging cervical fluid day after day is called a Basic Infertile Pattern (BIP) and is very common in premenopausal women. In such a case, you may want to use the BIP Rules discussed in Appendix B. They allow women with a sticky BIP to count more days as infertile than would be possible under the standard FAM rules. However the BIP rules are admittedly more difficult to follow, and as you can read in Appendix B, they are somewhat riskier for premenopausal women.

Understandably, you might decide that using them is simply not worth the trouble. Yet before deciding anything definitively, I would encourage you to at least continue charting for several months. Aside from the fascinating record you'll have of your reproductive system going through the throes of biological angst, it is almost certain that your cycles will become both increasingly longer *and* dryer, making FAM easier than ever.

When all is said and done, each couple will have to decide what is best for themselves. You might decide that it's not worth waiting for easier cycles. If this is the case, you may want to consider more permanent forms of contraception. Personally, I feel that vasectomy is a better option than tubal ligation, because it is a cheaper and less invasive procedure with fewer possible complications. But whatever you choose, remember that *menopausal women are considered potentially fertile for a full year after their last period.*

✻ MAINTAINING YOUR SANITY THROUGH THE MENOPAUSAL YEARS

In the end, how easily you glide through menopause will be determined in large part by your expectations before you get there. While the various menopausal signs can be a nuisance, they certainly don't have to be traumatizing. Reasonable solutions are available. So keep a sense of humor, and know that you're hardly alone.

Charting your cycles will offer you a unique opportunity to observe your body in a wondrous period of transformation. As your cycles veer from less than 3 weeks to 3 months or more, you'll always be on top of the hormonal turbulence within you. One day when you're about 50, after having gone all summer long without menstruating, you may have the opportunity to impress a friend. You'll be able to tell her that you know that you still have at least one more period to go, starting the following week. "How can you be sure?" she'll ask. "I know," you'll say, "because it says so on my chart."

CHAPTER 20

Enriching Your Self-Esteem Through Knowledge About Your Body

*Once we are old enough to have had an education, the first step
toward self-esteem for most of us is not to learn but to unlearn.*

—ANONYMOUS

> Luteal phase defect
> Hostile cervical mucus
> Incompetent cervix
> Inadequate pelvis
> Senile gravida
> Habitual aborter

*H*mm . . . let's see: defect, hostile, incompetent, inadequate, senile, aborter. Doesn't *that* paint a pretty picture? Regrettably, the list above merely describes women with fairly common conditions such as those with a short luteal phase, nonfertile cervical fluid, a weak cervix, a narrow pelvis, a pregnancy after 35, and a tendency to miscarry. If you'd like to be further entertained, you can review the entire list of medical terminology still used in women's health today (see Appendix J).

You may think that this type of language doesn't affect self-esteem, because most women aren't even aware that these descriptions are recorded in their medical records. But many are matter-of-factly informed that they have the above conditions by well-meaning doctors who are oblivious to how insulting this terminology can be. These phrases reflect an antiquated medical system that is often insensitive to women and out of touch with their needs.

275

Instead of identifying with the above vocabulary, picture an altogether different scenario. Imagine growing up being told that your body is a marvel of biological beauty that will orchestrate amazing changes every cycle. Rather than thinking that you keep producing infectious discharges, you'd know to identify healthy cervical secretions as a reflection of the remarkable hormonal system working within. Imagine going to the doctor and feeling knowledgeable rather than vulnerable. And instead of succumbing to douche commercials that diminish self-confidence by implying that women are dirty, you could simply disregard them, knowing that just showering with soap and water will keep you clean and feminine.

What if teenagers acquired practical knowledge about their cycles and fertility even before the first day they menstruated? Not only would it increase their self-assurance, but it would enable them to identify both medical problems and normal biological occurrences, sparing them so much of the fear and confusion that comes with adolescence. And although FAM should not be promoted as a method of birth control among adolescents, the reality is that the practical knowledge it affords could reduce unplanned pregnancies in a population that, unfortunately, still believes among other things that you can't get pregnant the first time.

Imagine being able to utilize your body's own fertility signs to provide you with a completely natural, safe, and effective method of birth control that promotes shared responsibility and communication between you and your partner. Or envision what it would be like to know your own hormonal symphony so well that you could plan every aspect of your pregnancy, from the month you want to deliver your baby, to perhaps increasing the odds of conceiving the gender of your choice.

And if by chance you or your partner really do have a fertility problem, picture a dialogue of truly informed participants. Imagine you, your partner, and your doctor using your own charts to find the least invasive strategy first, before deciding that IVF or other high technologies are your last and only solution. Yes, it may be, but at least you would understand why.

On a more mundane note, wouldn't it be nice to experience PMS in a whole new light, finally understanding why you develop symptoms on a cyclical basis? Knowing there are steps you can take to alleviate the various pains and discomforts will always help, particularly if you take preemptive steps based on conveniently predictable patterns. In such a case, your fertility charts could serve as a biomedical databank, perhaps helping you stave off that particularly unpleasant bloated feeling 3 days before your period.

And what if menopause was finally perceived for what it is—an inevitable, natural transition in a woman's life. If women were actually taught what to anticipate in the years leading up to their last period, they certainly wouldn't feel so confused and mystified by all the new changes. Indeed, women in their late 40s are hormonally like 13-year-old kids. Their bodies may create the biological equivalent of a Hollywood mystery, but like their adolescent daughters, these women can eliminate the confusion and take control as they enter the last phase of this long and curious journey.

There is a popular cliché that is as truthful as it is applicable:

Knowledge is power.

Unfortunately, so much of what people usually want to know is locked away in the secret papers of governmental, corporate, and academic bureaucracies. But there is also a treasure trove of eminently practical information that in many ways serves to define your womanhood, and that knowledge is available to you whenever you want. Yes, it does take a couple of minutes a day to access, but it requires no particular job connections, or even a computer. Fertility Awareness is certainly not high tech. But for all of you who are of reproductive age, the education it provides can reveal an entire world about which you may know so very little: yourself.

Epilogue to the Revised Edition:

The Women's Health Movement and the Missing Piece of the Puzzle

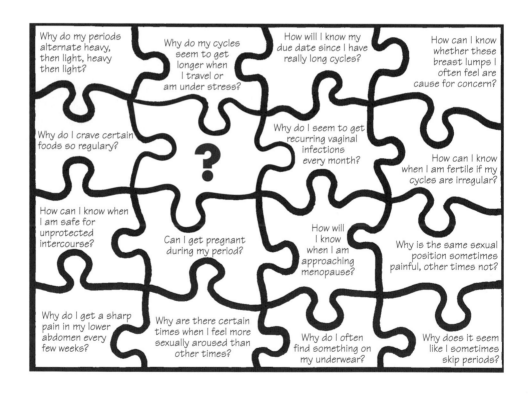

Many anthropologists are aware of a universal tradition among the Bantu women of East Africa, passed down from grandmother to granddaughter, generation after generation. In order to teach their descendants about the relationship of cervical fluid to fertility, the elder woman takes a smooth stone in order to gently wipe the outer lips of her granddaughter's vagina. She then explains to the maturing adolescent that it is in the secretions found on that stone that the key to her future fertility will come and go, magically, cycle after cycle.

*S*ince *Taking Charge of Your Fertility* was first published in 1995, I have had the opportunity to talk to hundreds of readers about the impact Fertility Awareness has had on their lives. What has been most gratifying to me is learning of their almost unanimous view that every woman should know its basic scientific principles. Not just to maximize their odds of conception, or to avoid pregnancy, but perhaps most important, to finally demystify the everyday riddles of their own bodies. Quite simply, these women have confirmed my own long-held belief that Fertility Awareness education could well become one of the most important chapters in the amazing multigenerational history of the American women's health movement, a history that is worth briefly noting in order to put the information contained in this book into some basic historical context.

✤ THE SEARCH FOR VIABLE CONTRACEPTION AND THE RAMIFICATIONS OF THE PILL

Of all the health-related struggles confronting women, perhaps the longest-lasting and most universal has involved the often contentious issue of birth control. Indeed, it is well known that various societies throughout history have acted to prohibit whatever contraceptive technologies were available to them, and of course the United States was no exception. In fact, it was only thanks to the courage of Margaret Sanger in the early twentieth century that Americans first enjoyed the lawful and widespread availability of condoms and diaphragms.

Sanger herself was arrested and harassed, both for publishing newsletters that demanded such access and for opening America's first birth control clinic in Brooklyn, New York, in 1916. (The clinic was abruptly closed by police.) Yet her actions struck a chord with women throughout the country, and by the early 1920s, the American Birth Control League (a forerunner to Planned Parenthood) had 37,000 members. The power of this and other organizations overcame both legal obstacles and resistance from the male-dominated medical establishment.

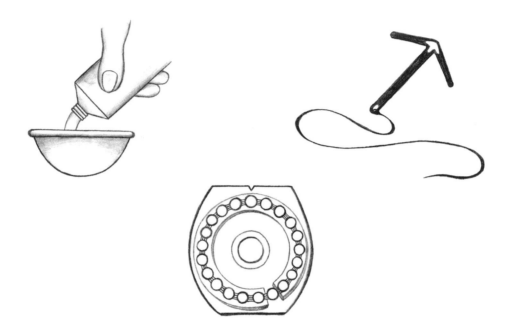

Of course, the most dramatic developments in modern contraceptive history came a couple of generations later, with the arrival of the Pill. Ironically, it was the difficulties that women initially faced in exposing its dangerous side effects (most of which have since been resolved) that helped lead to the first truly organized movement devoted to women's health itself. It's no coincidence that less than a year after activists disrupted a 1969 U.S. Senate hearing on the Pill (because not a single woman was called to testify as to their own negative experiences in taking it!), the Boston Women's Health Book Collective published the first version of what soon evolved into the landmark book *Our Bodies, Ourselves.*

By the time access to legal abortion was finally guaranteed in 1973, grass-roots activism devoted to a variety of women's health issues had taken hold, from the backlash against the overuse of radical mastectomies for breast cancer to the demand for more information about DES and its devastating effects on a genera-tion of girls born to mothers who had used it. Yet given the well-publicized risks of both the Pill and later the IUD, the movement as a whole remained most con-cerned with access to safe and effective contraceptive choices, and for many, this still remains one of the key women's health issues today.

๕๑ RETURNING CHILDBIRTH TO THE MOTHER'S CONTROL

The general tenor of the women's movement of the 1960s would soon have a powerful impact on other fundamental areas within women's health. In the de-cade or so following the release of the Pill, a highly visible campaign began to spread in reaction to what was seen as the general overreliance on medical tech-nology in the delivery room. Although most women had come to expect some form of modern anesthesia, many began to forcefully reject the routine use of labor-inducing drugs, surgical rupturing of membranes, forcep deliveries, epi-siotomies, and even the usual practice of whisking the baby off to the nursery as soon as it was delivered.

In 1972, Suzanne Arms's book *Immaculate Deception* made perhaps the most persuasive call for rehumanizing the entire process of childbirth, including stan-dard postpartum practices. Her book was a landmark that sparked great debate among both ordinary women and the medical community, in large part for her claim that the American hospital was often not the best or most logical place for childbirth to occur, and for her assertion that midwives should take the primary role over doctors in those routine births where medical intervention was not necessary.

As a result of Arms and other pioneers, many American women today ac-tively plan the type of birth they want, including such decisions as whether it should be at home or in a hospital, with a midwife or an OB/GYN, using Lamaze or Bradley childbirth preparation, and finally, whether it should be experienced naturally or with drugs. And though it is obvious that most women today don't choose to have a completely natural childbirth, the shift of decision-making power from the doctor to the mother appears to be one of the most significant ways in which women have taken control of a fundamental aspect of their repro-ductive lives.

℘ THE "OUTING" OF MENOPAUSE AND OTHER FEMALE TABOOS

In contrast to childbirth, societal developments concerning menopause have been marked not so much by any definitive social movement or medical breakthrough, as by simply an increase in candid and informed discussion. The fact is that until the late 1960s, most women rarely if ever broached the topic of menopause with even their closest friends. But as in other areas, the standard practices of the medical establishment began to draw increasingly vocal criticism. Specifically, a few courageous activists began to object to the prevailing view of menopause as a disease that needed to be treated (either psychologically or hormonally), and soon many were attacking the routine use of hormone replacement therapy, which at that time seemed to have as many negative drawbacks as benefits.

Still, the real breakthrough only came in the early 1990s, with Gail Sheehy's classic, *The Silent Passage*. This work clearly struck a nerve with millions of women and swept away the notion of menopause as a taboo topic. Not only did many women begin to see it as a potentially positive gateway to a newly energized phase of life (as opposed to merely the symptom-filled conclusion to one's fertile years), but more than ever before, women began to talk with everyone about their menopausal-related hopes, fears, and concerns, from their doctors and friends to strangers on talk radio. And thus today, hormone replacement therapy and hot flashes are just two more typical subjects of media inquiry and women's social gatherings.

Of course, menopause has only been the most notable example of a women's health-related subject that has gone from taboo status to a mainstream topic of great general interest. Witness the formation of PMS and hysterectomy support groups, the explosion of mass education and grass-roots organizing for breast cancer research, or even widely popular books, which have explored everything from the history of menstruation to female anatomy. For those who remember the ignorance and isolation that prevailed just a generation ago, all of this is wonderful news.

℘ THE PROMISE AND TEMPTATION OF HIGH-TECH FERTILITY PROCEDURES

Still, the most compelling topic in reproductive health, and the one that has probably captured the most attention of both women and men, has been the continuing advances in reproductive technology. From the birth of Louise Brown in

1977 (the world's first "test tube baby"), to the development of such procedures as GIFT and ZIFT in the 1980s, to the most recent headlines on sperm micromanipulation and ovum transfer, the world has witnessed a staggering revolution in the potential options that are afforded those couples who are perceived as being infertile. Yet these high-tech advances are hardly reproductive panaceas. Their overall success rates remain fair but not great, and because of their high costs in money, time, and emotional energy, they are not an ideal choice for most couples.

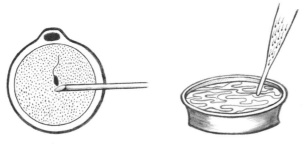

Of course, one can assume that assisted reproductive technologies will continue to improve, and that in the future their physical and financial costs may diminish to the point that many people will come to view them as just another routine alternative on the road to a successful pregnancy. To the extent that these technologies present ever greater choices *for those who truly need them,* this can only be seen as a positive development. Yet there is also a possibility that the progress to which I'm referring could have a very real downside—specifically, if future couples glibly turn to the latest technological advancements before seeking the knowledge with which so many of them could *naturally* become parents. And given the missed opportunities for self-edification that such knowledge would bring, this would be unfortunate, no matter how cheap and easy high-tech pregnancies become.

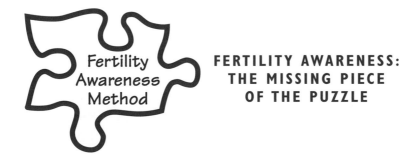

FERTILITY AWARENESS: THE MISSING PIECE OF THE PUZZLE

As we have seen, women over the last few generations have taken ever-greater control of their lives, and in so doing have often become substantially more in tune with their own bodies. Nevertheless, the progress they have made has been sporadic and piecemeal, with each new movement or breakthrough applying only to a relatively small part of life's great menstrual mystery. Indeed, the advances made in both childbirth and menopause have dramatically improved their physical welfare, but it's worth noting that childbirth usually occurs during the primary reproductive years of 20 to 40, while menopause only arrives in the decade or so that follows.

Likewise, women now have a variety of fairly decent alternatives for avoiding pregnancy, and every year yields new technologies and hope for those struggling couples trying to conceive. But birth control methods and high-tech fertility treatments reflect specific goals of different women at different times, and even though they are the flip side of the same menstrual coin, the pursuit of the final objective teaches women virtually nothing about how or *when* conception occurs in any given cycle.

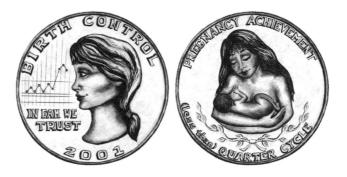

Given the exciting evolution of the various women's health movements discussed above, it is worth briefly mentioning the historical development of the Fertility Awareness Method (FAM), which is a comprehensive body of knowledge that is applicable to *all* menstruating women, for the entire duration of their reproductive years. As noted earlier, *Our Bodies, Ourselves* was a major step forward, but even this amazing source paid scant attention to FAM's initial development and validation, even though it had begun to gain a sizable number of adherents in Europe as early as the 1960s, the majority of whom used it as a form of birth control.

In fact, the first comprehensive studies to show the scientific validity of using both cervical fluid and waking body temperature as a way of accurately detecting ovulation occurred in the 1950s. Yet because Fertility Awareness would remain widely confused with the essentially useless Rhythm Method, it did not, alas, become a widely known contraceptive choice during that inspiring time in the 1970s when so many American women began to take so much of their physical well-being into their own hands.

By the time I wrote the first edition of this book in the mid-1990s, more and more women were beginning to hear that FAM was natural and effective, while its dubious association with the Rhythm Method and related religious doctrine was finally beginning to weaken. Of course, it still hadn't achieved the grass-roots impact that other women's health movements had, yet I was evermore confident that it was only a matter of time.*

What most of my readers now know is that the Fertility Awareness Method is not the antiquated Rhythm Method or just a system for maximizing the odds of conception. Nor is FAM the exclusive domain of strict Catholics or flower children of the 60s. They are thrilled to discover that it also serves as a wonderful window into all facets of a woman's gynecological well-being, and that it is basic knowledge that every woman should possess, no matter what she ultimately chooses to do with it.

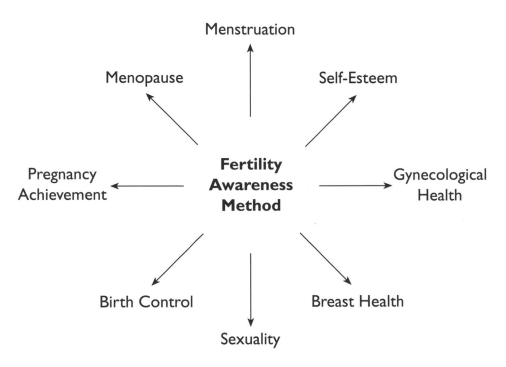

* It's important to note that FAM had been gaining increasing credibility due to the work of many people both within the United States and abroad. In this brief epilogue, though, it's not really feasible to write a thorough history of all of its "great founders." Nevertheless, I would like to briefly acknowledge the groundbreaking role of Australian doctors John and Evelyn Billings, whose development of the Billings Ovulation Method in the 1960s was perhaps the most critical factor in later popularizing the idea that a woman's body did indeed produce useful and reliable fertility signs.

✄ COMING FULL CIRCLE

Although I wrote *Taking Charge* with a clear vision of educating all women of reproductive age, the success of the first edition was primarily due to the large majority of readers who were seeking to *conceive*. Initially, I was puzzled as to why this was, because before I wrote it, my own seminars were still much more popular with those seeking to avoid pregnancy. Perhaps the very title of this book misleads people into thinking that it is strictly about getting pregnant.

Regardless, I find it fascinating that the continuing advances in high-tech reproductive technologies are perhaps most responsible for popularizing fertility awareness in general. This is because as increasingly more couples muster the financial and emotional resources to try high-tech reproductive options, they often discover that FAM should be the first step they take in their efforts to conceive, *before* they begin the invasive tests and procedures that drain so much of their money and energy. My vision is to still transform FAM into a body of knowledge that is a basic component of all sex education, but if it takes the determination of those struggling with infertility to propel it into broader society, then so be it.

I believe Fertility Awareness is drawing the women's health revolution full circle, and that its growing popularity may one day result in it being seen as important as the technological advances and grass-roots movements that have already come before it. This is because, as so many women are now learning, FAM is a truly liberating tool for understanding and maintaining basic reproductive health, and can function as such from an adolescent girl's first period to her last one, nearly four decades later. In fact, as we enter the twenty-first century, a growing critical mass of women have finally discovered that it is probably the most empowering information that women can be taught about the miraculous workings of their own bodies.

I feel privileged to play a role in the dissemination of such important and edifying knowledge, in large part because I have come to realize that if FAM continues to grow in popularity in the years ahead, it may one day be seen as the logical culmination of what has, in fact, been a series of women's health movements, from the first demands for access to contraceptives to the relatively recent and increasing interest in finding natural alternatives for menopausal symptoms. And yes, there is a certain irony in the fact that women considering high-tech pregnancy achievement procedures would be the group that is most responsible for bringing Fertility Awareness into the mainstream, for as you've learned in this book, the practice of using FAM to chart your cycles generally involves little technology. Still, the latest digital thermometers are wonderfully convenient, and because of the age we live in, it will probably become increasingly popular to use computerized fertility charting programs such as the one I developed to complement this book (TCOYF.com).

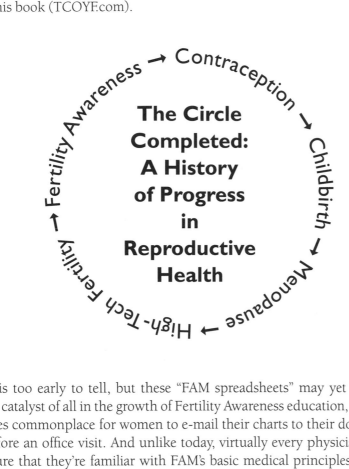

It is too early to tell, but these "FAM spreadsheets" may yet serve as the biggest catalyst of all in the growth of Fertility Awareness education, as it one day becomes commonplace for women to e-mail their charts to their doctors on the day before an office visit. And unlike today, virtually every physician would be darn sure that they're familiar with FAM's basic medical principles, in part because if they weren't, they would know less than your average teenage girl.

APPENDIXES

Troubleshooting Your Cycle: Expecting the Unexpected

After you have started to chart, you may come across situations in which you need more clarification or guidance. What follows is a list of what I believe to be the most likely problem areas, based on my twenty years of practice. They are categorized both by symptom or fertility sign and by when the problem occurs in the cycle. I hope these pages serve as a valuable resource that addresses any additional concerns or questions you may have.*

ᘓᕞ CATEGORIZED BY SYMPTOM OR FERTILITY SIGN

Bleeding

Waking Temperatures

* Many of the physical problems discussed in this appendix have potential solutions that you may wish to explore in Marilyn Shannon's *Fertility, Cycles, and Nutrition*.

Cervical Fluid

Cervix

Intercourse

✺ CATEGORIZED BY WHEN IT OCCURS IN THE CYCLE

Anytime in Cycle

SPOTTING BEFORE MENSTRUATION
(AT THE END OF THE LUTEAL PHASE)

Spotting before menstruation can be considered normal if it follows at least 10 days of high temperatures without spotting. Otherwise, it can be an indication that the corpus luteum is starting to break down too early, which in turn causes a premature shedding of the capillaries in the uterine lining. Either way, Day 1 of the cycle is considered the first day of a true menstrual flow.

Regardless, if the spotting consistently lasts longer than a few days, you should see a physician to rule out a number of conditions, including thyroid problems, fibroids, endometritis, or endometrial polyps. Assuming you have ruled out the above, for pregnancy *avoiders*, this type of spotting is generally just a nuisance. But for pregnancy *achievers*, it may be a potential problem since it could indicate an insufficient luteal phase necessary for implantation of the egg to occur (see page 151). The most common remedies to support the luteal phase are the following:

- progesterone cream, vaginal suppositories, or capsules, all given throughout the luteal phase and often continued through the first trimester once pregnancy is established
- HCG injections, which, when given during the luteal phase, act like LH to stimulate the ovary to produce more progesterone and oestrogen
- the oral ovulatory drug Clomid, which acts to correct the preovulatory *and* postovulatory phases of the cycle

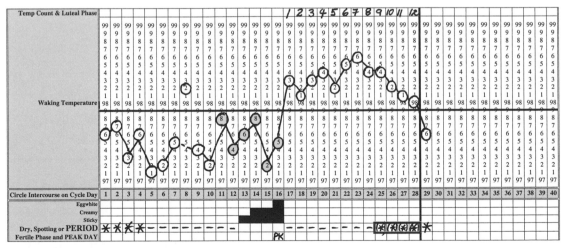

Chart A.1. Premenstrual Spotting.

VERY LIGHT OR HEAVY PERIODS

Exceptionally light or heavy periods can be the result of an anovulatory cycle—that is, a cycle in which an egg was not released. (This type of bleeding is especially common as women approach menopause.) It is critical that you differentiate between anovulatory bleeding and ovulatory spotting. You can determine if you ovulated by whether you had a thermal shift 12 to 16 days before this type of period. If there wasn't, you can be fairly certain that the bleeding you are experiencing is anovulatory. Technically, this is not a true menstrual period, since it did not follow the release of an egg. However, to maintain a point of reference, you would still consider it Day 1 of a new cycle. (See page 225 for other possible causes of bleeding.) Regardless, you may want to see a doctor if you are trying to conceive and have any of the following:

- *consistently* heavy periods, which may be due to fibroids, among other conditions
- several days of either premenstrual or postmenstrual spotting beyond Day 5, which may be a sign of a luteal phase problem
- very light periods, which may be due to an insufficient endometrial build-up

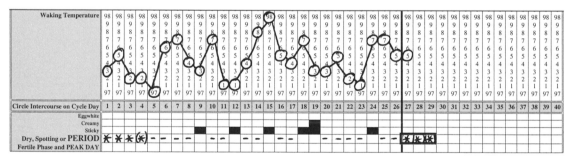

Chart A.2a. Anovulatory bleeding. Usually occurs after an absence of a thermal shift.

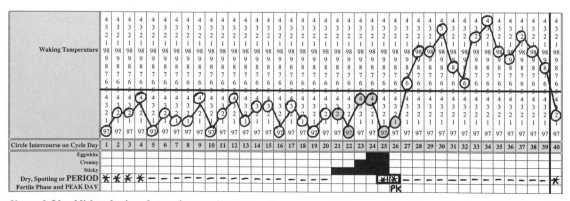

Chart A.2b. Midcycle (ovulatory) spotting. Usually occurs within a couple of days of a thermal shift, and is considered extremely fertile.

UNEXPLAINED BLEEDING

Once you know your cycle well, you won't need to be concerned if you occasionally get spotting in the day or so before your period or around ovulation. But if you have red blood at inexplicable times, you should probably be checked by a doctor. (See page 224 for causes of bleeding.)

You should also be aware that if you become pregnant, you may have implantation spotting due to the fertilized egg burrowing into the lining. So if you have reason to think you might be pregnant, pay special attention to spotting that might occur from about a week or so after your thermal shift. Your temperatures will verify whether you are indeed pregnant if they remain above the coverline for at least 18 days. Of course, anytime you suspect pregnancy, you should see a clinician to confirm it.

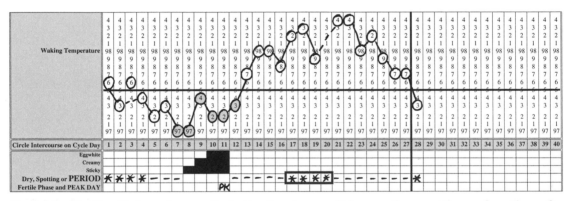

Chart A.3. Bleeding that requires medical attention, because it is more than spotting, and continues for a number of days.

MIDCYCLE SPOTTING

About 10% of women will notice that they occasionally have a day or two of spotting about midcycle, right around ovulation. In fact, they may even notice that the fertile cervical fluid (especially the eggwhite quality) is tinged with brown, pink, or red. This is a result of spotting mixed with cervical fluid. It is considered extremely fertile. It's usually due to the sudden drop in oestrogen that precedes ovulation and is nothing to be concerned about. If anything, it is a good secondary sign to record on your chart. It's typically more common in long cycles.

You can tell that it is ovulatory spotting because it occurs *within a couple days of* a thermal shift (Chart A.4a). If, however, the spotting lasts more than a couple days, is bright red, or you notice spotting at other times in the cycle that do *not* coincide with ovulation or the approach of your period, it could be an indication of a problem requiring medical attention (Chart A.4b), or possibly an early sign of pregnancy (see Chart A.5, next page).

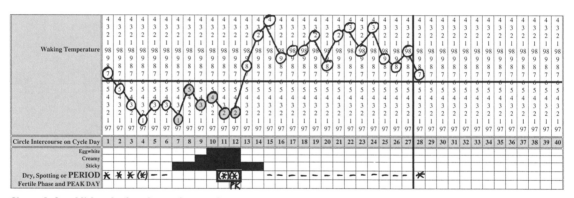

Chart A.4a. Midcycle (ovulatory) spotting.

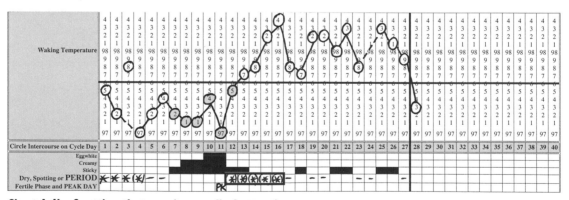

Chart A.4b. Spotting that requires medical attention.

SPOTTING ANYTIME FROM WEEK AFTER OVULATION TO EXPECTED PERIOD

If you experience spotting anytime from about a week after your temperature rises to the expected date of your period, it may be a sign of pregnancy. When the fertilized egg burrows into the uterine lining, it can cause implantation spotting. If you have reason to think you might be pregnant, pay special attention to your temperatures to see whether they remain above the coverline for at least 18 days (see page 157).

If you prefer to take a pregnancy test, even the most sensitive ones won't be valid until you've had at least 10 high temperatures. You should be aware that store-bought tests generally require a few more days because they are not as sensitive to the minute amounts of HCG that the embryo initially emits.

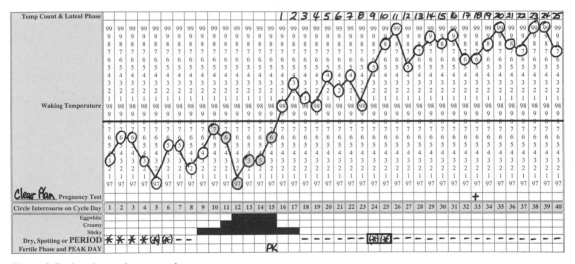

Chart A.5. Implantation spotting.

NO THERMAL SHIFT

Now and then you may have an anovulatory cycle. If this occurs, you won't see a shift in temperatures from low to high because no progesterone will have been released to cause the temperatures to rise.

In addition, you could be one of the small percentage of women whose bodies don't respond to the effects of progesterone, and therefore don't show a thermal shift even if you have ovulated. As discussed in Chapter 14, one of the only ways to definitively determine if ovulation has occurred in this case is through ultrasound. Short of that, you could get a blood test in the second phase of the cycle to determine the presence of progesterone.

You also may be experiencing a temporary cause of anovulation such as illness or stress. If you notice many anovulatory cycles, you may have a medical problem such as Polycystic Ovarian Syndrome (PCOS) (see page 204). Finally, you could be starting to approach menopause, in which case you will stop ovulating as often as you used to. Chapters 7, 14, 19, and Appendix B discuss these problems in more detail.

If you are using FAM for birth control and have established that you are indeed one of the few women whose temperatures simply do not reflect ovulation, you can use the Billings Method, which involves checking cervical fluid alone. While not as effective as the Fertility Awareness Method taught in this book, you can increase the effectiveness of the method by also charting cervical position, thus providing another sign to cross-check in cases of ambiguity.

If you do choose to use the Billings Method, you should be aware that you *cannot* use the First 5 Days Rule, because you can't prove that the bleeding you experience is menstruation and not ovulatory spotting. This is because you won't have the thermal shift to show that ovulation occurred 12 to 16 days before. Unfortunately, this may require you to apply the Peak Day Rule more than once per cycle. And because you can't confirm that you've already ovulated, I strongly recommend that you treat any wet cervical fluid or bleeding at *any* time during the cycle as fertile.

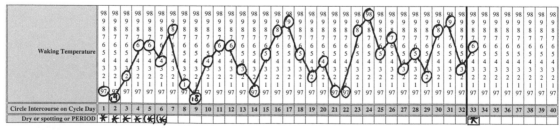

Chart A.6. In a cycle without a thermal shift, pregnancy avoiders should treat any bleeding as potentially fertile.

AMBIGUOUS THERMAL SHIFTS

Not all thermal shifts are obvious. A way of clarifying whether ovulation has most likely occurred is if one of the 3 high temperatures is at least three-tenths above the coverline (rather than just one-tenth above).

For those practicing birth control, the standard Temperature Shift Rule states that you are safe the evening of the third consecutive day that your temperature is above the coverline (see page 129). But if you have an ambiguous or "weak" thermal shift, you may prefer the somewhat more conservative rule, as discussed in Chart A.7b below.

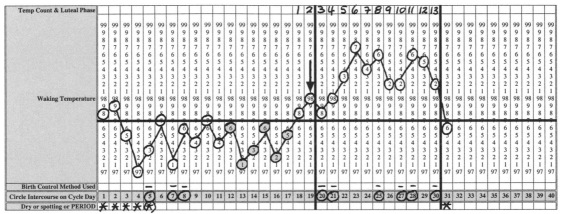

Chart A.7a. Note that in this cycle, her thermal shift is not as obvious as she might prefer, but it still meets the criteria of the more conservative approach. This is because Day 19 is in fact three-tenths above the coverline.

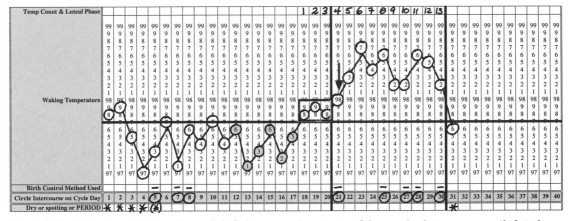

Chart A.7b. Note that while her thermal shift does meet the criteria of the standard Temperature Shift Rule on days 18 to 20 (since all 3 temps are at least one-tenth above the coverline), she chooses to be a bit more cautious, and thus does not consider herself past her fertile phase until one temperature is at least three-tenths above. In this case, this means that she would consider herself infertile only on the evening of Day 21, and not of Day 20.

ERRATIC TEMPERATURES

Some women may find that their temperatures do not seem to follow the classic pattern of lows and highs. For these women, consider trying any of the following:

1. If using a digital thermometer, verify that the battery is not low.
2. Consider trying a glass basal body thermometer, since digitals may be less accurate for some women.
3. If you do use a glass basal body thermometer, be sure to take your temperature for a full 5 minutes.
4. Regardless which type of thermometer you use, consider taking your waking temperature *vaginally* rather than orally. (Of course, be consistent in how you take it throughout your cycle.)
5. Remember that certain factors can definitely increase waking temperatures, such as fever, drinking alcohol the night before, or not getting 3 consecutive hours of sleep.
6. Try to take your temperature about the same time every day. For every half hour that you sleep *later* than normal, your temperature may tend to creep up about one-tenth of a degree. For every half hour that you wake up *earlier* than normal, it may tend to drop by about one-tenth of a degree. You should note the time you take it in the appropriate column. You should use the Rule of Thumb to discount aberrant temperatures that may result from sleeping late. (This will prevent you from attributing a high temperature to a thermal shift before it has actually occurred.)

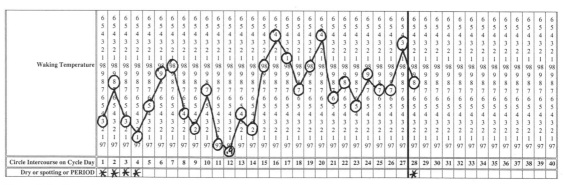

Chart A.8. Erratic temperatures.

OUTLYING TEMPERATURES

If you have temperatures that are clearly out of line (for example, from fever, drinking alcohol the night before, or having slept in and taken your temperature late) just use the Rule of Thumb, covering any outlying temperatures with your thumb. Remember to draw a dotted line between the correct temperatures on either side of the outlying temperatures. In calculating the coverline, you count the 6 low temperatures before the rise, *not* including the outlying temperature (see page 78).

If you have an outlying low temperature after your thermal shift, you may apply the same principle of the dotted line. But if you are using FAM for birth control, you should never ignore a low temp if it is within one of the first 3 days after the thermal shift. To be safe, you must count 3 temperatures above the coverline before you consider yourself infertile, as you can see in chart A.9b.

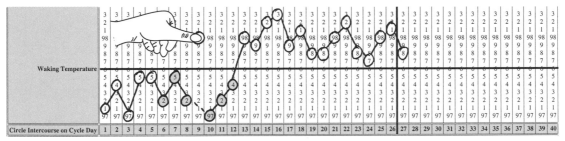

Chart A.9a. Outlying temperature within the 6 days before the thermal shift. Note that she counts back 6 temperatures before the thermal shift, passing over the outlying temperature in order to draw the coverline.

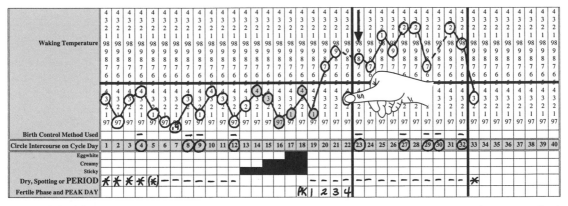

Chart A.9b. Outlying temperature within the first 3 days after the thermal shift. Note that as a method of birth control, she only considers herself safe Day 4 of the thermal shift, since one of her temperatures dropped below the coverline during the 3-day count. *If she wanted to be ultra conservative, she could wait until the third night in a row of high temps above the coverline. But in this case, her Peak Day was so obvious that she was able to use cervical fluid to corroborate the temps, and considered Day 23 the first safe evening.*

HIGH TEMPERATURES DURING PERIOD

It is fairly common for women to experience several days of high temperatures during their period. This is usually the result of residual progesterone from the last cycle or fluctuating hormones that occur during menstruation. Draw a dotted line from the high temperatures during your period down to the normal range temperatures. The high temperatures will probably be above the coverline, but you can simply disregard them by using the Rule of Thumb (see page 78).

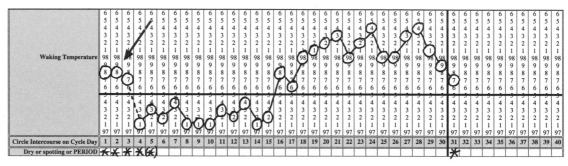

Chart A.10. High temps during period due to residual progesterone.

HIGHER- OR LOWER-THAN-AVERAGE WAKING TEMPERATURES THROUGHOUT CYCLE

One of the most obvious symptoms of a possible thyroid problem is a pattern of very high or low waking temperatures. (Most preovulatory waking temperatures range between 97.0 to 97.5 degrees and postovulatory range between 97.6 to 98.6 degrees.) If you find that you have any of the combination of symptoms below, you may want to see your doctor.*

Hyperthyroidism, or excessively high thyroid activity:
Symptoms of hyperthyroidism include high waking temperatures, scant menses, long cycles, and infertility.

Hypothyroidism, or low thyroid function:
Symptoms of hypothyroidism include low waking temperatures, unusually long cycles, anovulatory cycles (with no thermal shift), prolonged phases of fertile-quality cervical fluid, heavy menses, or unexplained infertility.

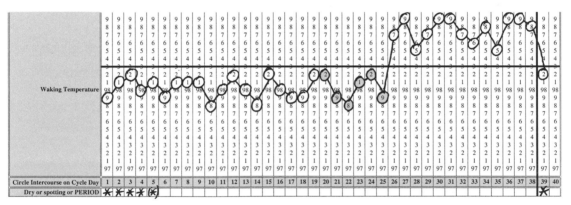

Chart A.11a. Possible hyperthyroid temperatures (high thyroid activity).

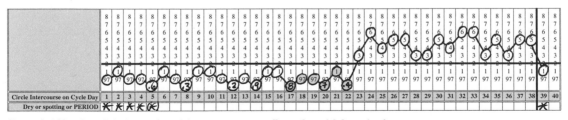

Chart A.11b. Possible hypothyroid temperatures (low thyroid function).

* For a more thorough discussion of thyroid conditions, see *The Thyroid Solution,* by Dr. Ridha Arem (1999).

TEMPERATURE DIP BEFORE THE RISE

You may be one of the few women who consistently have a temperature pattern in which you see a conspicuous dip before your thermal shift. Or you may only occasionally notice this pattern. Either way, it is believed that it usually occurs on the day of ovulation and is the result of high levels of oestrogen pushing your temperatures down.

For pregnancy avoiders, the dip does not affect your adherence to the pre-ovulatory rules of contraception. For pregnancy achievers, this would be an excellent day to time intercourse (assuming, of course, your cervical fluid is fertile that day).

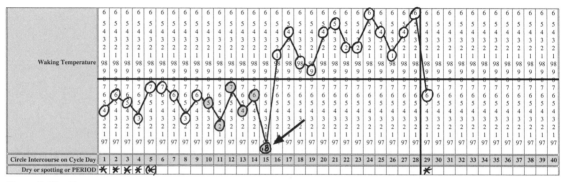

Chart A.12. Temperature dip. Note the plunge in temperature well below other preovulatory temps, often indicative of ovulation.

TEMPERATURES RISE IN SPURTS (STAIR-STEP PATTERN)

One of the more common types of temperature patterns are those where the thermal shift occurs in an initial spurt of several days, followed by a type of bell curve. In other words, you will probably notice a cluster of 6 low temperatures followed by a shift of at least two-tenths higher for perhaps 3 or 4 days, followed by the final bell curve. The coverline is always drawn after the *first* shift of at least two-tenths higher than the cluster of 6 preceding low temperatures.

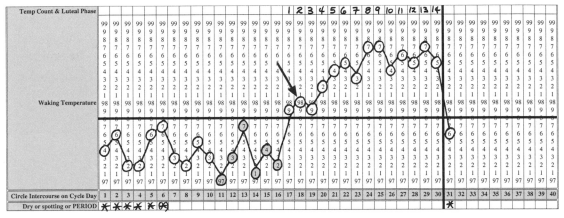

Chart A.13. Stair-step temperature pattern. Note the initial spurt of 3 high temperatures on Days 17, 18, and 19.

TEMPERATURES RISE ONE-TENTH DEGREE AT A TIME (SLOW-RISE PATTERN)

Some women will notice that instead of their temperature shifting by at least two-tenths of a degree higher than the previous 6 lows, their temperatures rise by merely one-tenth of a degree at a time. While this type of shift may seem fairly confusing to interpret, it can be done.

Wait for the first time your temperature rises at least one-tenth degree above the highest of the last 6 temperatures. On this chart, you would highlight Days 10 to 15 before the one-tenth-degree rise and draw the coverline straight through the elevated temperature on Day 16. Also note that in this particular case, Day 16 is in fact two-tenths of a degree above the previous day, but only one-tenth of a degree above the cluster of the previous 6 days. It is this latter fact that distinguishes the pattern as a slow-rise.

Once your temperature remains *above* the coverline for at least 4 days, you can be quite certain that you have ovulated. (Note that for pregnancy avoiders, to be conservative with this fairly rare temperature pattern, you should wait 4 days rather than 3 to consider yourself infertile. *C'est la vie.*) In addition, you should never consider yourself safe during such slow-rising temperatures unless you can corroborate your infertile phase with the Peak Day Rule (see page 131).

If you are using FAM for *achieving* pregnancy, you should consider the post-ovulatory phase to be all the temperatures above the coverline, but realize that your ovulation probably occurred a day or more earlier. Remember that ovulation most likely occurs the day of, or the day after the Peak Day, which is the last day of eggwhite-quality cervical fluid or lubricative vaginal sensation.

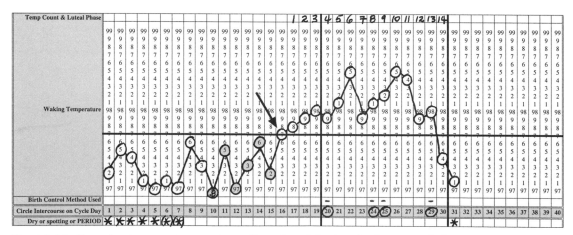

Chart A.14. Slow-rise temperature pattern. Note the subtle rise of only one-tenth degree on Day 16.

DROP IN TEMPERATURE DAY 2 OF THE THERMAL SHIFT
(FALL-BACK PATTERN)

Some women notice that they tend to have a pattern of a temperature drop on Day 2 of their thermal shift, followed by a sustained rise in temperature until their period. Unfortunately, to be conservative for birth control, you would want to start the count over again after the second sustained rise to be absolutely sure that the egg(s) are dead and gone.

If you don't want to wait the extra 2 days, you might rely on the Peak Day Rule to signal the start of the infertile phase. Admittedly, this could compromise contraceptive efficacy. However, if you verify that you are once again dry, and that your cervix has also returned to its infertile state, the increased risk of conception is quite small.

For pregnancy achievers, you should assume that you ovulated about the day of or day after your Peak Day, the last day of wet-quality cervical fluid or lubricative vaginal sensation.

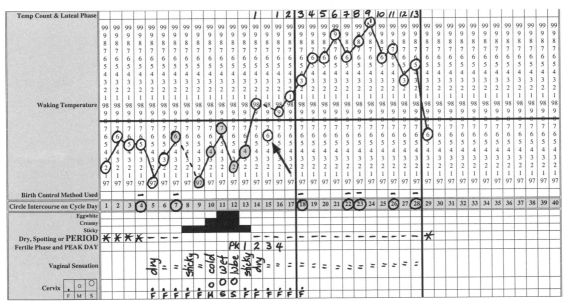

Chart A.15. Fall-back temperature pattern. Note the drop in temperature below the coverline on Day 15.

TEMPERATURE BELOW COVERLINE WELL AFTER OVULATION

After ovulation (during the luteal phase), there is a second smaller surge of oestrogen, which may cause a temporary drop in temperature and often coincides with a day or two of creamy cervical fluid. You need not get confused, though, because it is not an indication of returning fertility. The egg is already dead and gone by then (see page 326).

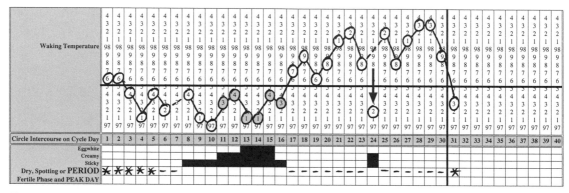

Chart A.16. Temperature drop mid-luteal phase.

DROP IN TEMPERATURE DAY BEFORE PERIOD BEGINS

Occasionally, you may notice an obvious drop in temperature the day before you get your period. While this is less common than when it occurs the day of menstruation itself, it is still considered part of the luteal phase (this sudden premenstrual drop is caused by the disintegration of the corpus luteum). Day 1 of the new cycle is not determined by the day of the drop, but by the first day of bleeding. This means that the luteal phase length is determined by the first day of the rise in temperature through to and including the last day before the red menstrual flow.

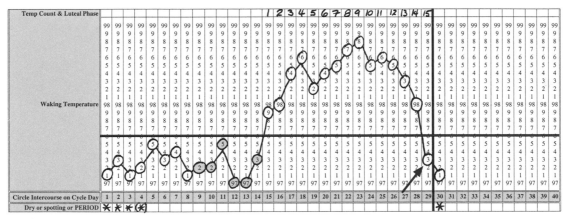

Chart A.17. Note that the luteal phase here is 15 days long because it goes from Day 15 through to and including Day 29, despite the fact there was a temperature drop on that day. Day 1 of the new cycle begins with the bleeding on the following day.

FEVER

You will inevitably have a fever now and then while charting. Practically speaking, it is best handled by using the Rule of Thumb. Assuming the temperature is off the chart, you can simply record the higher temperature above the 99, noting the fever and other symptoms of illness in the miscellaneous row. Be sure to draw a dotted line between the normal temperatures on both sides of your fever. (Also, remember that if you're using a glass BBT thermometer, you'll need to switch to a digital or fever thermometer for the days that you are sick.)

Depending on the intensity of the fever and when it occurs in the cycle, there are three possible impacts that it could have:

1. It could have no effect.
2. It could delay ovulation (causing a longer than usual cycle).
3. It could suppress ovulation (causing an anovulatory cycle).

If the fever occurs after you've already ovulated, it will almost certainly have no effect. If it occurs before you've ovulated, any of the three listed above are possible.

Regardless, you can continue to use FAM as birth control using all the rules described in Chapter 9. However, if your illness is preovulatory, you obviously have to eliminate the temperatures discounted by the fever, and thus *you cannot begin the 3-day count for the Temperature Shift Rule until you are no longer sick. Never assume you've entered your postovulatory infertile phase until you can clearly verify a thermal shift of 3 consecutive high temperatures without the interference of any fever.* And before assuming that you're safe, verify that your other fertility signs also reflect continued infertility (Chart A.18a).

The one time in the cycle when this can be a bit tricky is if you get sick in the few days immediately leading up to ovulation (Chart A.18b). Still, you should be able to verify that ovulation has occurred, since once you're no longer sick, your temperatures will drop down to the higher range of temperatures that you would normally have after ovulating. If the fever delayed (or suppressed) ovulation, your temperatures would drop all the way to their lower preovulatory range.

When using FAM as a method of birth control, just remember that the most effective way to use the method is to be sure *at least two signs coincide.* By doing this, you won't misinterpret the fever for a thermal shift, because if it really was a (preovulatory) fever, you have not yet entered your infertile phase.

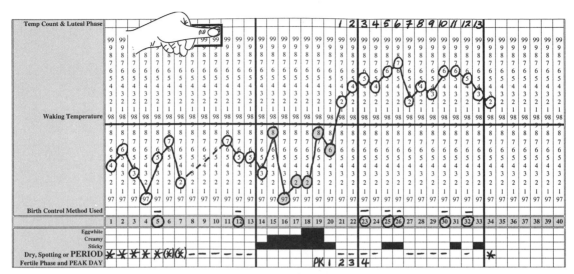

Chart A.18a. On Day 8 of her cycle, Cindy awakens to a bad flu, which pushes her temperatures off the chart for 3 days. She uses the Rule of Thumb for Days 8 to 10, in this case omitting those temps that are 99 or above. After recovering, she is able to verify that she still has not ovulated, since her temperature returns to its lower preovulatory range on Day 11. As she continues to chart, her signs reflect a delayed ovulation, which in this case probably occurs about Day 20.

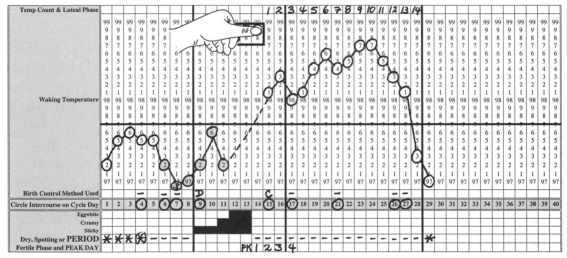

Chart A.18b. Eva awakens to a cold and low-grade fever, starting on Day 12. She uses the Rule of Thumb to discount Days 12 to 14. Completely well by Day 15, she carefully records her temperature and notices that it has only fallen to her relatively high postovulatory range. Thus she is able to start her temp count on Day 15, and by Day 17 she confirms through her two primary fertility signs that she has already ovulated. (Had her illness been intense enough to delay her ovulation, her temperature would have returned to its lower preovulatory range.)

10 OR FEWER DAYS OF HIGH TEMPERATURES ABOVE THE COVERLINE

If you have 10 or fewer days of postovulatory high temperatures above the coverline, it may indicate one of two things:

1. You have a short luteal phase (Chart A.19a).
   (For pregnancy achievers, this could be a problem. See page 174.)
2. Your temps may take a few days to reflect ovulation (Chart A.19b).

The way to determine what is occurring is to identify your Peak Day before the rise in temperature. Ovulation usually takes place within a day or so of that last day of wetness. If there is a large discrepancy between the Peak Day and the thermal shift, you can probably assume your temperature takes several days to increase following ovulation. But the only way to definitively confirm that is through ultrasound, which would obviously be very impractical.

If you are using FAM for birth control and would like to take advantage of more safe days than your temperature would otherwise allow, you could choose to depend on the cervical fluid and cervical position to determine your safe postovulatory phase. But, of course, this is not as conservative as also relying on the temperature.

And notice that if you only rely on cervical fluid and position, you can't assume that you've already ovulated. Thus any cervical fluid at any time in the cycle should be considered fertile, at least until a thermal shift verifies that ovulation has come and gone.

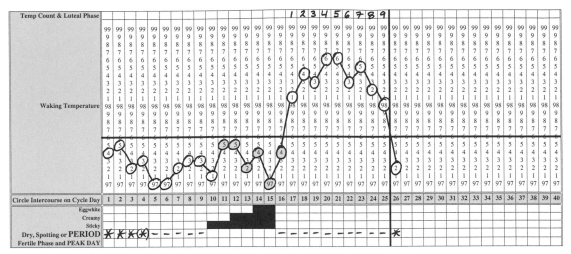

Chart A.19a. Short luteal phase. Note that her temperatures are probably an indication of a true short luteal phase (9 days in this case), because the shift coincides with her cervical fluid. She most likely ovulated about Day 16 on this chart, since ovulation usually occurs the day of, or the day after, the Peak Day.

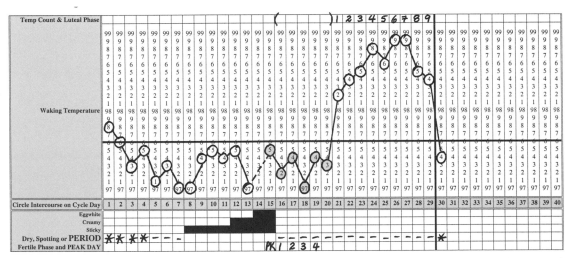

Chart A.19b. Probably normal luteal phase. By contrast, this chart shows that ovulation probably occurred earlier than the temperature reflected, because the Peak Day of cervical fluid was on Day 15, but the thermal shift wasn't until Day 21. Thus her body probably takes a few days to respond to the postovulatory progesterone, and she therefore does not really have a short luteal phase.

18 OR MORE HIGH TEMPERATURES AFTER OVULATION

If you have 18 or more consecutive high temperatures above the coverline with no sign of a period, it is almost always an indication of pregnancy. The sustained high temperatures are due to the corpus luteum continuing to live and release progesterone beyond its typical 12 to 16 day life span. In fact, in many pregnant women, the pattern of high temperatures even increases to a third level caused by the additional progesterone in their body (see next page).

Remember that most women will have a consistent luteal phase (the time from ovulation to menstruation). So, for example, if your own luteal phase is typically about 13 days, and your temperature remains high for 16 days, there is a good chance that you are pregnant. The point is to determine if the temperatures are staying high longer than what is normal for you.

Another possible reason for 18 high temperatures is an ovarian cyst, either from LUFS (see page 206), or a corpus luteum cyst. The latter is a rare condition in which the corpus luteum continues to live beyond the normal 12 to 16 days—even when the woman isn't pregnant. (Many women will have at least one such cyst in their lifetime.) If this should happen, the temperature may continue to remain high due to the progesterone that is still being emitted from the persistent corpus luteum. Of course, if the progesterone doesn't drop, the uterine lining is not shed during menstruation. It would therefore *appear* that you are pregnant.

You may also notice light spotting and mild pain about the time your period is due. A pregnancy test combined with a manual exam and ultrasound of the uterus may be warranted to rule out a corpus luteum cyst. If it turns out that you do have one, the good news is that they usually dissipate on their own.

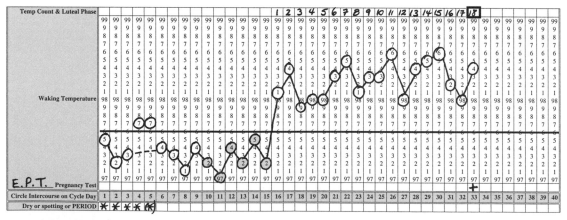

Chart A.20. High temps reflecting pregnancy.

TWO LEVELS OF HIGH TEMPERATURES AFTER OVULATION (TRIPHASIC PATTERN)

As mentioned in the previous section, a triphasic pattern of temperatures is virtually always caused by pregnancy. It is thought to be the result of additional progesterone circulating in the woman's body, and increases about the time of implantation of the egg. While there appears to be no discussion of this phenomenon in the medical literature, my professional experience is that this triphasic pattern seems to occur in most pregnant women who chart.

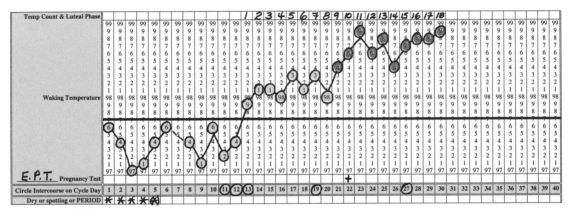

Chart A.21. Triphasic pregnancy pattern.

DROPPING TEMPERATURES AFTER EITHER 18 HIGH TEMPERATURES OR A POSITIVE PREGNANCY TEST

If you begin to experience sharply dropping temperatures after you have confirmed that you are pregnant through either 18 high temperatures or a pregnancy test, you should contact your doctor as soon as possible. The plummeting temps are often a strong indication that you are in danger of having a miscarriage. In healthy pregnancies, your postovulatory temps will almost always remain high due to the continued effects of progesterone.

Bleeding in itself is not necessarily a sign of danger, and indeed, many women notice normal implantation spotting in the week to 10 days following ovulation (see page 299). However, any significant bleeding beyond that should probably be checked by your physician.

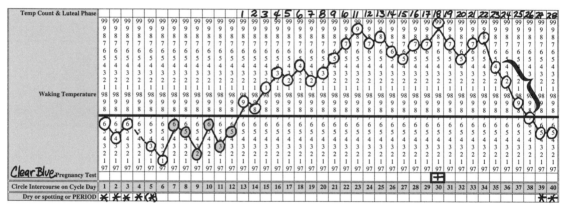

Chart A.22. Signs of a potential miscarriage.

WHEN TAKING ACCURATE TEMPERATURES IS NOT ALWAYS POSSIBLE

There are certain women who will be unable to take their waking temperatures at a consistent time. This may be because they have to work rotating shifts, or perhaps travel frequently across time zones. If you are ever in a situation where it is essentially impossible to obtain accurate waking temps, you can still use a modified form of the natural birth control method taught in this book. Unfortunately, it will require more days of abstinence or barriers.

This modified version relies exclusively on the Dry Day and Peak Day Rules as taught in Chapter 9. However, even after you have passed your Peak Day and counted your fourth evening beyond, you should not assume that you are infertile unless you are dry. This is because without a thermal shift to verify the passing of ovulation, you risk being misled by the cervical fluid into thinking that you have ovulated when you may actually have not. (This is often referred to as a "split peak," as discussed on page 132.)

To be most conservative, you should treat the presence of all cervical fluid and bleeding, including menses, as potentially fertile, no matter when it appears in the cycle. Unfortunately, this may mean using the "Peak + 4" rule more than once per cycle, although if the later patches of cervical fluid are only sticky and not wet you can get away with counting "Peak + 2" with little increase in risk. If you are able to verify that your cervix remains in its most infertile state (low and closed with no wet cervical fluid at the cervical tip), your increased risk from intercourse during any sticky days should be quite small.

For pregnancy achievers, inability to observe a thermal shift will unfortunately prevent you from learning about numerous facets of your fertility. However, the basic goal of timing intercourse for your most fertile cervical fluid days remains the same. (See Chapter 11.)

CONTINUAL STICKY CERVICAL FLUID DAY AFTER DAY (BASIC INFERTILE PATTERN)

Some women notice that they have a continuous nonchanging cervical fluid even during their infertile phase. You may want to get it checked to rule out any type of infection or cervical problem. If there is none, you should than consider such cervical fluid part of your Basic Infertile Pattern (BIP).

With a BIP, you will usually experience day after day of sticky cervical fluid at times in your cycle when you are not near ovulation. In order to establish a Basic Infertile Pattern, you must observe your cervical fluid very carefully for two weeks without the interference of semen, spermicides, douches, or anything else that may make your observations difficult.

Once you have established your BIP, any days with this pattern are treated as if they were dry, whether you are trying to avoid or achieve pregnancy. The trick is to learn to detect the *change* to a wetter, fertile-quality cervical fluid. For complete instructions on how to use FAM for birth control while you have a BIP with normal ovulatory cycles, see Appendix B.

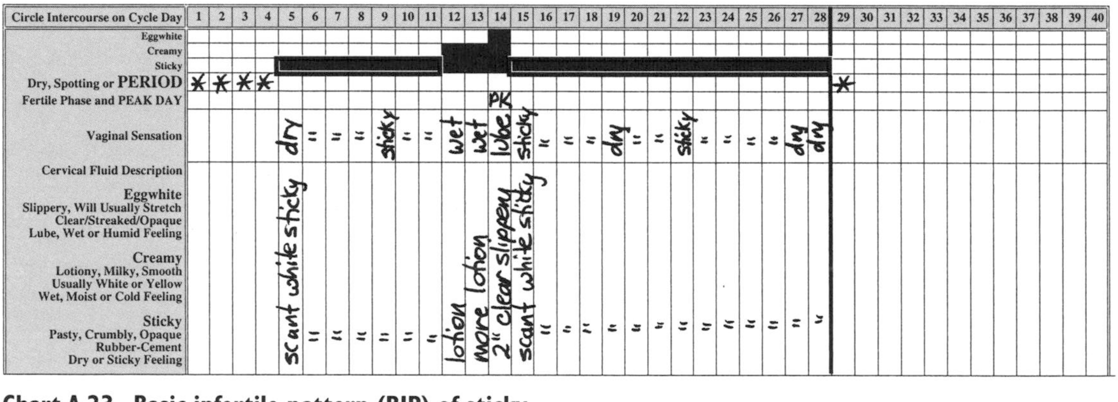

Chart A.23. Basic infertile pattern (BIP) of sticky.

CONTINUAL WET-QUALITY CERVICAL FLUID DAY AFTER DAY

If you notice continuous creamy or eggwhite-quality cervical fluid that extends for weeks at a time, it could be an indication of excessively high levels of oestrogen due to, among other conditions, PCOS (see page 204) or low thyroid function (see page 305). Some of the other symptoms of the latter condition include unusually long cycles with low waking temperatures. If you suspect you have either of these problems, you should consult a doctor.

Another common condition that may cause a prolonged phase of wet cervical fluid, often with a delayed Peak Day, is ovarian cysts. They are follicles in the ovary that stop developing before ovulation, forming fluid-filled cysts on the ovarian wall that usually last for a few weeks before disappearing on their own. Although they often have no symptoms, they can cause a chronic dull ache (usually on just one side), painful periods, or even pain during intercourse. Fortunately, physicians can usually diagnose them through a pelvic exam or ultrasound, and in most cases, they can be easily treated through a progesterone injection which disrupts the oestrogen dominance, dissipating the pain and allowing for bleeding 5 to 10 days later.

Prolonged wet cervical fluid could also be caused by stress. The classic stress-induced pattern usually consists of patches of wet cervical fluid as your body keeps attempting to ovulate, causing what appear to be split-peak days. Of course, a thermal shift will confirm when you ultimately *do* ovulate.

If you are breastfeeding, your body could be making numerous attempts to start ovulating again, thus extending your normal fertile pattern for longer than usual.

Finally, you could have a vaginal infection. If you have any of the following symptoms in addition to continual wetness, you should see a health practitioner for a proper diagnosis:

- abnormal discharge
- itching, stinging, swelling, and redness
- unpleasant odor
- blisters, warts, and chancre sores

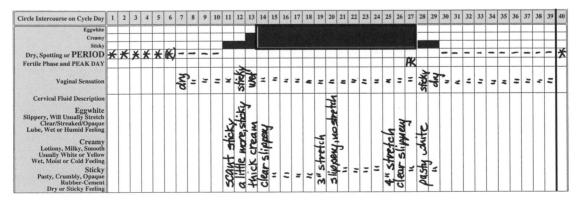

Chart A.24. Excessively wet cervical fluid.

WATERY CERVICAL FLUID RATHER THAN CREAMY

Occasionally, you may only have a watery cervical fluid that is either completely clear or the consistency and look of nonfat milk. In either case, consider it wet when charting. Fill in the "creamy" row, but then be sure to record the actual consistency in the Cervical Fluid Description row, treating it as fertile, just as you would creamy or eggwhite-quality cervical fluid.

For pregnancy achievers, however, this quality of cervical fluid may not have the viscosity necessary to allow sperm to swim. If this is the case, you might be able to benefit from one of the remedies discussed on page 173, or from IUI (intrauterine insemination) as described on page 207.

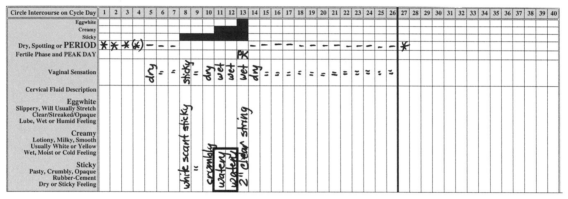

Chart A.25. Watery cervical fluid.

ABSENCE OF ANY EGGWHITE-QUALITY CERVICAL FLUID

You may find that you rarely if ever notice eggwhite-quality cervical fluid. Or you observe stretchy cervical fluid, but it is opaque rather than clear. Remember that fertile-quality cervical fluid is on a continuum, from dry to extremely wet, with the most fertile quality being the wettest. The wettest you produce may be just creamy. Either way, your Peak Day of fertility is always your last day of wet cervical fluid or a lubricative vaginal sensation, as described on page 91.

Women who have had cryosurgery or cone biopsies taken from their cervix may find that they don't produce much cervical fluid altogether. This is because many of the cervical crypts that produce the cervical fluid may be removed during these procedures. In addition, cervical infections may compromise cervical fluid production.

It is still possible to get pregnant without eggwhite, assuming you produce *some* wetness capable of sustaining sperm. However, cycles that do not produce eggwhite are not as fertile as those that do. In the end, if you are trying to get pregnant, and don't produce enough cervical fluid to conceive naturally, you have several options:

1. You can try plain Robitussin to increase the fertility of your cervical fluid. (See page 173.)
2. You can ask your doctor about taking a prescription of Estrace (not available in the UK) or Premarin. (See page 201 and Appendix I.)
3. You can have intrauterine insemination (IUI), the process in which sperm are deposited beyond your cervix directly into your uterus, bypassing the potential impediment of no cervical fluid. (See page 207.)

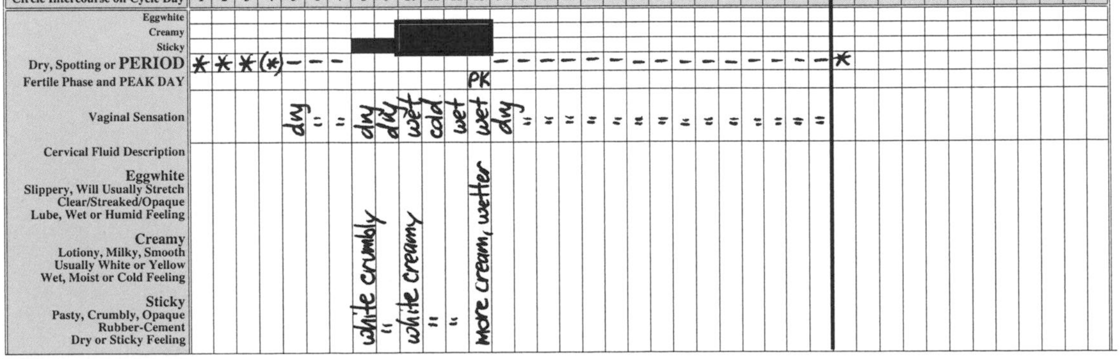

Chart A.26. No eggwhite-quality cervical fluid observed.

PATCHES OF WET CERVICAL FLUID INTERSPERSED OVER LONG CYCLES

Whether you are trying to avoid pregnancy or get pregnant, you should consider being checked for medical conditions such as PCOS if you have highly irregular or long cycles interspersed with long patches of slippery or stretchy cervical fluid (see page 204). In any case, you are still considered fertile during wet days as long as you have not seen your temperature rise.

Regardless, during the various phases in your life in which ovulation occurs less frequently, your body may go through episodes of trying to ovulate before it actually does. Eventually, after weeks or months of experiencing "false starts" in the form of patches of cervical fluid, you should be able to verify that ovulation took place by the arrival of a thermal shift.

For contraceptors, this transitional pattern can be frustrating in that the sympto-thermal rules require you to abstain or use barriers every day from the first day that you get your initial patch of cervical fluid. Technically, this would even include the first dry days that follow (as long as there is no thermal shift to show that ovulation has passed).

However, if you have this pattern, you can apply the Billings Method with only a slightly increased risk. This method allows you to discard the Temperature Shift Rule and simply apply the Peak Day Rule (meaning you are safe the evening of the 4th day after your Peak Day, as described on page 131). If you do this, though, remember you must continue to carefully check your cervical fluid every day, at least until you can observe a thermal shift that verifies you have ovulated. And with every *new* patch of cervical fluid, you must apply the Peak Day Rule again.

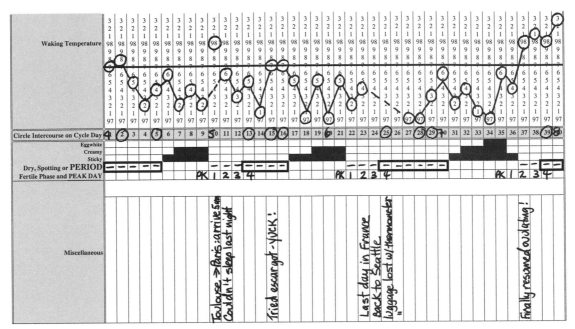

Chart A.27. Cervical fluid patches. When Courtney traveled to France for the summer, her cycle was thrown off kilter, and thus she actually didn't ovulate until about Day 76 (note that this chart starts with cycle Day 41). Several times over the summer her body "prepared" to ovulate, but then stopped short, as seen by the sporadic patches of cervical fluid in the weeks leading up to her thermal shift. With this extended cycle, she chose to use the Billings Method, which does not use the Temperature Shift Rule. Thus she considers herself infertile the evening of the fourth day after *each* one of her Peak Days, through to the following patch of cervical fluid. (Infertile evenings are boxed in red.)

WET, CREAMY CERVICAL FLUID WELL AFTER OVULATION

After ovulation, there is a second smaller surge of oestrogen well into the luteal phase, which occasionally causes a day or two of creamy cervical fluid. This often coincides with a temporary drop in temperatures. It is not an indication of returning fertility. So pregnancy avoiders need not be concerned, assuming the Temperature Shift and Peak Day rules have clearly shown ovulation has already occurred. If you're not sure, don't take risks. (See page 310.)

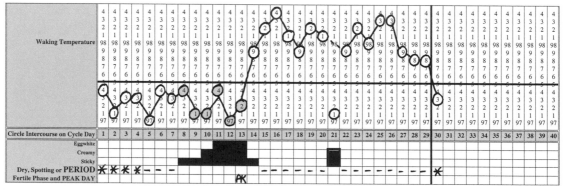

Chart A.28a. Creamy cervical fluid mid-luteal phase.

WET SENSATION OR EGGWHITE BEFORE MENSTRUATION

Having a very wet, watery sensation, or even an eggwhite-quality substance about a day or two before your period is absolutely normal. It is merely an indication that the corpus luteum has disintegrated, as it does before menstruation. The first part of the lining that typically flows out when progesterone drops is the water that composed part of the endometrial lining. This watery substance is not to be confused with fertile-quality cervical fluid. It has no bearing on your fertility. By definition, if it comes out just before your period and after you have established that you are in your infertile phase, than you are indeed not fertile on that day.

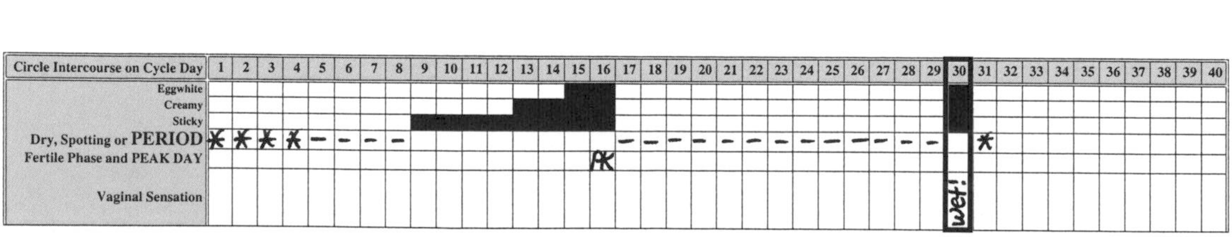

Circle Intercourse on Cycle Day	1	2	3	4	5	6	7	8	9	10	11	12	13	14	15	16	17	18	19	20	21	22	23	24	25	26	27	28	29	30	31	32	33	34	35	36	37	38	39	40
Eggwhite																																								
Creamy																																								
Sticky																																								
Dry, Spotting or PERIOD	✗	✗	✗	✗	–	–	–	–									–	–	–	–	–	–	–	–	–	–	–	–	–		✗									
Fertile Phase and PEAK DAY															PK																									
Vaginal Sensation																														wet!										

Chart A.28b. Lubricative feeling or substance on day or so before period.

INFECTION MASKING CERVICAL FLUID

Vaginal infections produce many aggravations, including their ability to mask cervical fluid. What typically differentiates most infections from healthy cervical fluid is that infections usually have at least one of the following symptoms:

1. True discharge, which is perhaps gray, green, foamy, or even like cottage cheese
2. Itching or irritation such as stinging
3. An unpleasant or unusual odor
4. Discoloration of the vagina, such as redness
5. Potential swelling of the vagina and vaginal opening

If you suspect that you have an infection, you should record a question mark in the Cervical Fluid Description row. It is imperative that you abstain from intercourse during this time in order to allow your body a chance to heal, and to prevent passing it back and forth between you and your partner. If nothing else, it can be extremely painful to have sex when you have an infection!

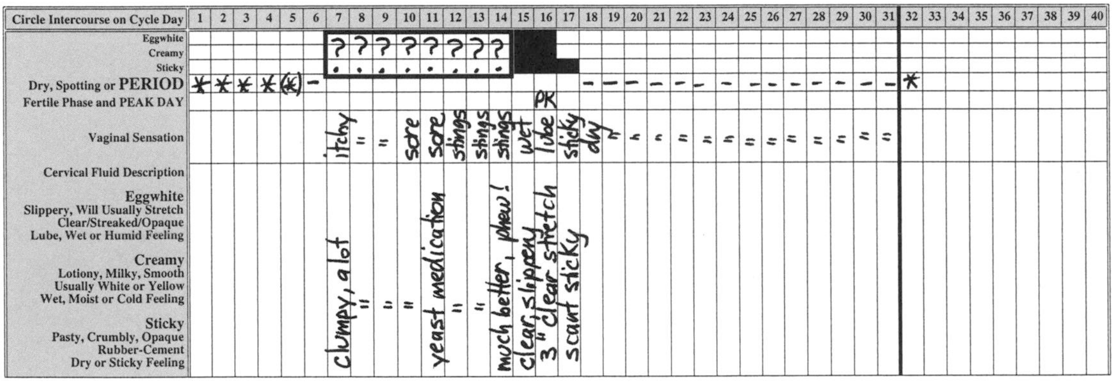

Chart A.29. Vaginal infection.

WET CERVICAL FLUID FOUND AT THE CERVIX BUT NOT AT THE VAGINAL OPENING

Women who check their cervical fluid at the cervical tip may notice that it sometimes seems wetter or more abundant than what they simultaneously observe at the vaginal opening. This is logical, since it can take a few hours for the cervical fluid to trickle down.

Remember to keep in mind that if you check internally, you will always have at least a slight moisture or film on your finger that should not be confused with cervical fluid. Simply wave your finger in the air for a few seconds. If the dampness dissipates, then you know it was only the moisture from the vagina itself.

If you find a slight, white filmy substance on your finger but your vaginal sensation is *dry,* you may then consider that day a dry day. This is because women will usually have such a substance internally even when it appears as if they are dry externally. This would still be considered low fertility.

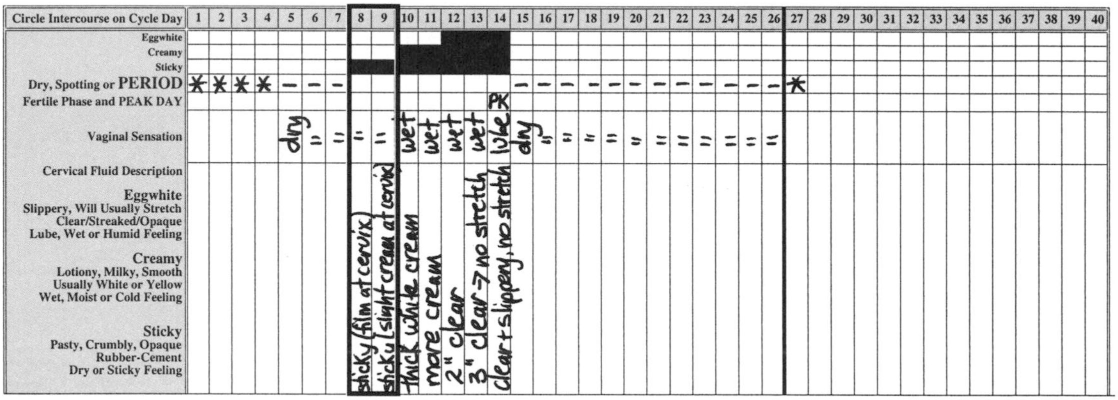

Chart A.30. Note that cervical fluid that is wetter at the cervical tip than externally, as well as any filmlike substance, can be recorded in the Cervical Fluid Description row. But the shading you record in the Cervical Fluid row should reflect what you observe at the external vaginal opening. You may prefer to use the Master Chart at the back of the book that is labeled in the bottom right-hand corner "Birth Control (internal and external cervical fluid checking)."

CERVIX THAT CAN'T BE FOUND

Although at times you may think your cervix has migrated up your body and out your ear, surprisingly, it is still there. When a woman is approaching ovulation, her cervix rises, often becoming so high it feels inaccessible. If this is the case, trust your body. If you have been able to feel it before, it probably means that you are just very fertile at that time. In such a case, simply record a question mark in the Cervix row on the days you can't actually feel it.

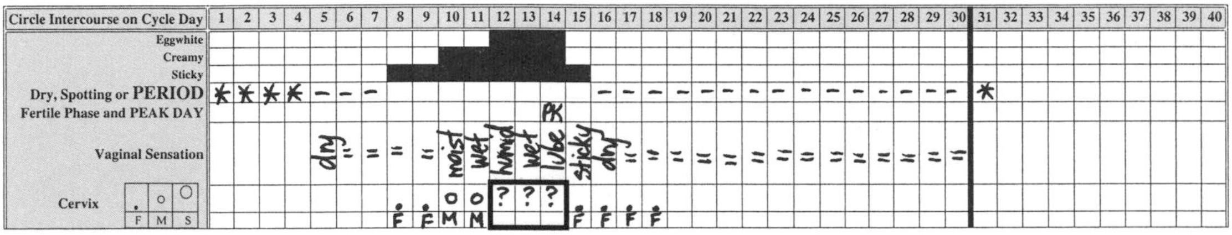

Chart A.31a. Missing cervix.

CERVIX THAT NEVER FULLY CLOSES

Women who have delivered a child vaginally usually have a cervix that never completely closes during the infertile phase. On infertile days, rather than feeling a tiny dimple, it feels more like a horizontal, slight opening. The trick is to learn how to differentiate between the subtle changes in the oval-shaped opening as ovulation approaches.

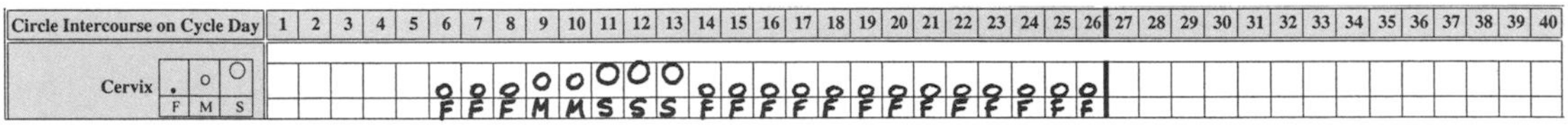

Chart A.31b. Partially open cervix.

BUMPS ON THE SURFACE OF THE CERVIX

You may notice bumps that feel like large, hard granules of sand just under the skin of the cervix. They are called nabothian cysts. Usually considered harmless, they tend to disappear on their own. Still, you may want to have a clinician confirm your suspicion the first time you feel one. Some women notice that they come and go with the cycle. Of course, a woman would probably never realize she had them unless she checked her cervix.

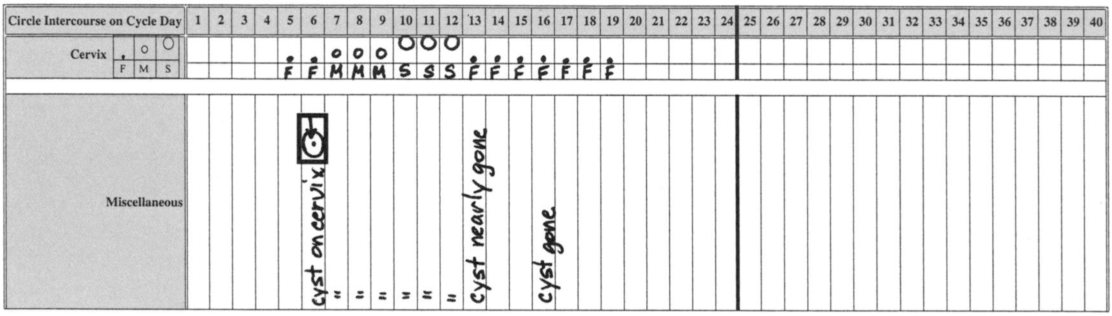

Circle Intercourse on Cycle Day	1	2	3	4	5	6	7	8	9	10	11	12	13	14	15	16	17	18	19	20	21	22	23	24	25	26	27	28	29	30	31	32	33	34	35	36	37	38	39	40
Cervix					•	•	o	o	o	O	O	O																												
					F	F	M	M	M	S	S	S	F	F	F	F	F	F																						

Miscellaneous — cyst on cervix / cyst nearly gone / cyst gone

Chart A.32. Nabothian cysts on cervix.

PAIN OR STINGING DURING INTERCOURSE

You may occasionally feel a deep pain during intercourse, depending on where you are in your cycle, and the sexual position you use. One of the causes of such pain may be the height of the cervix in your vagina at the time. When a woman is not in her fertile phase, the cervix is at its lowest point and can actually be tapped by her partner's penis during intercourse, especially if she straddles atop him. This is because that position tends to push the cervix down to its lowest point. To remedy the problem, simply be aware of how high your cervix is on any given day and avoid the position that causes discomfort.

Another cause could be from even the slightest tapping of the already tender ovary about to release an egg. Even a full bladder could cause pain during intercourse. However, if the pain is deep and intense, it could be a sign of an ovarian cyst or a more serious condition such as endometriosis.

Finally, if you feel vaginal pain or stinging, the causes may include a vaginal infection (symptoms are listed on page 223), a lack of lubrication, an allergy to latex, spermicide, or soap, or even vulvodynia, an increasingly recognized condition which can cause intense pain at the opening of the vagina.

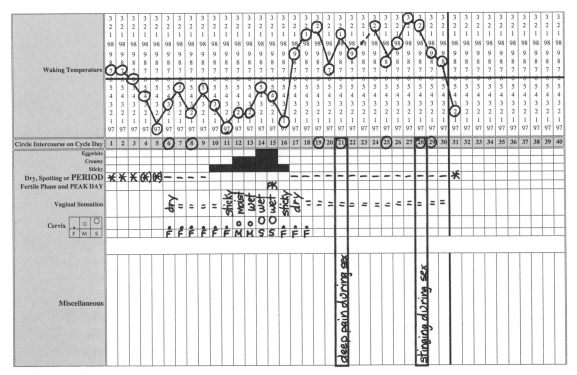

Chart A.33. Uncomfortable intercourse.

SPOTTING AFTER INTERCOURSE

Some women will notice occasional spotting after making love. It is usually due to the cervix being tapped by the penis. This is especially likely when the cervix is lowest and most vulnerable to being hit, especially postovulatory. If this occurs, it may be caused by such conditions as cervicitis (an inflammation of the cervix), cervical polyps (a common benign, protruding growth from the cervix), or a vaginal infection. Any of these conditions is easily remedied through an office visit. Finally, if the bleeding is heavy or occurs often, you should consult a physician to make sure it isn't anything more serious, such as cervical cancer.

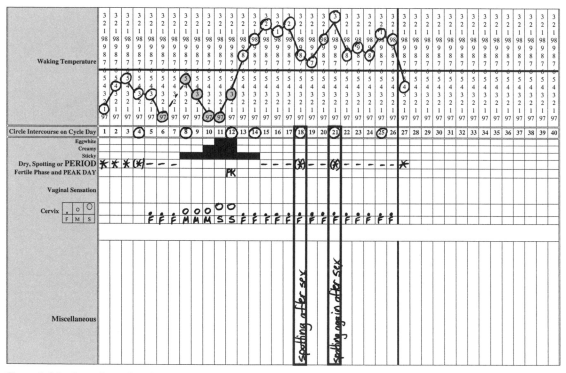

Chart A.34. Spotting after intercourse.

Using FAM for Birth Control During Special Circumstances (Stress, Breastfeeding, Premenopause, etc.)

> Please note: Before reading this appendix, you should have internalized the basic principles of Chapters 6 and 9. However, there is no reason to read these pages if your charting has revealed that you are ovulating normally. Breastfeeding women should read this appendix as well as the following one specifically devoted to using FAM while nursing. You should also be aware that FAM is a more difficult method to learn while you are going through these menstrual transitions.

The typical woman will experience about 400 periods in her lifetime. (OK, OK, kvetch and moan, if you must.) But remember, not every bleeding episode is preceded by ovulation, and therefore, technically, such anovulatory bleeding is not menstruation. Teenagers and breastfeeding or premenopausal women may go months without ovulating but may still experience menstrual-like bleeding.

Even excluding these groups, it is possible that the average woman may have an anovulatory cycle about once every year or two. And, occasionally, women may go for months without any bleeding at all. What all of this means is that if you bleed, it may or may not imply that you ovulated, but if you ovulate, you will bleed (unless, of course, you get pregnant.)

When a woman isn't ovulating, it would seem obvious that she isn't fertile, right? Well, yes and no. When women don't ovulate, of course they aren't fertile. But ironically, anovulatory cycles can be a little more challenging to interpret, because the obvious patterns of fertility don't occur. In essence, then, the woman must act as if she is continually in a preovulatory phase, since ovulation *could* still occur. This situation is very different from a typical cycle in which the fertility signs reflect the obvious approach and passing of ovulation.

Anovulation can be a temporary phase lasting no more than a month or two, or it could last up to several years. As described above, long periods of time without menstruation often occur during phases such as adolescence, breastfeeding, and premenopause. In addition, women coming off the Pill or other hormones, or those who exercise strenuously and whose body fat is extremely low, may also go for a long time without ovulating. There may also be physiological conditions that affect the hormone system. And finally, other factors that could delay ovulation for short or long phases are situations such as stress, illness, or travel.

✎ YOUR BASIC INFERTILE PATTERN (BIP) WHEN NOT OVULATING

During anovulatory cycles, you will usually experience a *Basic Infertile Pattern* (BIP) unlike what you are normally used to. Many women who experience a long phase of anovulation are continually dry, day after day. Other women may notice that instead of experiencing dry days when not ovulating, they have the same type of sticky cervical fluid, day after day. (This is usually normal, though you may want to check with a clinician to rule out the possibility of cervical inflammation.)

Regardless, if you also have a dry vaginal sensation, these days are treated *as if* they were dry days, but only after you have clearly established your BIP. While this modification is considered safe, there may be a small increase in risk, and therefore I strongly suggest that if you have a sticky BIP, it is best to check your cervical tip before intercourse to verify that there is no *wet* cervical fluid present. If there is, do not consider yourself safe.

✎ ESTABLISHING YOUR BASIC INFERTILE PATTERN

In order to establish a BIP, you must observe your cervical fluid very carefully for 2 weeks without the interference of semen, spermicides, douches, or anything else that may mask its observation. Ideally you should abstain during this time.

Once you have charted your cervical fluid for 2 consecutive weeks, and have established that you are continually dry, or have the same sticky-type cervical fluid, you have established your Basic Infertile Pattern. *Only then may you apply the two anovulatory rules listed in the two pink boxes on the following pages.*

UNCHANGING DAY RULE

If your 2-week Basic Infertile Pattern (BIP) is dry or the same-quality sticky cervical fluid day after day, you are safe for unprotected intercourse the evening of every dry or unchanging sticky day. (Women with a BIP of wet cervical fluid must consider themselves fertile.)

The Unchanging Day Rule Applied

Thus, if your 2-week BIP is *sticky* day after day, you are safe to have intercourse the evenings of sticky days (as if they were dry), as shown in Chart B.1 below.

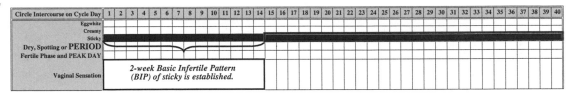

Chart B.1. Basic Infertile Pattern of sticky days. (Infertile evenings are boxed in red.)

A Basic Infertile Pattern of Both Dry and Sticky Cervical Fluid

You may observe a pattern of dry *and* sticky over the 2-week observation time in which you determine your BIP. If you are a new user of FAM, I would encourage you to consider only the evening of a dry day as safe. For experienced users of FAM, you may choose to use such a combination pattern as your BIP, paying special attention to any *change* to a wet-type cervical fluid. But you should be aware that you are taking a slightly greater risk when you consider a combination of dry and sticky as a Basic Infertile Pattern. If you have this type of BIP, I would particularly urge you to verify that you have no wet cervical fluid at your cervical tip before having intercourse.

A Word About Semen Masking Cervical Fluid

If there is semen or spermicide present the day after intercourse, you should note it with a question mark since it could mask cervical fluid. The day of semen is then considered potentially fertile.

As mentioned near the bottom of the box on page 88, a trick to eliminate the semen from your body following intercourse is to do SETs, or Semen Emitting Technique. If the day after intercourse you experience the same unchanged cervical fluid, you are safe for unprotected sex again that evening.

℘ SIGNS OF IMPENDING OVULATION

Occasionally, during the various phases of your life in which ovulation doesn't occur, your body may go through episodes of trying to ovulate before it actually does. During this time, after weeks or months of experiencing the same BIP, you may notice *patches* of more fertile cervical fluid interspersed with the dry or sticky days. It is critical to be attentive to such changes because it is your body's way of reflecting hormonal activity that may lead to ovulation again. So if you notice patches of more fertile cervical fluid interspersed among the dry or sticky phases, you must follow the rule below.

> ### PATCH RULE
>
> You are safe the evening of every day that your 2-week Basic Infertile Pattern remains the same. But as soon as you see a change in your BIP, you must consider yourself fertile until the evening of the fourth consecutive nonwet day after the Peak Day. The Peak Day is the last day of the more fertile patch of cervical fluid or lubricative vaginal sensation in your BIP. Obviously, any type of wet cervical fluid or bleeding must be considered a fertile patch.

The Patch Rule Applied

So, for example, if your 2-week BIP is dry day after day, you are considered safe the evening of any dry day. But if you get a patch of any type of cervical fluid following the 2-week observation time, you must consider those days potentially fertile through to the evening of the fourth consecutive nonwet day after your Peak Day (Chart B.2, below).

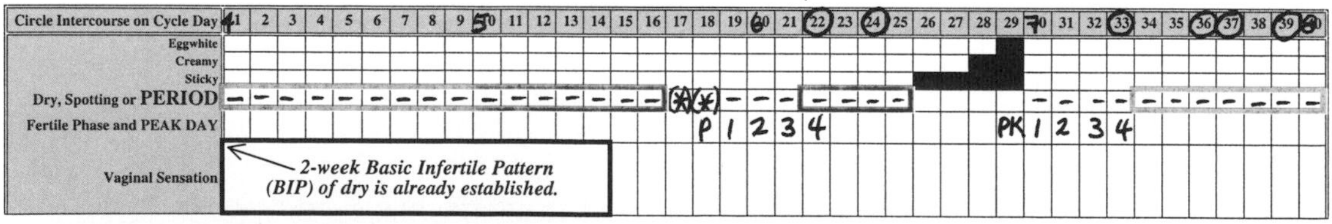

Chart B.2. Patch Rule with Basic Infertile Pattern of dry days. When she developed patches of spotting, sticky, or wet cervical fluid interspersed throughout her dry days, she considered herself fertile until she could identify the Peak Day plus 1,2,3,4. So in this chart the first patch she considered fertile started on Day 57 and continued through until Peak plus 4, or the evening of Day 62. She then considered herself safe all the dry evenings of dry days until her next patch on Day 66. Also note that if cycles extend beyond 40 days, you can renumber Day 1 of the chart as 41, as seen above. (Infertile evenings are boxed in red.)

If your 2-week BIP is sticky day after day, you are considered safe the evening of any sticky day. But if you get a patch of any type of wet cervical fluid following the 2-week observation time, you must consider those days potentially fertile through to the evening of the fourth consecutive nonwet day after your Peak Day (Chart B.3, below).

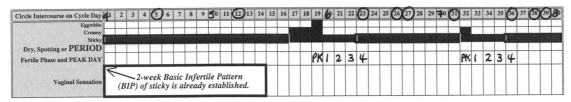

Chart B.3. Patch Rule with Basic Infertile Pattern of sticky days. When she developed patches of spotting or wet cervical fluid interspersed throughout her sticky days, she considered herself fertile until she could identify the Peak Day plus 1,2,3,4. So in this chart the first patch she considered fertile started on Day 57 and continued through until Peak plus 4, or the evening of Day 63. She then considered herself safe all the evenings of sticky days until her next patch on Day 72. (Infertile evenings are boxed in red.)

A Less Conservative Approach

Some clinicians believe if the patch is of a *sticky*- rather than wet-quality cervical fluid, you need only wait until the evening of the second nonwet day (rather than the fourth) beyond your Peak Day (Chart B.4, below).

This less conservative approach is still considered very safe, but if you absolutely can't risk a pregnancy, you should either wait until the evening of the fourth consecutive nonwet day beyond your Peak Day, or verify that there is no cervical fluid at the cervical tip before having intercourse.

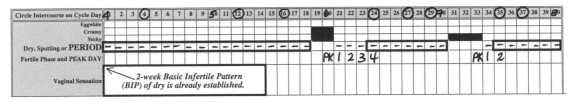

Chart B.4. Less conservative Patch Rule with Basic Infertile Pattern of dry days. She still counts 4 days after any patch of wet cervical fluid (or spotting), and thus with the cervical patch of Days 59 and 60, she does not consider herself safe until the evening of Day 64. However, she chose to be a little less conservative with patches that were only *sticky,* and thus with the patch ending Day 73, she considers herself infertile on the evening of Day 75, just 2 days after it ended. (Infertile evenings are boxed in red.)

Bleeding During Anovulatory Phases

When women experience episodes of bleeding during phases of anovulation, it is imperative that they treat those particular days as *potentially fertile*. The bleeding could be an indication of either ovulatory spotting or the start of hormonal activity preparing for ovulation. The key to determining *true* menstruation is the observation of a thermal shift 12 to 16 days prior.

Deciding what to call Day 1 of the cycle can be somewhat confusing when the bleeding is not true menstrual bleeding. You can either choose to start a new chart each time you have an episode of bleeding or continue as if you are experiencing one continuous, potentially months-long cycle with intermittent phases of bleeding. The critical point is to be able to identify when the bleeding is true menstruation.

Of course, this is where the basal temperatures will indicate once you've really ovulated. Remember that you normally have a thermal shift about 12 to 16 days prior to true menstruation. But when you are starting to resume cycling for the first time in months, your luteal phase may initially be shorter until your cycles get back to normal.

Changes in Your BIP

If a new cervical fluid pattern continues to be the same day after day for at least 2 weeks, that patch now becomes your *new* Basic Infertile Pattern, from which you must be on the lookout for yet another change. So, for example, if you had been dry day after day, then had a patch of sticky cervical fluid that lasted more than 2 weeks, that sticky quality would become your new BIP. You would then be considered safe all of those subsequent evenings until you observe a more fertile-quality patch (such as creamy) or experience spotting or bleeding. You must treat those patches as possibly fertile until you can apply the Patch Rule described earlier on page 336.

A Word of Caution for Premenopausal Women

Unfortunately, premenopausal women who follow the BIP rules could be at somewhat greater risk of pregnancy than their younger peers. While it is true that women are less fertile in their 40s, ironically, their cervical fluid can become wet more quickly during premenopause. Thus a woman who has a BIP pattern of sticky days may find herself becoming creamy or eggwhite faster than before, when a gradual transition occurred over a few days. As a result, the body may progress faster toward ovulation than in earlier years. Therefore, some FAM experts feel that a premenopausal woman should limit preovulatory intercourse to the evening of *dry* days only, since sperm will die in just a few hours in that environment.

I agree that premenopausal women may be taking a slightly greater risk in following the BIP rules. However I believe that the increased risk can be kept to a minimum *if you check your cervical fluid internally at the cervical tip to verify that there is no wet fluid present before having intercourse.* By taking this precaution, you are minimizing the possibility of a quick transition to the fertile wet cervical fluid needed for sperm survival.

❧ CONCLUDING REMARKS ON FAM AND ANOVULATORY PHASES

The most important point to remember when experiencing anovulation is to constantly be on the lookout for a change in cervical fluid that could indicate approaching ovulation. Ideally, you should continue to take your temperature to confirm that you are not ovulating. However, if you find this tedious during long months of not seeing a thermal shift, you could choose to wait to take your temperature until you see your cervical fluid change. Either way, remember that you always have the benefit of checking your cervix during times of uncertainty.

These rules are admittedly more complex than the standard FAM rules, and thus I encourage you to study the pink summary box on the back of this page. Until you internalize them, you can always use the rules discussed in Chapter 9, but this means that in doing so, you may have to consider yourself fertile more days than you would probably care to.

Finally, you should know that you will usually have ample warning of cycles resuming by the buildup of patches of cervical fluid as your body tries to ovulate. Just keep in mind that phases of anovulation can be confusing, so you need to be on the lookout for changes. And while it may be frustrating at times, remember that anovulatory phases will probably be a very small part of your reproductive life.

❧ SUMMARY OF NATURAL BIRTH CONTROL RULES WHILE EXPERIENCING ANOVULATION

UNCHANGING DAY RULE

If your 2-week Basic Infertile Pattern (BIP) is dry or the same-quality sticky cervical fluid day after day, you are safe for unprotected intercourse the evening of every dry or unchanging sticky day. (Women with a BIP of wet cervical fluid must consider themselves fertile.)

PATCH RULE

You are safe the evening of every day that your 2-week Basic Infertile Pattern remains the same. But as soon as you see a change in your BIP, you must consider yourself fertile until the evening of the fourth consecutive nonwet day after the Peak Day. The Peak Day is the last day of the more fertile patch of cervical fluid or lubricative vaginal sensation in your BIP. Any type of wet cervical fluid or bleeding must be considered a fertile patch.

Using FAM While Nursing Your Baby

> Please note: This appendix will be confusing if you haven't internalized the basic principles and rules discussed in the preceding appendix.

For those optimists who think you'll actually have *time* for lovemaking after having a baby, this appendix is for you. While breastfeeding is a wonderful and gratifying experience for most women, it can be difficult to identify when fertility will return, especially for those who haven't charted before. So let's set the record straight right from the beginning: Women *can* get pregnant while breastfeeding!

So why all the confusion over whether or not women are fertile while breastfeeding? Everybody has a neighbor, friend, or relative who swears they did or didn't get pregnant while nursing. These nursing women then become the standard by which people judge the effectiveness of breastfeeding for birth control.

Actually, the answer to the question of fertility during breastfeeding lies in how we define breastfeeding. It's true that the majority of women who breastfeed "on request," meaning throughout the day and night and every time the baby is hungry, may not see their periods resume for as long as a year or more. However, most women's fertility will only be suppressed by such intense breastfeeding if they also limit pacifiers and supplements, including water. It's simple biology.

This is because every time a baby suckles at the breast, it indirectly suppresses the hormones that trigger ovulation. But in order for breastfeeding to efficiently prevent the release of eggs, the baby must suckle at least every 4 hours during the day and every 6 hours at night. Thus, the key to determining when your cycles will return is to remember that *the longer and more often your baby is away from your breast, the sooner you will start ovulating again.*

341

&Fa; LEVEL OF BREASTFEEDING THAT AFFECTS FERTILITY

The table on page 346 is a simple synopsis of the factors that will determine which rules of natural birth control to use until your cycles resume after childbirth. As a new mother, you will choose to do one of the following:

- fully or nearly fully breastfeed on request
- partially breastfeed
- not breastfeed at all

Full or Nearly Full Breastfeeding

One of the best gifts you can give your baby is the life-long health benefit provided by breastfeeding. Not only is it excellent nourishment, but it offers important immunological protection against disease and allergies. Yet to fully attain such advantages, you should breastfeed around the clock, whenever your baby is hungry. Ideally, no supplements should be given during the first six months.

While such a disciplined regimen may be difficult to maintain, nature will reward you with one of the simplest and most effective forms of natural contraception available. You will be able to use the Lactational Amenorrhea Method (LAM)* if you meet the following three criteria:

LACTATIONAL AMENORRHEA METHOD (LAM)

- your menses have not returned
- you are fully or nearly fully breastfeeding
- your baby is less than 6 months old

The first criterion of LAM is that you have not resumed menstruating. What this means in practice is that any vaginal bleeding before the 56th day after giving birth is almost always anovulatory (and therefore can be ignored), assuming you are fully or nearly fully breastfeeding. However, any bleeding after the 56th day should be considered a sign of resumed ovulation.

---

* "Lactational" means pertaining to the production of milk and "amenorrhea" means lack of menstruation.

Full breastfeeding means that you are not giving your baby *any* supplements or pacifiers. However, the Institute of Reproductive Health at Georgetown University has shown through extensive studies that the contraceptive effectiveness of LAM is maintained even if your breastfeeding is *nearly* full, meaning that you supplement no more than 15% of all feedings. Of course the risk of resumed ovulation is on a continuum, and thus you should try to breastfeed as close to fully as possible. In addition, full or nearly full breastfeeding means that intervals between feedings should not exceed 4 hours during the day or 6 hours at night.

With LAM, you may prefer not to chart if you meet the boxed criteria, since it has a method failure rate of less than 2% per year. This is a tremendous advantage because charting while breastfeeding can be somewhat challenging. However, if you do not meet the LAM criteria, you will need to follow the FAM rules for breastfeeding discussed below.

Partial Breastfeeding

Partial breastfeeding means that supplements such as juices and solids are regularly given. It also means that you are nursing less frequently than every 4 hours during the day, and less than every 6 hours at night. Charting while partially breastfeeding is particularly challenging because it's harder to know when you will resume ovulating. Basically, you should follow the two anovulatory rules discussed in the preceding appendix (Unchanging-Day Rule and Patch Rule). But keep in mind that ovulation may return soon, since any supplements or long periods between nursing can lead to the early resumption of cycling. Of course, once true menstruation resumes, you should revert back to the four standard rules covered in Chapter 9.

When you are establishing your Basic Infertile Pattern discussed on page 334, chart your cervical fluid for 2 weeks following the stopping of lochia, the postchildbirth spotting. Ideally, you should abstain during this time in order to get an accurate reflection of what type of cervical fluid you produce while breastfeeding. (Chances are, if you've just had a baby, intercourse isn't top on your list of favorite activities, anyway.)*

---

* In fact, one of the most common complaints of breastfeeding mothers is that their vaginas tend to be dry, often making intercourse uncomfortable. This is due to the low levels of estrogen indirectly caused from circulating prolactin. But as your body gets closer to finally resuming cycling again after childbirth, this condition should dissipate on its own.

Once you start introducing supplements to your baby's diet, especially at about 6 months of age, you should breastfeed your baby *before* giving the supplement. The benefit of this approach is that your breast milk provides your baby with protection against disease while nursing helps to suppress the return of your ovulation.

Not Breastfeeding At All (Strictly Bottle Feeding)

Women who don't breastfeed find that their cycles resume very quickly—as early as 4 to 10 weeks after childbirth. If you aren't breastfeeding following the birth of your baby, you should start charting shortly after birth, since you can be fairly sure that your cycles will soon return. Note that in following the standard FAM rules, you must assume that you are in a preovulatory state until a temperature shift confirms that you have ovulated that first time after childbirth.

℘ THE TRANSITION TO RESUMED FERTILITY FOR ALL BREASTFEEDING WOMEN

Breastfeeding women will almost always have a warning of returning fertility through their cervical fluid. In fact, the episodes of cervical fluid may tend to be somewhat longer than normal as the body attempts to finally ovulate after months of anovulation. You will probably notice quite a few "false starts" in which you see longer and longer patches of fertile-quality cervical fluid as your body tries to finally pass over the oestrogen threshold necessary to release an egg.

One of the most important points to understand regarding the transition to fertility relates to what is considered fertile-quality cervical fluid. Once your cycles resume (as reflected by a thermal shift), *any* preovulatory cervical fluid is considered fertile. In other words, the type of sticky cervical fluid that may have previously reflected infertility (your Basic Infertile Pattern) must now be considered fertile *once you start cycling again*. The bottom line is that you must go back to the four standard rules used for normal cycles discussed in Chapter 9.

✌ CONCLUDING REMARKS ON NATURAL BIRTH CONTROL WHILE BREASTFEEDING

The most important point to remember when experiencing the transition from childbirth to resumed cycling is to constantly be on the lookout for a *change* in cervical fluid that could indicate approaching ovulation. You may prefer to not take your temperature until you see that change. And, of course, you can always have the benefit of checking your cervical position during times of uncertainty.

You should also not be surprised if you go through weeks or even months of wet cervical fluid before you return to normal cycles. (In such a case, you'll need to decide whether you want to abstain or use a barrier method.)

Remember that your body has not ovulated in a long time, and it may take a while for it to get back into its usual pattern of fertility. This can be frustrating, but try to keep it all in perspective. Before you know it, your baby will be dating and you'll be dealing with bigger issues than your *own* contraceptive concerns!

NATURAL BIRTH CONTROL RULES WHILE BREASTFEEDING

Degree of Breastfeeding	Natural Birth Control Method	Natural Birth Control Rules	When to Resume Taking Waking Temperatures	Comments
Not Breast-feeding at All	FAM with: *Standard* rules	First Five Days Rule Dry Day Rule Temp Shift Rule Peak Day Rule	By Day 14 after baby's birth	Cycles may resume within 4 weeks of child-birth. You must consider your-self preovulatory until you can confirm that ovulation has resumed by temperature shift prior to menstruation.
Partial Breastfeeding Partial breastfeeding means that sup-plements such as bottlefeeding, juices, and solids are fre-quently given. It also means nurs-ing less frequently than every 4 hours during the day or every 6 hours at night.	FAM with: *Anovulatory* rules	Unchanging Day Rule Patch Rule	• When you notice a change in your Basic Infertile Pat-tern of cervical fluid or • When you have a bleeding episode or • When your baby suddenly de-creases suckling or • When you intro-duce solid foods (whichever comes first)	Partial breastfeeding is the most challenging to chart because it is harder to predict when you will resume ovulating. You must consider your-self preovulatory until you can confirm that ovulation has resumed by temperature shift prior to a menstruation.
Full or Nearly Full Breastfeeding Full breastfeeding means not giving supplements at all, whereas *nearly* full means that supple-ments are given, but for no more than 15% of feedings. It also means nurs-ing at intervals of at least every 4 hours during the day and at least every 6 hours at night. (A critical point: for contraceptive pur-poses, the first two criteria listed to the far right must also apply.)	Lactational Amenorrhea Method (LAM)	None, so long as the LAM criteria in the right column are met.	• When you have your first bleed-ing episode which is over 56 days since childbirth or • When the baby is 5 to 6 months old or • When you in-crease the use of solids or supple-ments to more than 15% of feed-ings or no longer nurse your baby at least every 4 hours during the day and every 6 hours at night (whichever comes first)	LAM has a method fail-ure rate of less than 2% per year so long as you meet the following three criteria: 1. Menses has not yet re-sumed (you can ignore bleeding before 56 days postpartum). 2. The baby is under 6 months old. 3. You are fully or nearly fully breastfeeding, as defined by first column. If any of these three cri-teria are no longer met, you'll need to use the appropriate FAM rules listed in the above rows.

The Contraceptive Effectiveness of Natural Birth Control

Why do mice have such small balls? Because only 10% can dance!
—A JOKE TOLD AMONG BIOSTATISTICIANS WHO
NO DOUBT GOT IT QUICKER THAN THE REST OF US

Before any couple decides to use a method of contraception, they should know its rate of effectiveness. The only "guaranteed birth control" is abstinence, and thus, for any sexually active woman of reproductive age, there is always some risk of pregnancy. A critical question in selecting a contraceptive is ascertaining the *degree of risk* you personally find acceptable.

The Fertility Awareness Method as taught in this book, *if understood thoroughly and always used correctly,* is extremely effective in preventing pregnancies. Indeed, it is so effective that the weakest link will be the barrier method you use, if you choose to have intercourse during your fertile phase. If used perfectly *and* you abstain during your fertile phase (as is done with Natural Family Planning), the chance of becoming pregnant would be approximately 2% over the course of a typical year. According to the 1998 edition of *Contraceptive Technology,* this is a lower failure rate than any barrier method. If you correctly use a barrier throughout the fertile phase, then the chance of your becoming pregnant would be close to the method failure rate of the barrier you use. The table on page 355 will help to put this data in context.

Indeed, putting contraceptive data into proper social and biostatistical perspective is an important undertaking that is worth the few minutes it takes to read this appendix. You should know that when scientists discuss the efficacy of a contraceptive, there are in fact two different types of effectiveness ratings. One is called *method failure* rate, and refers specifically to the ability of a given form of birth control to prevent pregnancies when that method is *used correctly for every act of intercourse.* What is considered correct usage is usually defined by set guidelines, often spelled out by contraceptive manufacturers. For the Fertility Awareness Method, correct usage is detailed in Chapter 9 of this book.*

In many ways, what is more important than the method failure rate of any contraceptive is the *user failure* rate, for that is where you can see what occurs in the real world. User failure is generally defined as the rate of unwanted pregnancies for the population as a whole, taking into account both correct and incorrect usage. For example, the method failure of the condom is estimated by *Contraceptive Technology* at 3%, but user failure is closer to 14%, in part because men sometimes fail to put it on in a way that avoids leakage. This means that over the course of the first year of use, 14% of regular condom users will become pregnant. Fortunately, user failure rates for almost all contraceptives tend to drop after the first 12 months.

As you can imagine, there are some birth control methods in which the method and user failure rates are nearly identical, for the method chosen does not rely on the behavior of the user. Male and female surgical sterilization is the best example of this, with both method and user failure at or below .5%. Their disadvantages aside, it's true that long-term hormonal treatments such as Norplant and Depo-Provera are also exceptionally effective, with both method and user failure rates even lower than sterilization!

Standard birth control pills have a method failure rate of .5% or lower, but typical user failure rises to 5% or higher, depending on the study. This is primarily because women may forget to take the Pill for a few days. As the table shows, the condom has a lower method failure rate than the other barrier methods, with all barriers showing user failure rates substantially higher than their corresponding method rates. This is because some people are not sure how to use the particular contraceptive or, more likely, because people are somewhat careless in their employment of the various devices.

---

* "Method effectiveness rates," as opposed to "failure rates," are expressed as a positive number showing how many sexually active women would *not* become pregnant over the course of a year were the method in question used perfectly (correctly, every time). Thus if a diaphragm manufacturer claims a method effectiveness of 94%, it is another way of saying that over the course of that year, 6% of women using that method are likely to get pregnant, assuming they use it perfectly.

It should be noted that while manufacturers certainly prefer to express the positive (94% effective), rather than the negative (6% failure), it is more accurate to discuss contraceptive statistics in terms of *failure* rates rather than *efficacy* rates. This is because in the real world, a 6% failure rate does not actually translate into a 94% success rate. Why? Because only about 85% of sexually active women of reproductive age would get pregnant over the course of a year even if they used *no* method. Also, given that women are fertile only a few days per cycle, it is clear that barrier method effectiveness rates will always be overstated. In this discussion, I will use the more statistically accurate failure rates.

Where does this leave NFP among the major contraceptive methods? (For the rest of this appendix, I will usually refer to NFP and not FAM, unless dealing specifically with barrier method issues. This is because research on the effectiveness rates of natural methods should be uncompromised by barrier method failures.) As I have already stated, the method failure rate of the rules as taught in this book is estimated at 2%. However, the user failure rates are much harder to pinpoint, because quite frankly, the medical literature is filled with studies showing such rates ranging widely, from 1%, to certain studies claiming user failure as high as 20%.*

With such a wide discrepancy in data, is it possible to use the rules with the confidence you need? In fact, yes, very much so, but first you need to know where the data arise and why the discrepancy in reported rates is really not such a mystery. Finally, you need to really think about what the data *do* imply in terms of the type of people who should, and should not, use NFP or FAM as their contraceptive choice.

✌ NATURAL FAMILY PLANNING: HIGHLY EFFECTIVE, HIGHLY UNFORGIVING

NFP is highly effective when used correctly, but more than any other method, it is extremely unforgiving of improper use, or more specifically, of "cheating." The reason for this is really quite logical. If, for example, you misuse a diaphragm or condom or even forget to take a pill, the chances are that for any individual act of intercourse it probably wouldn't matter anyway since you most likely wouldn't be in the fertile phase of your cycle. NFP, of course, is the exact opposite, in that if you disregard the rules, you are by definition having unprotected intercourse precisely when you *are* potentially fertile. To use NFP effectively, you need to understand this, and most important, you need the necessary motivation to avoid pregnancy. As the major studies make clear, if you lack the latter, you will indeed be taking substantial and foolish risks.

As mentioned, various studies show that in the real world, NFP user failure rates vary greatly. Still, 10 to 12% per year seems close to the average reported in the medical literature for the sympto-thermal rules taught in Chapter 9. But what

---

* These data refer specifically to the sympto-thermal method, the technical name given for the natural birth control rules detailed in Chapter 9. It involves observing *both* waking temperature and cervical fluid as well as the option of observing cervical position. Generally, other methods of natural birth control only observe waking temperature or cervical fluid. And the Rhythm Method (often referred to as the Calendar Method) doesn't involve observing any fertility signs.

is equally important is that all these studies clearly suggest that in a large percentage of pregnancies that occur while "using" NFP, the cause of conception was due to *intentional violation of the method rules*. Simply put, many couples without sufficient motivation did cheat, and many of those paid the price*

Ultimately it is a question of semantics as to whether those couples are reflective of user failure or simply should be considered nonusers, but you can see why NFP and FAM instructors get frustrated when they hear that the method is "not really considered effective." Indeed, a man using a condom who gets his wife pregnant because he remains inside her too long after ejaculation can certainly be included in the user failure rate. But if just one day he gets lazy and leaves the condom in the drawer, is this seriously a user failure if a pregnancy results? I would suggest that for any contraceptive, intentional, and complete abandonment of the method in question reflects a category of nonusage that simply cannot be seen within the user failure classification.

More than any method, motivation to avoid pregnancy dramatically affects the user failure results. Some of the studies have in fact separated the test groups into motivational categories such that, for example, couples who used NFP to avoid pregnancy were put in one group whereas those who used NFP merely to better space their children were put in another. Not surprisingly, the "spacers" would invariably take greater chances, resulting in user failure rates substantially higher than the "avoiders," who showed user failure rates as low as 2%. (In fact, user failure rates well below 1% have been documented, but usually when intercourse is limited to the postovulatory infertile phase.)

℘ NFP, MOTIVATION, AND RESPONSIBILITY

I write all of this not simply to tell you that the medical literature (and mainstream media) is inherently biased against NFP in reporting its effectiveness. The fact is that the numbers do tell us something quite valuable, that each one of you

---

* One major study in the *American Journal of Obstetrics and Gynecology* (October 15, 1981, p. 368) reported without irony that "Couples who stated that they had used the fertile phase of the cycle in an attempt to achieve pregnancy accounted for 9.8% . . . of pregnancies. Since these couples did not give advance notification of their desires to attempt pregnancy, these . . . were attributed to the respective method." (!) It's also clear that a significant percent of the other failures, while not trying to get pregnant, were quite happy to take chances during the fertile phase. In fact, this particular article is actually a good and quite representative example of the numerous studies cited in the medical and scientific journals. In this report, over a hundred women representing more than 1,600 total cycles of sexual exposure were monitored for contraceptive failure rates in use of the sympto-thermal method used in this book. Perhaps the most interesting result reported was that the authors concluded after intensive follow-up interviews that there were *no method failures whatsoever.*

should contemplate before deciding whether NFP is the right method for you. Simply stated, the wide variance in user and method failure rates show that the very "device-free" nature of the method means that it is extremely easy to slip into a "taking chances" mentality. Indeed, NFP is not a difficult method to learn, and learn well, but it is unfortunately an easy method to practice poorly, which by its very nature really means to not practice it at all.

The bottom line on NFP as a contraceptive choice is this: *No one truly wishing to avoid pregnancy should be using it if they do not thoroughly understand the rules of the method, and most important, have the necessary discipline to follow those rules correctly and consistently.* If you do not completely understand the method as presented in this book, I urge you to get training through one of the institutions listed in Appendix M before relying on NFP as a contraceptive choice. Ultimately, natural methods of contraception are only appropriate for those couples with the maturity and self-respect necessary to not take foolish risks.

❧ FERTILITY AWARENESS, BARRIERS, AND THE FERTILE PHASE: ASSESSING THE ODDS

There are a number of tangential issues related to Fertility Awareness efficacy rates that should be briefly addressed so that all couples can make the most appropriate contraceptive decisions. As I have mentioned, studies have shown that the method failure of NFP is estimated at 2%. However, you should realize that there is a higher risk of pregnancy for those couples who use barrier methods rather than abstain when the woman is fertile.

The statistical reality is actually quite intuitive. For those couples who choose to use a barrier method over abstinence *throughout* the fertile phase, the method and user failure rates of FAM will always be at least as high as the failure rates of the barrier they choose to use. It is for this reason that I suggest that couples who do not abstain use a condom as their method of choice. At approximately 3% method failure and 14% estimated user failure, it is a better barrier than any of the others, as seen in the table on page 355. (Of course the very fact that you'll know that you are fertile should encourage the type of diligent behavior necessary for keeping your own user failure rate to a minimum).

For those couples who are determined to absolutely minimize their risk yet do not want to practice abstinence for the *full* fertile period, there are very reasonable compromises. In reality, the vast majority of conceptions will occur from intercourse that takes place when the woman has creamy or eggwhite cervical fluid. This is the time not only closest to ovulation, but also the time that sperm have the best odds of survival. If a barrier failure is going to result in pregnancy, it is very likely to happen at this point in the cycle. Fortunately, for most women this phase lasts five days or less. Thus for those determined to avoid pregnancy, I suggest you consider alternatives to intercourse for that short period of time.

✑ FAM/NFP AND THE RISK CONTINUUM

In discussing the contraceptive rules and the temptation to stray from them, it should be clear that there is in fact a range of possible acts that make up the entire pregnancy-risk continuum. Given this, I would like to address the increased risks associated with what I know to be the specific times most couples are tempted to "cheat."

Unprotected Intercourse When the Two Postovulatory Rules Don't Coincide

Some women may notice that the Temperature Shift and Peak Day rules do not always reflect infertility on the same day. The safest approach is to consider yourself fertile until both rules say that you are not (the line "farthest to the right" as described on page 133). However, it is also true that you run only a slightly increased risk in using the following modified guideline: If your temperatures clearly reveal that you're safe on one day, but your cervical fluid reveals you're not safe until a day or so later, you may shave off the last day that the cervical fluid says you are still fertile. It should be stressed that the reverse does not apply. This is because three high temperatures are stronger evidence than "Peak + 4" that the egg(s) are already dead and gone. If you would like to use this modified guideline but are still a bit hesitant, you can always check your cervix. If it is at its lowest, most closed position, your increased risk of pregnancy is virtually nil.

Unprotected Intercourse on Preovulatory Dry Days
Before 6 P.M.

One of the most common questions I am asked is what risk is associated with unprotected intercourse on preovulatory dry days *before* 6 P.M. As you know, the 6 P.M. rule is there in order to give the cervical fluid a chance to descend to the vaginal opening, lest unprotected intercourse that morning be greeted by unseen cervical fluid wet enough to nurture the sperm that noon. Unfortunately, I have not found any studies on this particular issue (you could imagine the logistical problems in organizing such a survey).

However, my years of teaching this method have convinced me that the increased risk is very small, *if you can verify before intercourse that there is no cervical fluid at your cervical tip and your cervix remains in the lowest infertile position.* The physiological possibility that sperm can survive in such a dry vaginal environment long enough for the cervical and hormonal changes that are necessary for their survival must be remote, and thus I personally would not consider this to be an unreasonable risk. But until studies verify my personal beliefs, unprotected intercourse at such times in the cycle must still be considered abandonment of the rules taught in this book.

Unprotected Intercourse on Preovulatory Sticky Days

The risk of unprotected intercourse during the preovulatory sticky cervical-fluid phase is a directly related issue. In reality, the only women who can have unprotected sex during this time with only a small rise in risk are those who have clearly established that they have a Basic Infertile Pattern of sticky days, as discussed in Appendix B.

For all other women, you should not take the risk. The truth is that you are not extremely fertile at this time, because sperm need wet cervical fluid to survive beyond a few hours, and anyone with stickiness is probably still a few days from ovulation. However, it is also a fact that if you're just a little unlucky, sticky fluid can turn to wet in the few hours before sperm will die, thus preparing the way for a conception in the days to follow.

Unprotected sex at this point is therefore the type of cheating that significantly increases the "user failure" rates in all Fertility Awareness studies. I would argue that such acts are incorrect use of the method. But if you still decide to take the increased risk, I strongly urge you to verify that there is no *wet* cervical fluid at the cervical tip before having sex. If there is, intercourse without a barrier would be downright foolish.

❧ A FINAL WORD ON CERVICAL POSITION AND CONTRACEPTIVE EFFICACY

By now, it should be obvious that your cervical position can play an important role in confirming your fertility status. Indeed, for those of you determined to take the absolute lowest risk of pregnancy while still using natural birth control, I suggest that you continue to use the standard rules but limit intercourse to when your cervix is in its lowest, most infertile position (with no wet cervical fluid at the cervical tip). Although no studies have been done, I believe that if women did this, NFP method failure would fall from 2% to well below 1% per year. Admittedly, you may find that such a guideline results in an extra day or so of abstinence, but this may be a trade-off that you're happy to accept.

🖎 A NOTE ABOUT THE BILLINGS METHOD

Finally, I should mention here that many people around the world practice a simplified form of Fertility Awareness called the Billings Method. The primary way that it differs from the Fertility Awareness Method used in this book is that it relies exclusively on observing cervical fluid to determine the fertile phase. Because it does not use basal body temperature to verify the occurrence of ovulation, failure rates are somewhat higher, though method failure is still listed at only 3% by *Contraceptive Technology*. The problem is with *user* failure, which is generally quite a bit higher than the corresponding sympto-thermal rates. For this reason, I personally urge you to use a basal body thermometer in order to maximize both contraceptive efficacy as well as the number of days considered safe for unprotected intercourse.

CONTRACEPTIVE METHOD EFFECTIVENESS TABLE*

Method	Typical User Failure	Method Failure
Chance	85%	85%
Spermicides (foams, creams, vaginal suppositories, etc.)	26	6
Cervical cap† (w/spermicidal cream or jelly)	20	9
Sponge‡	20	9
Diaphragm (w/jelly/foam)	20	6
Withdrawal	19	4
Female Condom (Reality)	21	5
Male Condom (without spermicides)	14	3
The Pill§	5	≤.5
IUD**	≤2	≤1.5
Sterilization (male and female)	≤.5	≤.5
Depo-Provera/Norplant	≤.3	≤.3
NFP‡‡ (FAM w/sympto-thermal rules and abstinence during fertile phase)	(see footnote ‡‡)	2

* All data in this table are adapted from *Contraceptive Technology*, Seventeenth Revised Edition, 1998.

† For women who have given birth, the failure rates are substantially worse, at 40% and 26%, respectively.

‡ For women who have given birth, the failure rates are substantially worse, at 40% and 20%, respectively.

§ Method failure rate varies with type of Pill chosen.

** Method failure rate varies with type of IUD chosen.

‡‡ *Contraceptive Technology* puts NFP *method* failure of the sympto-thermal rules taught in this book at 2%. The sympto-thermal *user* failure rate is not listed. Based on the various studies throughout the medical literature, the traditionally calculated user failure rate appears to be about 10 to 12%. However, when *intentional violation of the method rules* is factored out, this number falls substantially.

The Menstrual Cycle: A Summary of Events Through the Use of a 28-Day Model

> Note: You should refer to page 5 of the color insert while reading this appendix.

The main text of this book provided a brief overview of how the female reproductive system works. Still, I believe it is worth taking a few pages here to give a somewhat more detailed description of the typical menstrual cycle. For those of you who have often wondered how and why your body does what it does, this summary can offer a more complete introduction to the topic. Should you find it interesting, I would encourage you to explore a more thorough discussion of the subject in biology and medical texts, especially if you experience gynecological conditions that stray considerably from the norm.

Like so much in nature, your body is a highly complex system of continuous feedback loops. If they are functioning smoothly, the menstrual cycle's hormonal influences will ultimately create an intricate self-correcting thermostat. Of course, the principle goal of the system is a much more ambitious project than keeping a room at 72 degrees. Every cycle, your body works to produce an egg capable of being fertilized and the conditions necessary to nurture it for the duration of a pregnancy.

In order to explore how this happens, I'll take the prototype 28-day cycle and analyze the hormonal developments that occur in chronological progression. I will also overlay the major fertility signs so that you can review how the pieces all fit together. *Please remember that what will follow is a description of a per-*

fectly functioning 28-day cycle, but as you certainly know by now, what is 28 days for Jane Doe may be a completely normal 24 to 36 days for you. In fact, studies show that less than 15% of cycles are precisely 28 days, and it is equally rare for ovulation to occur on exactly Day 14.*

✌ THE KEY HORMONES

Before beginning, it's advisable to review the primary function and sources of the five most important female sex hormones. While your reproductive system has more than a dozen hormones, these are the five key ones that I think women should know. They are:

1. Oestrogen: The most potent of the three main types of oestrogen is estradiol, the type that is produced by the follicles that develop within your ovaries as you progress from menstruation to ovulation. Each cycle it is responsible for maturing eggs and uterine lining and developing a wet, fertile-quality cervical fluid as you approach ovulation. In addition, it is responsible for promoting the maturation of female sex organs as well as secondary sexual characteristics. There is very little oestrogen in your system as a new cycle begins.

2. Progesterone: The heat-producing hormone primarily manufactured by the corpus luteum, beginning immediately following ovulation. It is the hormone most responsible for nurturing and maintaining the endometrium in the postovulatory phase. As you have learned, the corpus luteum is the follicular body on the interior of the ovarian wall that is left behind by the ovulated egg. The immediate cause of menstruation is the cessation of progesterone production, triggered by the disintegration of the corpus luteum a couple of days earlier.

3. Follicle Stimulating Hormone (FSH): The hormone most responsible for the initial development of a select few follicles each cycle. Under the influence of FSH, a dozen or so follicles evolve from tiny and immature (primordial) to relatively large and partially matured (vesicular). As this occurs, the eggs within each follicle gradually approach the capacity to be ovulated. FSH is produced in the anterior part of the pituitary, but absorbed by FSH receptor cells on the follicular wall. The pituitary is a gland at the base of the brain located between the brain stem and the hypothalamus. There is little FSH in the system as menstruation begins.

---

* Even the *mean* average cycle length among fertile women is believed to be 29.5 days, and not 28. This is based on what is thought to be the most extensive study ever done on this topic, by Dr. Rudi F. Vollman, a Swiss gynecologist whose name is synonymous with research in this field.

4. Luteinizing Hormone (LH): The other major hormone produced in the anterior pituitary, LH is responsible for both stimulating and completing follicular growth (with FSH), as well as the luteinization of the ruptured follicle in order to transform it into a corpus luteum following ovulation. LH is best known for the "LH surge," that dramatic increase in LH production that serves as the immediate trigger to ovulation, which follows a day or so later. Together, FSH and LH are called the pituitary or gonadotropin hormones. There is little LH in the system as menstruation begins.

5. Gonadotropin Releasing Hormone (GnRH): The hormone produced in the hypothalamus, which when secreted, causes the anterior pituitary to increase production of the gonadotropin hormones, specifically FSH and LH. The hypothalamus is located just above the pituitary, and essentially forms the floor and lower walls of the brain. It is for this reason that some speculate stress and other environmental factors can play such havoc with the length of menstrual cycles. It is believed that stress directly affects the hypothalamus and its manufacture of GnRH, which in turn changes output of FSH, LH, and so on down the cyclical line.

It should be pointed out that knowledge of GnRH is somewhat more speculative than that of the other hormones. This is because it is harder to monitor since it operates between the hypothalamus and pituitary within the brain. It is known that it is released in pulses that last about an hour or so, and that various experiments have shown that it is indeed these GnRH pulses that stimulate FSH and LH production within the anterior pituitary. However, there is still some uncertainty as to the intensity and timing of GnRH production within the hormonal system. (It is for these reasons that GnRH is not charted on the graph in the color insert.)

❧ THE ROAD TO OVULATION

Day 1 of any cycle is the first day of menstruation. As you've learned by now, it is hardly the most important day, for that distinction belongs to the day of ovulation. Yet for women the world over, it certainly is the most noticeable event. The majority simply accept their menstrual fate, and some (though I suspect not most) have even learned to celebrate it. In any case, why the bleeding, and why now?

Like any recurring cycle, you can't simply pick a given day, call it the first, and then explain what is going on, without at least acknowledging that what happens on Day 1 is a direct result of what happened on the last days of the previous cycle. In this case, it was the sudden plunge in progesterone, the hormone that had kept the endometrial wall nourished and in place, which now causes the dramatic menstrual events that mark the first phase of the reproductive cycle. It is also worth noting that as menstruation begins, none of the key hormones are present in significant quantity.

In the days before you begin to menstruate, the uterine wall, or endometrium, has reached its full maturity, approximately 5 to 6 millimeters thick. Cellular proliferation in the endometrium has been accompanied by swelling and secretory development, as well as an increased supply of nutrients and blood vessels that have built up over the previous cycle. In brief, the endometrium has reached the goal necessary for its only purpose: to provide the appropriate conditions to nurture a fertilized ovum.

Now, on Day 1, with neither progesterone nor the HCG (human chorionic gonadotropin) that an implanted embryo would supply, the endometrial wall begins to disintegrate. Over a period of approximately 5 days, the uterine lining is gradually washed away as the blood vessels that supply it with nutrients and oxygen begin to constrict. Menstrual blood begins to flow from the uterus through the cervix and out the vagina. The secretion that results also contains matter from the collapsing endometrium. Over the course of your period, you will generally lose anywhere from 1 to 8 ounces of blood and other fluids, though 2.5 ounces appear to be more typical.

As soon as you have begun to menstruate, your body's endocrine system has started to take action. Even before the first day of the new cycle, the pituitary gland has already begun to secrete small but ever increasing amounts of FSH, the hormone that begins to develop the dozen or so follicles in the ovary that will later compete for the prize of ovulation a couple of weeks later. It is generally believed that the plunging levels of progesterone and oestrogen in the last few days of the previous cycle is what allows for the increased production of FSH. In other words, it was the high levels of progesterone (and to a lesser extent oestrogen) that had been blocking FSH production.

By about Day 5, or just as menstruation is ending, the pituitary also begins to release small but increasing amounts of LH. It is believed that LH production within this stage of the cycle is about 3 days behind production of FSH. In fact, the gradual release of LH is a direct result of a positive feedback system triggered by the previous production of FSH. As the FSH begins to act on the handful of ovarian follicles that move toward ovulatory potential, they begin to develop a new coating of granulosa cells, cells which in turn begin to secrete the first amounts of oestrogen for the new cycle.

It is this new oestrogen that apparently signals the hypothalamus to release GnRH, which in turn triggers the gradually increasing secretion of LH. This newly released LH, working in biochemical unison with FSH, continues to develop those follicles whose growth now extends this positive feedback system of follicular development for the next several days. As your period ends, the hormonal game plan is now well on its way to creating the conditions necessary for ovulation. Indeed, follicular growth during menstruation has already doubled the size of the several primordial follicles that have started to mature for that cycle.

By Day 7 or 8, and for reasons not completely understood, one of the follicles begins to emerge as dominant, while the others begin to disintegrate in a process called atresia. Many endocrinologists believe that the dominant follicle has begun to secrete so much oestrogen in the week or so following menstruation (Days 6 to 12) that LH and FSH production is somewhat decreased. It is believed that the increased oestrogen begins to signal the hypothalamus to reduce production of GnRH, thus slowing the manufacture of LH and FSH. And it is this slowdown that leads to the atresia of most of the other primary follicles, though the dominant follicle continues to mature. (In cases of multiple ovulation, two or more follicles progress to complete maturation.)

While creation of FSH and LH is therefore reduced in Days 6 to 12, oestrogen production from the emerging dominant follicle begins to rise dramatically. This rising level of oestrogen begins to act on your uterus, in both noticeable and subtle ways. As the oestrogen rises, the endometrial cycle also begins anew, with the beginning creation of stromal and epithelial cells within the uterus. By about Day 12, this building process has resulted in an endometrial wall approaching 3 to 4 millimeters thick, whereas when menstruation had ended a week earlier, there was virtually no such structure in existence.

As this process moves forward, the rising levels of oestrogen are also beginning to produce the fertility signs that form the foundation of this book. Usually by about Day 8 or 9, their effect on cervical glands have triggered the first flow of cervical fluid, although this early in the process it is generally a sticky quality. But as oestrogen production from the developing follicles within the ovaries rises to its highest levels on Days 10 through 13, the cervical fluid gradually changes to creamy and then to eggwhite. Typically by Day 13, oestrogen levels have reached their peak, with the resulting cervical fluid having reached its most lubricative consistency. By now, the cervix itself is soft, high, and open.

On Day 12 or 13, something dramatic happens in the hormonal feedback system. As already stated, increasing levels of oestrogen are believed to be the reason FSH and LH production are kept relatively low in Days 6 to 13. But at a certain point, for reasons we don't truly understand, oestrogen production reaches a threshold level in which its hormonal effect on the pituitary abruptly reverses. LH secretion by the anterior pituitary gland suddenly surges six to ten times its normal rate, peaking about 12 to 16 hours before ovulation. Within hours of this LH surge, a less dramatic FSH surge follows. In combination, the two cause a negative feedback effect that suddenly shuts down the production of oestrogen in the remaining dominant follicle. The follicle has now fully matured, reaching a size of 1 to 1.5 centimeters. For this 28-day journey, you have now reached the halfway point, and thus ovulation is imminent.

On Day 14, under direct stimulation from the soaring levels of the gonadotropin hormones, the dominant follicle begins to ooze liquid from a protrusion that has formed on its surface. Simultaneously, it begins to swell, severely weakening the follicular wall. Sometime during the next few hours, the follicle ruptures, with the interior ovum being propelled through the ovarian wall into the abdominal cavity. Ovulation has now taken place.

Most likely, your cervical fluid has reached its last day of eggwhite (and in fact has already begun to rapidly dry up), your cervical position has reached its most fertile (i.e., soft, high, and open), and that morning, you had your last low basal temperature before the thermal shift. For many of you, Day 14 will also produce *mittelschmerz,* that secondary fertility sign in which an occasional sharp pain around your abdomen verifies indeed that ovulation is about to or has already occurred.

℘ COMPLETING THE CYCLE

The newly released ova now begins its long journey through the fimbria and down the fallopian tube. Assuming there are no sperm to fertilize it, it will disintegrate within the next 6 to 24 hours. Meanwhile, the body's own hormonal progression continues unabated into the next phase. Back in the ovary from which ovulation took place, the leftover granulosa cells of the dominant follicle are quickly being transformed into luteinizing cells by the high amount of LH. Within hours, these cells have formed the corpus luteum on the interior of the ovarian wall, and it in turn has already begun to secrete heavy doses of progesterone into the body. Waking up on Day 15, you can usually see the result, as this heat-producing hormone triggers your thermal shift.

From Day 15 until about Day 26, the corpus luteum continues to secrete large amounts of progesterone, as well as a modest amount of oestrogen. There are several things that immediately result from this combination of hormonal stimulants. With the dramatic fall of oestrogen production caused by the hormonal events immediately preceding ovulation, the fertile cervical signs quickly reverse. By Day 16, there is generally no more cervical fluid, and the cervical position has returned to firm, low, and closed. (In fact, cervical fluid dries up so quickly you are frequently already dry on the very day you are actually ovulating!)

Still, the corpus luteum continues to release enough oestrogen to continue building up the endometrial wall. In addition, progesterone both holds the wall in place as well as contributes to additional endometrial swelling and development, so that by Day 26 the endometrium has reached a thickness of 5 to 6 millimeters. Were a fertilized egg able to reach the endometrium any time from Day 21 onward (which is likely the first day it could have if ovulation was a week earlier), this uterine shelter would now be ready to house the new embryo.

In the days following ovulation, the combination of high progesterone and low oestrogen creates other hormonal effects. Most important, the anterior pituitary and hypothalamus are now alerted by the progesterone to sharply curtail production of GnRH, LH, and FSH. Thus production of these hormones will stay very low from ovulation until near the end of the cycle, or about Day 27. Meanwhile, the corpus luteum itself continues to grow under the initial influence of the LH surge, but peaks in size about a week after ovulation. By Day 21, it can be up to 1.5 centimeters, and has generally reached full maturity.

Without the continued presence of LH to sustain it, the corpus luteum now begins to deteriorate. It continues to secrete large but decreasing amounts of progesterone (thus sustaining the endometrium), but by about Day 26, its secretory function is extinguished and cellular degeneration occurs rapidly. Had there been a pregnancy, release of HCG from the developing fetus would have signaled the corpus luteum to remain viable for several more months.

Thus by Day 27, the body's release of progesterone (as well as oestrogen) has plummeted, setting the stage for the hormonal transition to the next menstruation, and the beginning of another cycle. As soon as the corpus luteum dies, the absence of ovarian hormones allows for the initial buildup of FSH. And most dramatically and as previously discussed, the plunge in progesterone production quickly triggers the disintegration of the endometrial wall, and the beginning of your next period. We are now once again where this voyage began.

> **COMMON TERMS TO DESCRIBE**
> **THE MENSTRUAL CYCLE PHASES**
>
> **Preovulatory:**   **Postovulatory:**
>
> Estrogenic Phase   Progestational Phase
> Follicular Phase   Luteal Phase
> Proliferative Phase   Secretory Phase

🙰 KEEPING TRACK OF THE MENSTRUAL JOURNEY

I would like to conclude by repeating what I hope this book has already made clear: While the prototypical 28-day cycle is a useful tool for charting chronological order and biological cause and effect, it is in fact not the cyclical experience of most women most of the time. As you have already learned, typical cycle lengths vary among women from 24 to 36 days, and of course within individual women, there are great variations over time due to stress, diet, and other influences. You already know that given these factors, it's not possible to predict the length of the preovulatory phase, and thus the preceding description was accurate as to the order of events, but not as to the actual day of occurrence. I hope that if nothing else, this book has taught you that in matters of fertility, you simply need to chart if you want to know where you are within your cycle.

Frequently Asked Questions (FAQs)

As a FAM instructor, I have been asked just about every possible question regarding fertility. I have chosen to address the most frequently asked among them in this appendix. They are categorized by subject, but are more thoroughly discussed in relevant sections of the book. These pages simply serve as a review, or perhaps as an introduction for your friends, who may want to know more about such a fundamental aspect of their lives.

✌ THE FERTILITY AWARENESS METHOD (FAM)

✿ OVULATION

✿ FERTILITY AND CYCLES

✿ THE FERTILITY AWARENESS METHOD (FAM)

HOW EFFECTIVE IS FAM FOR BIRTH CONTROL?

If *used correctly every cycle,* and you abstain during the fertile phase, the FAM rules taught in this book have a failure rate of approximately 2% per year for the typical couple. This is considered lower than any barrier method, including the condom. (Sterilization and chemical methods such as Norplant and the Pill have an even lower equivalent failure rate of 1% or less.) However, for those couples who choose to have sex throughout the fertile phase while using a barrier method, the overall failure rate will naturally be no lower than the rate of the barrier the couple chooses to use. The fertile phase is usually about 8 to 10 days per cycle.

In actual use, studies show that failure rates vary greatly, from about 1 to 20% per year, with most of the variance being a direct function of the *motivation* of the couples involved. For a more thorough discussion of Fertility Awareness and contraceptive effectiveness, see Appendix D.

WHAT IS THE DIFFERENCE BETWEEN THE FERTILITY AWARENESS METHOD AND THE RHYTHM METHOD?

Probably a more appropriate question is: What do they have in common? It is true that both are natural methods of birth control and pregnancy achievement. But the Rhythm Method is an obsolete, ineffective method of identifying the fertile phase using statistical prediction based on *past* cycles. The Fertility Awareness Method, on the other hand, is a scientifically validated method involving the observation of the three primary fertility signs: waking temperature, cervical fluid, and cervical position. Unlike Rhythm, FAM is considered very effective because the woman's fertility is determined on a day-to-day basis.

HOW MUCH TIME IS REQUIRED TO LEARN AND USE THE METHOD?

How long it takes to learn the method will vary with each woman. I hope that many of you will be able to assimilate all you need to know by thoroughly reading the relevant chapters of this book. Others may want to take a class from a qualified instructor, which typically involves two 3-hour sessions and an individual 1- or 2-hour follow-up consultation. It's also worth noting that it usually takes one or two cycles of observation to feel confident enough to rely on FAM for birth control.

Charting usually requires about 2 minutes per day: About 1 minute to take your temperature with a digital thermometer upon awakening, and about a minute or so to check and record the other fertility signs. If you eventually use the shortcut method as described in Chapter 10, you will need to chart about 10 days per cycle, for a total time commitment of about 20 minutes a month.

I should reiterate here that while it is true that the shortcut method does not compromise contraceptive efficacy, I personally recommend charting every day of your cycle (outside menstruation), especially for the first few cycles that you chart. I should also point out that some women may not be able to use the digital thermometers if they do not reflect an obvious temperature pattern reflecting ovulation. In that case, those women would have to use a glass basal body thermometer, which requires 5 minutes upon awakening.

IS FAM A GOOD METHOD FOR EVERYBODY?

No, not as a method of birth control. It is only appropriate for those women who have the discipline to learn the method well, and then to follow the rules once they have internalized them. In addition, it is only recommended for monogamous couples, given the danger of AIDS and other STDs.

However, as a method of pregnancy achievement, it is highly advised as the first step that every couple should take to maximize their chances of conception, and to determine if there may be anything impeding their ability to get pregnant. In addition, Fertility Awareness can be very effective in helping couples plan the timing of their baby's birth.

FAM is also highly beneficial for all cycling women who simply want to educate themselves about their own bodies. So even if you have no interest in using the method for avoiding or achieving pregnancy, it is an empowering means of taking control of your gynecological health.

HOW MANY DAYS DO YOU HAVE TO ABSTAIN WHEN USING FAM FOR BIRTH CONTROL?

You never have to *abstain* when using the Fertility Awareness Method. This is different than Natural Family Planning, which does require abstinence during the fertile phase. However, if you do have intercourse when you are potentially fertile, you must use a barrier method of contraception. The fertile phase will vary, but in practice this means that the average couple would have to use barriers about 8 to 10 days per cycle. The average cycle is 27 to 31 days, and thus for the typical couple, barriers (or abstinence) would be required for about 30% of the cycle.

DO WOMEN EVER HAVE TRULY "DRY" DAYS?

When a woman charts, she identifies her cervical fluid by various degrees of wetness, and records a dash if no cervical fluid is present at the vaginal opening. This symbol for dry refers to a lack of cervical fluid, and not to internal vaginal moisture, which is present to some degree all of the time. It's easy to distinguish between cervical fluid and vaginal moisture. Cervical fluid on your finger will stay moist for minutes or longer, whereas vaginal moisture, like that inside your mouth, will dissipate from your finger within seconds.

IS THERE REALLY A RISK OF PREGNANCY IF I ONLY HAVE STICKY (NONWET) CERVICAL FLUID?

Yes. While sticky cervical fluid is certainly much less fertile than creamy or eggwhite, it is still possible to conceive from preovulatory intercourse on a sticky day.

IS IT POSSIBLE TO GET PREGNANT WITHOUT OBSERVING EGGWHITE-QUALITY CERVICAL FLUID?

If you are trying to conceive, you shouldn't get discouraged if you don't see eggwhite-quality cervical fluid. It doesn't mean there is anything wrong with you. As long as you have some type of *wet*-quality cervical fluid, the sperm should still be able to swim through the cervix to ultimately reach the egg.

Think of cervical fluid on a continuum from the extremes of dry to eggwhite, with successively wetter cervical fluid in the middle. As you can imagine, the ideal quality would be the wettest and most slippery, since this is the type that most closely resembles the man's seminal fluid.

If you don't notice the eggwhite quality, it probably just means that your "window of fertility" is shorter than those women who do produce it. There are still a number of things you can do to increase your chances of conceiving. You want to be sure to time intercourse for the last day of whatever is your wettest day, even if that means simply creamy cervical fluid.

One practical way to increase the quality and fluidity of your cervical fluid is to start taking plain Robitussin, whose *sole* ingredient is *guaifenesin*. You should take 2 teaspoons, 3 times a day on the first day you notice sticky-quality cervical fluid and continue through to the first day of the rise in your waking temperature. The reason this often improves the quality of your cervical fluid is that it works systematically, meaning that it liquefies not only the mucus membranes in your lungs but in all areas of your body.

DO I HAVE TO WAKE UP EVERY DAY AT THE SAME TIME TO TAKE MY TEMPERATURE?

No, although you should try to be as consistent as possible. In general, waking temperatures tend to creep up about two-tenths of a degree for every extra hour you sleep in. Thus, if you take it substantially later than usual, it may result in a reading that is outside the range of your usual pattern. If you wake up *earlier* than usual, you should take your temperature upon awakening, so long as you have had at least 3 consecutive hours of sleep.

Regardless, an occasional aberrant temperature can easily be dealt with by following the Rule of Thumb. You should also be aware that if taking your temperature feels like a burden, you can, in fact, take it for only about a third of the cycle without sacrificing contraceptive efficacy, as described in Chapter 10.

HOW CAN TEMPERATURES BE RELIED UPON IF I SOMETIMES GET A FEVER?

There may be several factors, from fever to alcohol to lack of sleep, that could affect your waking temperatures. Yet this doesn't compromise your ability to rely on them while charting, because you ultimately want to identify a *pattern* of low and high temperatures, rather than focusing on individual ones. Outlying temperatures can be effectively dealt with by using the Rule of Thumb, which usually allows you to ignore them in interpreting your chart. In addition, you will always be able to rely on your other two signs to cross-check your fertility in situations such as these. (See page 312.)

IS IT WORTH CHECKING MY CERVICAL POSITION?

Although it is not necessary to check your cervix in order to practice FAM effectively, I urge you to learn how to do so. At a minimum, I think you should practice checking in the days leading up to and just past ovulation, for the first few cycles that you're learning the method. Once you recognize how your cervical position reflects your fertility, you will always be able to use it as a cross-check whenever you find the slightest ambiguity in your other two fertility signs.

The bottom line is that complete familiarity with the changes in your cervix will greatly increase the confidence with which you observe your fertility and overall gynecological health. And since it only takes *seconds* a day to check, my attitude is that for those few relevant days per cycle, you should just do it!

A distinct but closely related question is whether those women using FAM for contraception should ever check their cervical fluid at the cervical tip. The short answer is that it isn't necessary to do so, although if you want to be even more conservative than the FAM rules require, or if you simply want to know your cervical fluid status ahead of time, it certainly couldn't hurt. (Remember that the cervical fluid you normally check at the vaginal opening might have taken several hours to trickle down from the cervical tip.) Finally, checking this way may provide some couples with more time for unprotected sex.

℘ OVULATION

DO WOMEN ALWAYS OVULATE ON DAY 14 OF THEIR CYCLE?

No! The day of ovulation can vary among women as well as within each individual woman. However, once a woman ovulates, the time between ovulation and her menstruation is very consistent, almost always between 12 and 16 days. Within most *individual* women, this length of time generally doesn't change by more than a day or two. In other words, if there is going to be variation in the cycle, it is the first preovulatory phase that may vary. The second (postovulatory) phase generally remains constant.

CAN YOU "FEEL" OVULATION HAPPEN?

The most obvious outward sign of impending ovulation is increasing wet and slippery cervical fluid. In fact, it can be so abundant that women notice a string of cervical fluid literally hang down when they are using the toilet. (Yikes!) If a woman notices this, she should assume that ovulation is about to happen within a day or two. This is what is referred to as a primary fertility sign.

Some women are lucky enough to notice other signs on a regular basis, all of which are very helpful in being able to further understand their cycles. These signs are referred to as *secondary* fertility signs, because they do not necessarily occur in all women, or in every cycle in individual women. Yet they are still very practical for giving women additional information to identify their fertile and infertile phases.

Secondary signs as ovulation approaches may include:

- midcycle spotting
- pain or achiness near the ovaries and uterus (called *mittelschmerz*)
- increased sexual feelings
- fuller vaginal lips
- abdominal bloating
- water retention
- increased energy level
- heightened sense of vision, smell, and taste
- increased sensitivity in breasts and skin
- breast tenderness

CAN A WOMAN OVULATE MORE THAN ONCE PER CYCLE?

No. Have you ever heard of a woman getting pregnant on Monday, and then again that following Friday, and then two weeks later on Thursday? Certainly not, because once a woman ovulates, her body cannot release any more eggs that cycle. Ovulation may take place over approximately 24 hours, but just once per cycle. During those 24 hours, one or more eggs may be released (as in the case of fraternal twins). But once ovulation has occurred, it is virtually impossible for a woman to release another egg until the next cycle.

WHAT IS MULTIPLE OVULATION?

Multiple ovulation is the release of two or more eggs in a single cycle. It occurs within 24 hours or less, after which no more eggs will be released until the following cycle. It is responsible for the birth of *fraternal* twins, as opposed to identical twins, which are the result of a single egg that divides after fertilization.

Multiple ovulation appears to be more common than once thought. While it is true that about 1 in 80 naturally conceived births are fraternal twins, researchers now realize that there are many more fraternal *conceptions*. Most of these second fetuses miscarry in what is called the "vanishing twin phenomenon.'" Taking this into account, it is believed that multiple ovulation may actually occur as frequently as 5 to 10% of all cycles.

DO WOMEN FEEL MORE SEXUAL AROUND OVULATION?

Many women do. Because oestrogen peaks around ovulation, women typically experience a wet, slippery sensation due to the fertile cervical fluid they produce. This cervical fluid feels similar to sexual lubrication, and can therefore be experienced as a sexual feeling. A woman who practices FAM needn't worry about confusing the two, because cervical fluid is checked periodically throughout the day, and *not* when she is sexually aroused.

CAN ORGASM CAUSE OVULATION?

No. Orgasms and ovulation are unrelated. In order to ovulate, oestrogen must build up in the woman's system gradually, usually over a period of days. Orgasm can occur at *any* time in the cycle!

ɤ੭ FERTILITY AND CYCLES

WHAT PERCENT OF A WOMAN'S CYCLE IS FERTILE?

The answer to this question is somewhat tricky. The general answer is that most women are fertile for only a few days per cycle. However, there are several factors to consider:

1. The woman's egg can only live up to 24 hours. Two or more eggs may be released over a maximum of 24 hours. So, in a vacuum, a woman is fertile for only about a day or two. But the man's sperm can live up to 5 days, so the *combined* fertility of the two individuals is about a week.
2. For a couple trying to get pregnant, the woman's fertile phase is as long as she has fertile-quality cervical fluid, up through ovulation. That might be several days, or as few as one.
3. For a couple trying to prevent pregnancy, FAM adds a buffer zone of a few days to assure that an unplanned pregnancy does not occur. This usually amounts to about 8 to 10 days per cycle.

WHAT ARE YOUR CHANCES OF CONCEIVING IN ANY GIVEN CYCLE?

It is believed that the average fertile couple has about a 25% chance of conceiving for any given cycle, depending on their age, frequency of intercourse, and numerous other factors. Of course, if couples are taught precisely when to time intercourse based on when the woman is most fertile, those odds can be greatly increased.

CAN A WOMAN GET PREGNANT DURING HER PERIOD?

The answer lies in the wording of the question. More precisely, it is essentially impossible for a woman to get pregnant *during* her period, but on rare occasions it is possible for a woman to get pregnant from *intercourse* during her period. Since sperm can live for five days, a couple could have sex near the end of the woman's period, and the sperm could then live long enough to fertilize an egg several days later, if the woman had a very early ovulation. (Conception is more likely in these cases if intercourse occurs at the end of a 6- or 7-day menstruation.) It's also possible that women who think they got pregnant from intercourse during their period were actually having sex during ovulatory spotting.

IS IT TRUE THAT A WOMAN CAN GET PREGNANT ANYTIME?

No, it is not. It is true that ovulation can vary greatly from cycle to cycle, but once a woman ovulates, she cannot ovulate again for the remainder of that cycle.

CAN A WOMAN GET PREGNANT IF SHE HASN'T BEEN MENSTRUATING?

Yes. Since a woman releases an egg 12 to 16 days *before* menstruation, it is possible to get pregnant without actually having periods. Thus women who are not menstruating due to any reason, such as excessively low body fat, breastfeeding, or being premenopausal, are always at risk of ovulating at any point. This is because the underlying condition causing the lack of menstruation could change, thus unexpectedly triggering the release of an egg.

The bottom line is that women who don't menstruate cannot count on their condition as reliable contraception. In fact, the only practical way to know if ovulation is approaching is through charting your cycles, and more specifically, observing the change in your cervical fluid.

Of course for those couples *desiring* to get pregnant, the reality is that you will definitely want to resolve the underlying problem preventing menstruation. Until you do so, your chances of conception will be very low. (See Chapter 7.)

CAN YOU HAVE A CYCLE IN WHICH YOU DON'T OVULATE BUT YOU STILL GET YOUR PERIOD?

The quick answer is, "Yes, sort of." But the more enlightening and biologically correct answer is that if you fail to ovulate, you can only have anovulatory bleeding. The distinction is this: Technically speaking, a period is the bleeding that occurs about 12 to 16 days after the release of an egg. So, if no egg is released, it is not really a period that follows, but anovulatory bleeding.

There is a huge difference between cycles in which the woman ovulates but does not get her period, and one in which she gets her period but does not ovulate. What is that difference? In the former case, the woman is almost certainly pregnant! In the latter case, she has had an anovulatory cycle. (See Chapter 7.)

HOW DOES THE PILL WORK?

In essence, the Pill works by tricking the body into thinking it's already pregnant. It does this by manipulating the normal hormonal feedback system. The end result is that the body doesn't release the hormones necessary to stimulate the ovary to release an egg. As a back-up, every other facet of the woman's reproductive system is also altered. Most important, the uterine lining is obstructed from producing a rich site for egg implantation, and the cervical fluid is prevented from forming a wet, fertile quality necessary for sperm survival.

CAN STRESS AFFECT YOUR FERTILITY?

The role that stress plays on one's fertility is fairly complex. Stress, per se, does not prevent conception. However, it can delay ovulation by suppressing the hormones necessary for ovulation to occur. If a couple adheres to the myth of ovulation always occurring on Day 14, they then may inadvertently prevent pregnancy by timing intercourse at the wrong time, thus triggering a vicious circle of misperceived infertility causing more stress. Charting her cycle would allow the couple to regain control by correctly identifying the woman's fertile phase. (See pages 178–81.)

HOW MANY DAYS CAN SPERM SURVIVE?

Sperm can generally survive a maximum of 5 days in the fertile-quality cervical fluid that women produce around the time of ovulation. It is much more likely that sperm will survive a maximum of 3 days, and only a few hours in dryer, less fertile types of cervical fluid. If there is no cervical fluid present, the sperm will probably die within a couple of hours.

HOW LONG CAN A HUMAN EGG SURVIVE?

Most ova probably survive about 6 to 12 hours after ovulation. However, for the purposes of contraception, you must count on a 24-hour survival period, plus an additional 24 hours in case there is a multiple ovulation.

WHAT THINGS SHOULD I LOOK FOR NOW THAT MIGHT HELP IDENTIFY A POTENTIAL FERTILITY PROBLEM IN THE FUTURE?

If you plan to get pregnant someday and tend to experience any of the signs listed below, you should consult with your physician to rule out any possible problems:

- limited cervical fluid or completely dry (see page 173)
- excessive fertile-quality cervical fluid (see page 321)
- short luteal phases (see page 314)
- premenstrual spotting (see page 295)
- post-menstrual brown bleeding (see page 226)
- light periods (see page 296)

The Difference Between Natural Methods of Birth Control

	Rhythm Method	Billings (Ovulation) Method	BBT (Basal Body Temperature) Method	FAM/NFP* (Sympto-Thermal Method)
Fertility Signs That Are Observed	None	Cervical fluid	Waking temperature	Waking temperature and cervical fluid
Comments	An obsolete method based on a mathematical formula using past cycle lengths to predict future fertile phases.	Because only cervical fluid is observed, you do not have the benefit of a thermal shift to confirm that ovulation has indeed occurred.	Because only temperature is observed, the first day of your cycle that you are considered safe is not until the third night after an obvious temperature shift.	Because the two primary fertility signs are observed, as well as any number of secondary signs (such as cervical position, ovulatory pain, or midcycle spotting), this method is considered the most comprehensive and reliable.

* The difference between the Fertility Awareness Method (FAM) and Natural Family Planning (NFP) is that those who practice NFP choose to abstain during the fertile phase, whereas those who practice FAM allow themselves to use a barrier during this time.

Optional Coverline

There is an optional way of drawing the coverline from that taught on page 77. It is often simpler to use, but it unfortunately can't be applied in many cycles. *Draw the coverline one-tenth degree above the highest temperature during the first 10 days of your cycle.* Once your temperature passes over it and remains above for at least 3 consecutive days, you have presumably ovulated. For a lot of women, this system works well, but I personally don't like it because the only temperatures that are hormonally significant are the 6 or so that precede the thermal shift. In addition, many women have elevated temperatures during the first week or more of the cycle that precludes its effective use. If you would still prefer to use it, especially as a method of birth control, I encourage you to be especially attentive to your other fertility signs to corroborate ovulation (see next page for further clarification).

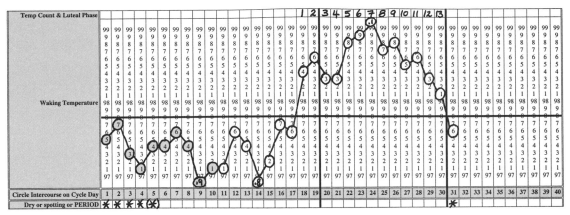

Chart H.1. The type of temperature pattern that allows for the simpler coverline rule. Because all of the temperatures in the first part of the cycle are conspicuously below those in the second part, you can easily draw the coverline one-tenth degree above the highest of the first 10 days.

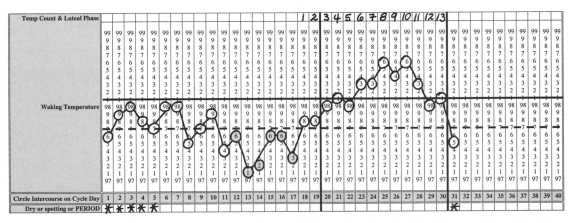

Chart H.2. The type of temperature pattern that would not allow for the simpler coverline rule. Note that many of the early temperatures are too high, preventing the drawing of an effective optional coverline (solid line) one-tenth of a degree above the highest of the first 10 days. Thus, this pattern requires the standard coverline (dashed line) drawn one-tenth degree above the highest of the previous 6 days.

Drugs That May Affect Your Fertility Signs or Cycle

This appendix lists common drugs that may affect your fertility signs or cycle. There are two ways to find a drug: in the categorized table below or in the alphabetical index on the next page. The extensive table that follows describes the effects of each. Please note that this list is not comprehensive. If you do not see the drug you are taking here, ask your pharmacist.

DRUGS LISTED BY CATEGORY	
Category	**Drugs**
1. Acne Relief Agents	Isotretinoin
2. Analgesics	Ibuprofen, Naprosyn, etc.
3. Antibiotics	Penicillins, Ampicillin, Tetracyclines, Erythromycin, etc.
4. Antidepressants	Selective Serotonin Reuptake Inhibitors (Prozac, etc.); Tricyclics (Elavil, Ludiomil, etc.)
5. Antiendometriosis Drugs	Danazol; Lupron Depot (Leuprolide); Buserelin
6. Antiestrogens	Tamoxifen, Clomiphene, Clomid
7. Antihistamines and Antihistamines with Antiserotonin Action	Dimetane, Sudafed, Claritin, Optimine, Seldane, etc.
8. Antipsychotics	MAO Inhibitors, Mellaril, Lithium, etc.
9. Antispasmodics	Atropine, Belladonna, Dicyclomine, Propantheline
10. Antitumor Drugs	Busulfan, Cyclophosphamide, Cyclotoxic Agents, Mercaptopurine, Chlorambucil, Actinomycin
11. Antivertigo Agents	Dramamine, etc.
12. Cough Mixtures with Antihistamines	Phenylephrine, etc.
13. Diuretics	Midamor, etc.
14. Expectorants with Guaifenesin	Robitussin Plain, Potassium Iodide, etc.
15. Hormones	Estrogens (Premarin, etc.); Progesterones (Provera, etc.); Thyroid Hormones (Synthroid, etc.)
16. Oral Contraceptives	"The Pill," Implants, Injections
17. Ovulatory Drugs	Clomid; Serophense; Clomiphene; Gonadotropins (Pergonal, Humegon)
18. Respiratory Drugs	Acetylcystene
19. Sleep Aids	Nytol, etc.
20. Steroids	Cortisone, Prednisone, etc.
21. Ulcer Drugs	Cimetidine (Tagamet)
22. Urinary Control	Bethanechol

DRUGS LISTED ALPHABETICALLY

Drug or Category of Drug	In table	Drug or Category of Drug	In table	Drug or Category of Drug	In table
Acetylcystene	18	Cyclotoxic Agents	10	*Ovulatory Drugs*	17
Acitnomycin	10	Danazol	5	Penicillins	3
Acne Relief Agents	1	Dicyclomine	9	Pergonal	17
Ampicillin	3	Dimetane	7	Phenylephrine	12
Analgesics	2	*Diuretics*	13	"The Pill"	16
Antibiotics	3	Dramamine	11	Potassium Iodide	14
Antidepressants	4	Elavil	4	Prednisone	20
Antiendometriosis Drugs	5	Erythromycin	3	Premarin	15
		Estrogens	15	Progesterone	15
Antiestrogens	6	*Expectorants with Guaifenesin*	14	Prolixin	8
Antihistamines	7			Propantheline	9
Antihistamines with Antiserotonin Action	7	Gonadotropins	17	Provera	15
		Hormones	15	Prozac	4
Antipsychotics	8	Humabid LA	14	*Respiratory Drugs*	18
Antispasmodics	9	Humegon	17	Robitussin Plain	14
Antitumor Drugs	10	Ibuprofen	2	Seldane	7
Antivertigo Agents	11	Isotretinoin	1	Selective Serotonin Reuptake Inhibitors	4
Atropine	9	Leuprolide	5		
Belladonna	9	Lithium	8	Serophene	17
Bethanechol	22	Ludiomil	4	*Sleep Aids*	19
Buserelin	5	Lupron Depot	5	*Steroids*	20
Busulfan	10	MAO Inhibitors	8	Sudafed	7
Chlorambucil	10	Mellaril	8	Synthroid	15
Cimetidine	21	Mercaptopurine	10	Tagamet	21
Claritin	7	Midamor	13	Tamoxifen	6
Clomid	6, 17	Midol	2	Tetracyclines	3
Clomiphene	6, 17	Mucomist	18	Tricyclics	4
Cortisone	20	Naprosyn	2	*Ulcer Drugs*	21
Cough Mixtures with Antihistamines	12	Nytol	19	*Urinary Control*	22
		Optimine	7		
Cyclophosphamide	10	*Oral Contraceptives*	16		

DRUGS LISTED BY EFFECT ON FERTILITY SIGNS OR CYCLE

	Drug	Usually Prescribed For	Type of Effect
1.	**Acne Relief Agents**	Severe acne	Can reduce and dry up cervical fluid.
	Isotretinoin		High risk of birth defects.
2.	**Analgesics**	Pain reduction	Can cause scanty or reduced cervical fluid.
	Midol, etc. *(Ibuprofen)*		Can cause delay in ovulation (and thus in temp shift).
	Naprosyn, etc.		May cause changes in menstrual bleeding and breasts.
3.	**Antibiotics**	To treat bacterial infections	Minimal effect on cycle, but it may cause yeast infections, which can mask cervical fluid.
	Penicillins, Ampicillin,		
	Tetracylines, Erythromycin, etc.		Could increase or thin cervical fluid.
4.	**Antidepressants**	To fight depression, anxiety, etc.	Could delay ovulation or cause weak temp rise.
	Selective Serotonin Reuptake Inhibitors		May dry up cervical fluid, or decrease quantity of fertile cervical fluid.
	Prozac, etc.		May cause hypothyroidism and menstrual irregularities including anovulation and amenorrhea.
	Tricyclics and Tetracyclics		Same as above plus may cause irregular bleeding, breast enlargement, or breast pain.
	Elavil, Ludiomil, etc.		
5.	**Antiendometriosis Drugs**	Endometriosis	Both suppress fertility and put women in temporary menopause.
	Danazol		Ovulation is suppressed.
	Lupron Depot (Leuprolide)		Can cause hot flashes, bleeding, irregularities, etc.
	Buserelin		
6.	**Antiestrogens**	Breast Cancer	Reduces or suppresses cervical fluid. May cause a variety of menstrual disturbances from menorrhagia to menopause.
	Tamoxifen		
	Clomiphene (Clomid)	To induce ovulation	See **Ovulatory Drugs.**
7.	**Antihistamines**	Coughs, colds, and allergies	May dry or thicken cervical fluid and diminish quantity.
	Dimetane, Sudafed, etc.		
	Antihistamines with Antiserotonin Action	Coughs, colds, and allergies	Same as above and can cause breast tenderness or pain.
	Claritin, Optimine, Seldane, etc.		
8.	**Antipsychotic Agents**	Mental illness	May act to dry cervical fluid. May cause an overall rise in BBT throughout cycle. Could cause breast engorgement, pain, or lactation.
	Prolixin, Mellaril, MAO Inhibitors etc.		
	Lithium	Mental Illness	Could lower or raise BBT throughout cycle, and could cause continual cervical fluid pattern with more fertile cervical fluid patches (see Appendix B).

	Drug	Usually Prescribed For	Type of Effect
9.	**Antispasmodics** *Atropine, Belladonna, Dicyclomine, Propantheline*	Used to treat epilepsy, seizure disorders	Can decrease amount of cervical fluid, plus cause thickening or dryness.
10.	**Antitumor Drugs** *Busulfan, Cyclophosphamide, Cyclotoxic Agents, Mercaptopurine, Chlorambucil, Actinomycin, etc.*	Used to treat tumors (*Actinomycin is also used for systemic fungus infection*)	Suppresses ovulation, induces menopausal (high) levels of FSH, LH.
11.	**Antivertigo Agents** *Dramamine, etc.*	Motion sickness	Can dry up cervical fluid, especially if taken for extended period.
12.	**Cough Mixtures with Antihistamines** *Phenylephrine, etc.*	Cough	Can decrease amount of cervical fluid, can cause thickening or dryness.
13.	**Diuretics** *Midamor, etc.*	Hypertension, high blood pressure, edema, etc.	Can dry up cervical fluid, especially if dry mouth is also a side effect.
14.	**Expectorants with Guaifenesin** *Robitussin Plain, Potassium Iodide, etc.*	Nasal congestion, common cold, sore throat, bronchitis, etc.	Can increase fertile-quality cervical fluid, and make it more stretchy or watery.
15.	**Hormones**		
	Estrogens *Premarin, etc.*	Lack of estrogen, Menopausal symptoms (hot flashes, vaginal dryness, etc.)	Can produce more fertile-quality cervical fluid. May slightly lower BBT levels. Could cause irregular menstrual bleeding, breast tenderness.
	Progesterones *Provera, etc.*	Hormonal imbalance, abnormal uterine bleeding, endometriosis, PMS, Menopausal symptoms, (hot flashes, vaginal dryness, etc.)	Can raise BBT levels. Can dry cervical fluid, or produce a thick, tacky cervical fluid quality.
	Thyroid Hormones *Synthroid, etc.*	Replace hormonal thyroid deficiency	Will improve fertility signs, increase fertile-quality cervical fluid, and raise temps throughout cycle.

	Drug	Usually Prescribed For	Type of Effect
16.	**Oral Contraceptives** *"The Pill," Implants, Injections*	To prevent pregnancy or regulate cycles	Prevents ovulation, produces elevated flat BBT pattern, and tends to greatly reduce cervical fluid.
17.	**Ovulatory Drugs** *Clomid, (Clomiphene), Serophene,* etc. Gonadotropins *Pergonal, Humegon,* etc.	Lack of ovulation	Dries up cervical fluid. Possible menopausal symptoms such as hot flashes. May enhance cervical fluid.
18.	**Respiratory Drugs** *Acetylcystene (Mucomist)*	Asthma, cystic fibrosis	If sufficiently absorbed, could increase or thin cervical fluid.
19.	**Sleep Aids** *Diphenhydramine (Nytol, etc.)*	Insomnia	May dry or thicken cervical fluid and diminish quantity.
20.	**Steroids** *Cortisone, Prednisone,* etc.	To alleviate symptoms in many types of disorders, including rheumatoid arthritis, severe asthma, and miscellaneous eye, skin and respiratory conditions.	Can significantly delay ovulation. May cause menstrual bleeding irregularities.
21.	**Ulcer Drugs** *Cimetidine (Tagamet)*	Used to treat peptic ulcers	A variety of menstrual disturbances ranging from menorrhagia to menopause. Inhibits histamine, also pituitary gonadotropins.
22.	**Urinary Control** *Bethanechol*	Cholinergic agent for urinary retention	Could thin secretions.

Interesting Terminology in Women's Health

> The following is a list of medical terms that are routinely used to describe common female conditions and functions. Cover the right side and quickly glance down the list of phrases on the left. After all these years, you'd think someone would have developed more appropriate means of expressing these concepts.

Advanced geriatric status — Women over 35

Senile gravida — Pregnant woman 35 or older

Elderly prima gravida — First-time pregnant woman 35 or older

Senile vaginitis — Dry vagina of (postmenopausal) woman after her oestrogen levels have subsided

Vaginal atrophy — Same as above

Vagina clean — Terminology recorded in a woman's medical records to indicate no infections (implication is that others are dirty)

Discharge — Used to describe healthy, cyclical cervical fluid, as well as a true infection with symptoms of unhealthy secretions

Hostile cervical mucus — Infertile-quality cervical fluid that doesn't support sperm survival

383

Irritable cervix	A cervix that is sensitive during pregnancy
Incompetent cervix	Cervix that tends to dilate prematurely during pregnancy
Infantile or juvenile uterus	Small, completely functional uterus
Inadequate pelvis	Pelvis considered too narrow to allow a vaginal birth
Expected date of confinement (EDC)	The due date for childbirth
Failure to progress (or arrested labor)	Labor that takes longer than average
Habitual aborter	A woman who tends to have recurring, spontaneous miscarriages
Spontaneous abortion	Miscarriage
Threatened abortion	Bleeding while pregnant
Missed abortion	A fetus that has miscarried or died, but has not emerged naturally
Products of conception	Fetus which is delivered dead
Pregnancy wastage	Same as above
Hysterectomy	In ancient Greek, literally means "removal of hysteria" (their word for "womb" came from the belief that disturbances in the uterus caused female insanity)
Fibrocystic breast disease	Fibrocystic breasts or breasts which tend to have benign lumps
Luteal phase defect	Short luteal phase (usually less than 10 days)
Dysfunctional uterine bleeding	Irregular or anovulatory bleeding
Premature ovarian failure	Early menopause

Some of the terms I've included here simply because their origins are particularly interesting. Obviously, I am not suggesting that words as embedded in the lay vocabulary, such as "hysterectomy," should be changed at this point. However, I don't think it's unreasonable to suggest that the English language is capable of producing more gender-sensitive terms than "senile vaginitis" or "incompetent cervix."

I suspect that no man is ever told he has a medically incompetent anything, but if he were, he might start to understand why these terms are simply inappropriate in this context. I don't mean to discredit the medical establishment, but only hope that one day these descriptions will be communicated in a more enlightened way. Empowering yourself and your doctor with the information in this book will help further that process.

Fertility Abbreviations

ACA	Anti-Cardiolipin Antibodies
ACR	Age of Child Requested (adoption term)
ACTH	Adrenocorticotropic Hormone
AH, AZH	Assisted Hatching
AHI	At-Home Insemination
AI	Artificial Insemination
AID	Artificial Insemination from Donor
AIH	Artificial Insemination from Husband
ALT	Alanine Aminotransferase
ANA	Anti-Nuclear Antibodies
AO	Anovulation
APA	Anti-Phospholipid Antibodies
APTT	Activated Partial Thromboplastin Time
ART	Assisted Reproductive Technology
ASA	Anti-Sperm Antibody
ASRM	American Society of Reproductive Medicine
ATA	Anti-Thyroid Antibody
BA	Baby Aspirin
BBT	Basal Body Temperature
BCP	Birth Control Pills
Beta, beta hCG	Serum pregnancy test: qualitative (yes/no) or quantitative (numeric level)
BG	Blood Glucose
BSE	Breast Self-Exam
BT	Balanced Translocation
BTB	Breakthrough Bleeding
BW, b/w	Bloodwork
C#	Cycle Number
CAH	Congenital Adrenal Hyperplasia

CASA	Computer-Assisted Semen Analysis
CAT	Computerized Axial Tomography
CAVD	Congenital Absence of the Vas Deferens
CCCT	Clomiphene Citrate Challenge Test (Clomid Challenge)
CD	Cycle Day
CD56+	Natural Killer Cells
CF	Cervical Fluid
CM	Cervical Mucus
CMV	Cytomegalovirus
CNM	Certified Nurse Midwife
COH	Controlled Ovarian Hyperstimulation
CP	Cervical Position
CRP	C-Reactive Protein
CVS	Chorionic Villus Sampling
D&C	Dilation and Curettage
D&E	Dilation and Evacuation
DE	Donor Eggs
DES	Diethylstilbestrol (a synthetic oestrogen)
DHEAS	Dihydroepiandrosterone Sulfate
DI	Donor Insemination
DIPI	Direct Intra-Peritoneal Insemination
DNA	Deoxyribonucleic Acid
DOST	Direct Oocyte-Sperm Transfer
DP3DT	Days Post-3-Day Transfer
DPO	Days Post-Ovulation
DPR	Days Post-Retrieval
DPT	Days Post-Transfer
Dx	Diagnosis
E2	Estradiol (Oestrogen)
EB, EMB	Endometrial Biopsy
EDC	Expected Date of Confinement (Due Date)
EDD	Estimated Due Date
ENDO	Endometriosis
EPT	Early Pregnancy Test
ET	Embryo Transfer
ETA	Embryo Toxicity Assay
ETF	Embryo Toxic Factor
EW	Eggwhite
EWCF	Eggwhite Cervical Fluid

EWCM	Eggwhite Cervical Mucus
FAST	Fallopian Sperm Transfer System
FBG	Fasting Blood Glucose
FET	Frozen Embryo Transfer
FHR	Fetal Heart Rate
FP	Follicular Phase
FSH	Follicle-Stimulating Hormone
GD	Gestational Diabetes
GIFT	Gamete Intra-Fallopian Transfer
GnRH	Gonadotropin Releasing Hormone
GP	General Practitioner
GTT	Glucose Tolerance Test
HbA1c	Glycosylated Hemoglobin (also called glycohemoglobin)
hCG, HCG	Human Chorionic Gonadotropin
HCP	Health Care Practitioner
HEPA	Hamster Egg Penetration Assay
hMG, HMG	Human Menopausal Gonadotropin
HPT	Home Pregnancy Test
HRT	Hormone Replacement Therapy
HSC	Hysteroscopy
HSG	Hysterosalpingogram
IBD	Immunobead Binding Assay
IBT	Immunobead Binding Test
ICI	Intra-Cervical Insemination
ICSI	Intra-Cytoplasmic Sperm Injection
IF	Infertility
IGTT	Insulin and Glucose Tolerance Test
IM	Intra-Muscular (injections)
IOR	Immature Oocyte Retrieval
IR	Insulin Resistant
ITI	Intra-Tubal Insemination
IUD	Intrauterine Device
IUFD	Intra-Uterine Fetal Demise
IUGR	Intra-Uterine Growth Retardation
IUI	Intra-Uterine Insemination
IVC	Intra-Vaginal Culture
IVF	In Vitro Fertilization
IVIg	Intravenous Immunoglobulin
LAD	Leukocyte Antibody Detection Assay

LAP	Laparoscopy
LH	Luteinizing Hormone
LIT	Leukocyte Immunization Therapy
LMP	Last Menstrual Period (1st day of red flow)
LP	Luteal Phase
LPD	Luteal Phase Defect
LSP	Low Sperm Count
LUF, LUFS	Luteinized Unruptured Follicle Syndrome
MC, m/c	Miscarriage
MESA	Microsurgical Epididymal Sperm Aspiration
MF	Male Factor
MIFT	Micro Injection Fallopian Transfer
MMR	Measles-Mumps-Rubella Vaccine
MRI	Magnetic Resonance Imaging
MSAFP	Maternal Serum Alpha-Fetoprotein
NEST	Nonsurgical Embryonic Selective Thinning
NK	Natural Killer Cells (Cd56+)
NORIF	Nonstimulated Oocyte Retrieval In (Office) Fertilization
NP	Nurse Practitioner
NSA	Nonsurgical Sperm Aspiration
O, OV	Ovulation
OB	Obstetrician
OB/GYN	Obstetrician/Gynecologist
OC	Oral Contraceptives
OCP	Oral Contraceptive Pill
OD	Ovulatory Dysfunction
OHSS	Ovarian Hyperstimulation Syndrome
OPK	Ovulation Predictor Kit
OPT	Ovulation Predictor Test
ORT	Ostrogen Replacement Therapy
OTC	Over the Counter
P4	Progesterone
PA	Physician's Assistant
PCAO	Polycystic Appearing Ovaries
PCO	Polycystic Ovaries
PCOD	Polycystic Ovary Disease
PCOS	Polycystic Ovarian Syndrome
PCP	Primary Care Physician
PCT	Postcoital Test

PESA	Percutaneous Epididymal Sperm Aspiration
PG	Pregnant
PGD	Pre-Implantation Genetic Diagnosis
PI	Primary Infertility
PID	Pelvic Inflammatory Disease
PIO	Progesterone in Oil
PLI	Paternal Leukocyte Immunization
PMS	Premenstrual Syndrome
PNM	Perinatal Mortality
POC	Products of Conception
POF	Premature Ovarian Failure
PROM	Premature Rupture of Membranes
PTSD	Post-Traumatic Stress Disorder
PZD	Partial Zone Dissection
RE	Reproductive Endocrinologist
R-FSH, R-hFSH	Recombinant Human Follicle Stimulating Hormone
RI	Reproductive Immunologist
RIP	Reproductive Immunophynotype
ROS	Reactive Oxygen Species
RPL	Recurrent Pregnancy Loss
RSA	Recurrent Spontaneous Abortion
Rx	Prescription
SA	Semen Analysis
SART	Society for Assisted Reproductive Technology
SB	Stillborn
SCORIF	Stimulated Cycle Oocyte Retrieval in (Office) Fertilization
SHG	Sonohysterogram
SI	Secondary Infertility
SIN	Salpingitis Isthmica Nodosa
SLE	Systemic Lupus Erythematosis
SPA	Sperm Penetration Assay
STD	Sexually Transmitted Disease
SubQ	Subcutaneous Injection
SUZI	Sub-Zonal Insertion
T4	Thyroxine
TeBG	Testosterone-Estradiol-Binding Globulin
TESA	Testicular Sperm Aspiration
TESE	Testicular Sperm Extraction
TET	Tubal Embryo Transfer

TL	Tubal Ligation
TNF	Tumor Necrosis Factor
TORCH	Toxoplasmosis, Other, Rubella, Cytomegalovirus, and Herpes test
TPA	Thyroid Peroxidase Antibodies; Antithyroid Antibodies
TR	Tubal Reversal
TRH	Thyroid-Releasing Hormone
TSH	Thyroid Stimulating Hormone
TUFT	Trans-Uterine Fallopian Transfer
Tx	Treatment
TZD	Thiazolidinediones
UR	Urologist
US, u/s	Ultrasound
UTI	Urinary Tract Infection
V	Vasectomy
VR	Vasectomy Reversal
WBC	White Blood Cells
WNL	Within Normal Limits
ZIFT	Zygote Intra-Fallopian Transfer

Sniglets

Sniglets are clever expressions devised by the creative brainpower of the numerous people of the alt.infertility community on the Internet. There are undoubtedly many more additions since the publication of this book.

The list was initially inspired by Rebecca Smith Waddell and Lisa A. Kramer, who have generously given permission to print it. As they explain it, sniglets are "funny made-up words or definitions for those things in life that just don't seem to have any 'official' terminology. The world of fertility provides lots of hilarious inspiration."

❧ GENERAL FERTILITY SNIGLETS

Psychosymptomatic syndrome	A psychosomatic condition afflicting women during the two-week waiting period; marked by a tendency to incorrectly attribute every bodily twinge and twitch to the early stages of pregnancy
Yearnation	The overwhelming urge to urinate while recording your morning basal body temperature reading
Peetience	What you learn to acquire when starting to chart your basal body temperature
Mucusology	The inexact science of attempting to determine the timing of ovulation

Basal instinct	An urge to shake down your basal thermometer *before* recording your temperature in a futile attempt to work up a sweat and boost your temperature; usually strikes late in the menstrual cycle about the time your temperature would be naturally plummeting to indicate the onset of your dreaded period
Coitus timeruptus	The practice of timing intercourse to correspond with the timing of ovulation
Doggus interruptus	When your dog interrupts sex
Cattus interruptus	When your cat interrupts sex
Coinus interruptus	The impact of infertility treatments on one's pocketbook
"The Sperminator"	Nickname for any friend of your husband's who insists on extended sauna sessions after playing squash
Freeballing	The step beyond boxers taken by truly devoted husbands with low sperm count
Briefectomy	Furtive removal of all tight-fitting briefs from your husband's underwear drawer
Rigorous mortis	Loss of interest in sex due to lack of spontaneity in timing
Transfurryence	Treating your pets like human babies
Furrtility	When your cat gets pregnant
"Looteal" phase	The period of time between cycles when all of the insurance statements/doctor's bills come in from the beginning of the cycle; also a time to save $$ for the upcoming cycle
Assincline	The odd-looking practice of elevating a woman's buttocks after intercourse in order to maximize the sperm's ability to swim for the egg

Gluteus unrelaximus	Side effect of the uncomfortable act of propping up the buttocks after baby-sex
Hindsight	Looking back to see what is happening as you get your shot!
Sperm washing	What you have to do to the sheets when hubby accidentally falls off the pillows at *just* the wrong moment and/or you cough/sneeze/laugh just after that precise moment
Climbmax	What you say to hubby (if his name is Max) as he prepares to ascend the mountain of pillows before him
Indifferent costimulus	The need during intercourse for her to concentrate on fertilizing and him to avoid all thoughts of fertility/infertility and just come
Monthus offalus	Taking a month off from baby-making sex, trying to remember what exactly "birth control" is, so you can be poked and prodded mercilessly with no hope of getting pregnant
Preconceived notion	The idea (before trying to get pregnant) that one will get pregnant within a month or two, three at the most
Hormonophobia	Dread fear of saying the wrong thing to your wife when she is on fertility drugs
Pitspermitis	The crick in your armpit that arises from carrying that plastic bottle of semen from home to the clinic
Preggozone	The magnetic area around all infertile women that draws expectant mothers into close viewing range; the first day of any cycle has the greatest magnetic field, closely followed by any day on which an infertile woman fails a pregnancy test
Pregnesia	The way pregnant women forget everything, sometimes even the fact that they were infertile

Inferguilty	How you feel when you're having a bad day and you read someone's post announcing their pregnancy and you are overcome with the urge to kill them
Perganoltory	The 2 week, in-between waiting time
Wining and complaining	Drinking *lots* of red wine while whining about another negative pregnancy test
Justwaition	The 2 weeks between ovulation and a pregnancy test or a period of time just before gestation
Hormotional	Easily rattled emotional state brought on by hormone surges; especially symptomatic of women on fertility drugs
Indijection	Getting sick to your stomach while getting Metrodin shots
Postcoital nest	The secret vaginal hiding place where sperm hide when they are faced with fertilization anxiety; especially frequented by sperm avoiding the cervix swab during a postcoital test
Petri dish	A womb with a view (for IVFers)

❧ EGG-THEME FERTILITY SNIGLETS

Egg retrieval	What some eggs do at the mere mention of sperm
Eggstatic	What a woman on fertility drugs hopes to feel
Eggspurt advice	What all the fertility books write about ovulation
Egg poaching	Indulging in extended hot-tub soaks during ovulation *or* having frozen eggs stolen from an IVF clinic
Eggsplotion	Hyperstimulation of ovaries induced by overdosing on fertility drugs

Eggsploitation	What drug companies do to women who need fertility drugs to ovulate or to produce enough eggs for IVF
Eggsplanation	Instructions on the label of a fertility drug bottle
Eggswhiteation	The incredible excitement one feels when finding eggwhite mucus when not even looking for it!
Eggspedition	The route an egg takes once it leaves the ovary
Eggspectation	The period of waiting prior to ovulation
Eggsaspirated	1) Eggs that have been aspirated; 2) the annoyed or irritated state of women on fertility drugs or men who have to supply a sperm specimen as they await results, an appointment, or an RE's phone call; 3) the way an infertile woman feels when forced to listen to another's insensitive comments
Eggsplosive	What a woman on fertility drugs is like
Eggscavation	The process of removing follicles from the ovaries
Eggsploited	What those undergoing any reproductive treatments are, by the insurance companies and clinics
Eggcessive	Another word for hyperstimulation
Eggsamination	The process of looking at follicular development via vaginal ultrasound
Eggsuberant	The joy you feel upon finding out that you ovulated!
Eggo	The correct path the ova follows through the female reproductive tract, as in "Eggo through the fallopian tube into the uterus."

Eggstra sensory perception	The certain knowledge that *this* time, sexual intercourse will result in pregnancy
Eggstravaganza	The three-ring circus that ensues when your doctor, his/her residents, interns, and medical students (not to mention several nurses and all the operating room personnel) are working on harvesting your egg(s) for in vitro fertilization
Truly eggscellent	High degree of egg quality, as in "A truly eggscellent egg is easily fertilized and results in a pregnancy."
Eggspress	The route an egg takes through the fallopian tubes, *nonstop!*
Eggscuse me!	What a polite egg says after bumping into a swarm of sperm
Eggsonerated	What an egg is after being told, "You're, not good enough to be fertilized," "You'll never implant," or "You'll never go to term" and then does all three, thank you very much!

✧ HOW DO YOU LIKE YOUR EGGS?

Over easy	Pregnancy resulting after only *one* treatment of any kind
Sunny side up	Checking egg in petri dish under light microscope for signs of cell division, meaning successful in vitro fertilization has occurred
Scrambled	Fertilized egg that wasn't viable due to genetic defects
Hard-boiled	Egg that is impervious to husband's sperm

Fertility-Related Resources

The organizations listed below should be able to help you locate a Fertility Awareness instructor in your area. The majority specifically teach Natural Family Planning, which as a method of birth control requires abstinence during the fertile phase. Ultimately, the information taught is virtually the same as the Fertility Awareness Method, but you should be aware that NFP instruction often comes with a religious orientation that you may or may not appreciate. If you would prefer to use barriers during the fertile phase, try to find a FAM instructor first. Both the NFP organizations themselves as well as some of the Community Resources listed afterward may be able to refer you to one.

✌ NFP/FAM ORGANIZATIONS

Whether you are trying to avoid or get pregnant, you may want to verify that they teach the sympto-thermal method, which involves the observation of both waking temperatures and cervical fluid. Many NFP instructors only teach the Billings Method, which relies exclusively on the observation of cervical fluid. The list below is in alphabetical order.

American Academy of Natural Family Planning
3680 Grant Drive, Suite O
Reno, Nevada 89509 USA
Phone: (775) 827 5408
Web: www.aanfp.org

Billings Ovulation Method Association – USA
PO Box 16206
St. Paul, Minnesota 55116 USA
Phone: (651) 699 8139
Fax: (651) 699 8144
Web: www.boma-use.org

Couple to Couple League (GB)
44 Park Street, Beeston
Nottingham NG9 1DF
Phone: 0115 8778310
Web: www.cclgb.org.uk

Diocesan Development Program for NFP
3211 4th Street NE
Washington, D. C. 20017-1194 USA
Phone: (202) 541 3240
Fax: (202) 541 3054
Web: www.nccbuscc.org/profile/issues/nfp/index.htm

Family of the Americas Foundation
PO Box 1170
Dunkirk, Maryland 20754-1170 USA
Phone: (800) 443 3395
Fax: (301) 627 0847
Web: www.familyplanning.net

Fertility Awareness Network
PO Box 1190
New York, New York 10009 USA
Phone: (800) 597 6267
Web: www.fertaware.com

Fertility UK
Bury Knowle Health Centre
207 London Road
Headington
Oxford OX3 9JA
Web: www.fertilityuk.org

Institute for Reproductive Health
Georgetown University Medical Center
3 PHC, Room 3004
3800 Reservoir Rd, NW
Washington, D.C. 20007 USA
Phone: (202) 687 1392
Fax: (202) 687 6846
Web: www.irh.org

Natural Family Planning Center of Washington, D. C.
8514 Bradmoor Drive
Bethesda, Maryland 20817-3810 USA
Phone: (301) 897 9323
Fax: (301) 571 5267
Email: hklaus@dgsys.com

Pope Paul VI Institute
6901 Mercy Road
Omaha, Nebraska 68106-2604 USA
Phone: (402) 390 6600
Fax: (402) 390 9851
Web: www.mitec.net/~popepaul/about1.htm

Serena Canada
151 Holland Avenue
Ottawa, Ontario K1Y 0Y2, Canada
Phone: (613) 728 6536; (888) 373 7362
Fax: (613) 724 1116
Web: www.serena.ca

World Organisation Ovulation Method Billings (WOOMB)
27 Alexandra Pde
North Fitzroy, Victoria 3068
Australia
Phone: (03) 9481 1722
Fax: (03) 9482 4208
Web: www.woomb.org

ɤ COMMUNITY RESOURCES

You might also try contacting any of the following, which may be able to point you in the right direction:
Catholic churches and dioceses
Family planning clinics
Health food stores and co-ops
Hospital education departments
Public health departments
University health clinics
Women's clinics

✌ CONTRACEPTIVE RESOURCES

Family Planning Association
2–12 Pentonville Road
London N1 9FP
Phone: (020) 7837 5432
Fax: (020) 78373042
Web: www.fpa.org.uk

✌ FERTILITY RESOURCES AND SUPPORT

If you are facing fertility problems and would like to be part of an organized community dealing with similar issues, I particularly recommend contacting RESOLVE, the wonderful organization listed below. In addition, there are scores of groups on the Internet, too many to list here, but all extremely helpful.

AceBabes
31 Hillview Road
Carlton
Nottingham NG4 1JX
Phone: (0115) 987 9266
or
8 Yarwell Close
Derwent Heights
Derby DE21 4SW
Phone: (01332) 832558
Web: www.acebabes.co.uk

BICA: British Infertility Counselling Association
69 Division Street
Sheffield S1 4GE
Phone: (01342) 843880
Web: www.bica.net

CHILD: National Infertility Support Network
Charter House, 43 St Leonards Road
Bexhill on Sea
East Sussex TN40 1JA
Phone: (01424) 732361
Fax: (01424) 731858
Web: www.child.org.uk

The Electronic Infertility Network
Woodlawn House, Carrickfergus
Co. Antrim
Northern Ireland BT3 8PX
Phone: (0)7885138101
Fax: (0)2893 350450
Web: www.ein.org

HFEA: Human Fertilisation and Embryology Authority
Paxton House, 30 Artillery Lane
London E1 7LS
Phone: (020) 7377 5077
Web: www.hfea.gov.uk

ISSUE: The National Fertility Association
114 Lichfield Street, Walsall
West Midlands WS1 1SZ
Phone: (01922) 722888
Web: www.issue.co.uk

MoreToLife
114 Lichfield Street, Walsall WS1 1SZ
Phone: (01922) 722888
Web: www.moretolife.co.uk

The National Endometriosis Society
Suite 50, Westminster Palace Gardens
1–7 Artillery Row
London SW1P 1RL
Freephone helpline: (0808) 8082227
Web: www.endo.org.uk

RESOLVE
1310 Broadway,
Somerville, MA 02144 USA
Phone: (617) 623 0744
Fax: (617) 623 0252
Web: www.resolve.org

✿ SOME WEB SITES OF NOTE

There are countless Web sites devoted to FAM, NFP, fertility, and women's health issues in general. Unfortunately, Web pages have a tendency to suddenly disappear, and thus I have chosen to list only a handful of the most useful ones that I think are most likely to exist well after this book has been published.

www.TCOYF.com
Official site of Ovusoft, which produces the *TCOYF* software specifically designed to supplement this book

dir.yahoo.com/Health/Women_s_Health
An excellent, regularly updated resource from Yahoo!, with links to sites on all major women's health issues

www.obgyn.net
A general women's health site for women and their doctors

www.4women.gov
Official site of the National Women's Health Information Center

www.medlineplus.gov
An extensive source of all types of medical information from the National Library of Medicine at the National Institutes of Health

www.ferti.net
A wide range of material on infertility

www.ivf.com
Extensive information on high-tech reproductive technologies

www.woomb.org
International site devoted to the teaching of the Billings Ovulation Method

www.fertilityuk.org
An excellent British site on Fertility Awareness education

www.mum.org
Official home of the Museum of Menstruation and Women's Health. Highly recommended!

Recommended Books

The following list of books is not comprehensive. There are excellent women's health and fertility-related books continually being written. I have simply chosen several that I've found particularly useful.

FERTILITY AWARENESS

Billings, Evelyn, M.D., and Ann Westmore. *The Billings Method: Controlling Fertility Without Drugs or Devices.* Australia: Life Cycle Books, 2000.

Clubb, Elizabeth, M.D., and Jane Knight. *Fertility: Fertility Awareness and Natural Family Planning.* United Kingdom: David and Charles, 1996.

Kippley, Sheila. *Breastfeeding and Natural Child Spacing.* Cincinnati: The Couple to Couple League International, 1999.

PREGNANCY ACHIEVEMENT

Aronson, Diane and the staff of RESOLVE. *Resolving Infertility.* New York: Harper-Resource, 1999.

Berger, Gary, M.D., et al. *The Couple's Guide to Fertility.* New York: Doubleday, 1995.

Douglas, Ann, and John Sussman, M.D. *Trying Again: A Guide to Pregnancy After Miscarriage, Stillbirth, and Infant Loss.* Dallas: Taylor Trade Publishing, 2000.

Lauersen, Niels H., M.D., and Colette Bouchez. *Getting Pregnant: What You Need to Know Right Now.* New York: Simon and Schuster, 2000.

Marrs, Richard, M.D. *Dr. Richard Marrs' Fertility Book.* New York: Dell Books, 1998.

Scher, Jonathan, M.D. *Preventing Miscarriage.* New York: HarperCollins, 1991.

Silber, Sherman, M.D. *How to Get Pregnant with the New Technology.* New York: Warner Books, 1998.

WOMEN'S HEALTH

Ammer, Christine, and Jo Ann E. Manson. *The New A to Z of Women's Health: A Concise Encyclopedia.* New York: Facts on File, 2000.

Boston Women's Health Book Collective. *Our Bodies, Ourselves for the New Century.* New York: Simon and Schuster, 1998.

Brody, Jane E. *The New York Times Book of Women's Health.* New York: Lebhar-Friedman Books, 2000.

Faelten, Sharon, editor. *The Doctors Book of Home Remedies for Women.* New York: Bantam Books, 1998.

Lauersen, Niels H., M.D., and Eileen Stukane. *Listen to Your Body: A Gynecologist Answers Women's Most Intimate Questions.* Fireside Books, 2000.

Northrup, Christiane, M.D. *Women's Bodies, Women's Wisdom.* New York: Bantam Books, 1998.

Stoppard, Miriam, M.D. *Women's Health Handbook.* New York: Dorling Kindersley Publishing Inc., 2001.

Turkington, Carol A., and Susan J. Probst, M.D. *The Unofficial Guide to Women's Health.* MacMillan Publishing Company, 2000.

Vliet, Elizabeth Lee, M.D., *Screaming to Be Heard: Hormonal Connections Women Suspect and Doctors Still Ignore.* New York: M. Evans & Co., 2000.

PMS

Hahn, Linaya. *PMS: Solving the Puzzle.* Chicago Spectrum Press, 1995.

Kallins, George J., M.D. *5 Steps to a PMS Free Life.* Laguna Niguel, CA: Village Healer Press, 2000.

MENOPAUSE

Gittleman, Ann Louise. *Before the Change: Taking Charge of Your Perimenopause.* San Francisco: HarperSanFrancisco, 1999.

Lark, Susan, M.D. *Menopause Self-Help Book.* Berkeley, CA: Celestial Arts, 1998.

Lee, John R., M.D. *What Your Doctor May Not Tell You About Premenopause.* Little, Brown & Company, 1999.

Love, Susan, M.D. *Dr. Susan Love's Hormone Book: Making Informed Choices About Menopause.* Random House, 1998.

Northrup, Christiane, M.D. *The Wisdom of Menopause.* New York: Bantam Books, 2001. HarperCollins, 1998.

Ojeda, Linda, Ph.D. *Menopause Without Medicine.* Alameda, CA: Hunter House Publishers, 2000.

Sheehy, Gail. *The Silent Passage: Menopause.* New York: Pocket Books, 1998. HarperCollins, 1994.

Vliet, Elizabeth Lee, M.D. *Screaming to Be Heard: Hormonal Connections Women Suspect and Doctors Still Ignore.* New York: M. Evans & Co., 2000.

MISCELLANEOUS

Angier, Natalie. *Woman: An Intimate Geography.* Virago Press, 1999.

Ballweg, Mary Lou. *The Endometriosis Sourcebook.* Chicago: Contemporary Books, 1995.

The Burton Goldberg Group. *Alternative Medicine: The Definitive Guide.* (2nd edition) Celestial Arts, 2002.

Castleman, Michael. *Sexual Solutions.* Simon & Schuster (revision/update) 1989.

Cutler, Winnifred, Ph.D. *Love Cycles.* Chester Springs, PA: Athena Institute, 1996.

Delaney, Janice, et al. *The Curse: A Cultural History of Menstruation.* Champaign, IL: University of Illinois Press, 1988.

Dr Foster. *Dr Foster Fertility Guide.* London: Vermilion, 2002.

Harris, Colette, and Adam Carey, M.D. *PCOS: A Woman's Guide to Dealing with Polycystic Ovarian Syndrome.* New York: HarperCollins, 2000.

Murray, Michael, N.D., and Joseph Pizzorno, N.D. *Encyclopedia of Natural Medicine.* Little, Brown, 1998.

Shannon, Marilyn. *Fertility, Cycles, and Nutrition.* Cincinnati: The Couple to Couple League International, 2001.

Shettles, Landrum, M.D., Ph.D., and David Rorvik. *How to Choose the Sex of Your Baby.* New York: Doubleday, 1997.

Sloane, Ethel. *Biology of Women.* Albany, NY: Delmar Publishers, 2001.

Wright, Jonathan V., M.D., and Morgen Thaler, John. *Natural Hormone Replacement.* Petaluma, CA: Smart Publications, 1997.

APPENDIX O

Tear-out for Your Clinician

Fertility Essentials You *and* Your Patients Should Know

by Toni Weschler, MPH,
author of *Taking Charge of Your Fertility*

If you are reading this tear-out, you are either:

- A health practitioner whose patient encouraged you to read *Taking Charge* because she is convinced that the information within it is something that all women and their clinicians should know.

- The type of medical professional women cherish—current, sensitive, and respectful of their desire to be fully informed about their bodies.

In any case, if you've had a chance to even skim my book, you've hopefully seen that my goal is to fundamentally empower women with the knowledge they need to truly understand their reproductive health. By learning the basic principles of the Fertility Awareness Method (FAM), they will be able to easily chart their menstrual cycles on a daily basis, providing them with information that will one day be as fundamental to a young woman's education as basic feminine hygiene. And in the process, they will be doing their part to help revolutionize the clinician-patient relationship.

What you will discover by reviewing the accompanying sample charts is that Fertility Awareness is a comprehensive means of allowing women to finally take control of *all* aspects of their cycles, from natural birth control and pregnancy achievement to PMS, premenopause, and basic gynecological health. As a medical professional, you'll quickly see the basis for this remarkable body of self-empowering knowledge that can only serve to benefit you and your patients. More specifically, it will make your job infinitely easier by giving you the tools to more efficiently diagnose potential problems listed in the box on the next page.

409

CONDITIONS FAM CAN HELP IDENTIFY

Fertility Conditions	Gynecological Conditions
anovulation	irregular or abnormal bleeding
delayed ovulation	vaginal infections
short luteal phases	urinary tract infections
unsuitable cervical fluid	cervical anomalies
hormonal imbalances	breast lumps
insufficient progesterone levels	premenstrual syndrome
miscalculated date of conception	
occurrence of miscarriages	

If you get a copy of *Taking Charge of Your Fertility,* I would encourage you to peruse the several specific sections listed below:

- color insert: eight color pages of photos and graphics on fertility, menstrual cycles, and FAM
- page 150: Fertility Factors You Can Detect Through Waking Temps
- page 135: Summary of the Four FAM Rules
- page 291: Troubleshooting Your Cycle: Expecting the Unexpected

& GENERAL FAM INFORMATION

What is the Fertility Awareness Method (FAM)?

The Fertility Awareness Method is a scientifically validated, natural form of contraception or pregnancy achievement. It is *not* the Rhythm Method, an antiquated and ineffective method of birth control based upon a strictly mathematical computation of the average of a woman's past cycle lengths, with no observations to determine impending ovulation for *each individual cycle.*

FAM involves the daily observation of the three primary fertility signs that indicate the fertile phase surrounding ovulation: basal body temperature, cervical fluid, and cervical changes. As a method of birth control, couples choose to either abstain (called Natural Family Planning) or use another method of contraception during the woman's fertile phase. The 1998 edition of *Contraceptive Technology* places the method failure rate of FAM at 2%, which is lower than any barrier.

BabyMad Basal Body Temperature and Cervical Mucus Chart (Fahrenheit) – www.babymad.com

Name: _____

Dates covered: ___/___/___ to ___/___/___

Cycle Day	1	2	3	4	5	6	7	8	9	10	11	12	13	14	15	16	17	18	19	20	21	22	23	24	25	26	27	28	29	30	31	32	33	34	35	36	37	38	39	40	41	42	43	44	45
Weekday																																													
Date																																													
Time																																													
99.1																																													
99.0																																													
98.9																																													
98.8																																													
98.7																																													
98.6																																													
98.5																																													
98.4																																													
98.3																																													
98.2																																													
98.1																																													
98.0																																													
97.9																																													
97.8																																													
97.7																																													
97.6																																													
97.5																																													
97.4																																													
97.3																																													
97.2																																													
97.1																																													
97.0																																													
96.9																																													
CM * Intercourse																																													
Cervical Mucus Textures																																													

*CM = cervical mucus; P=period, D=dry, M=mucus, E=egg white

Notes: (List any changes to your routine)

If you'd like an electronic copy of this chart so you can print off as required please email: info@babymad.com. I'll also send a very useful guide on BBT Charting

What other benefits does FAM provide?

In addition to helping identify when a woman is fertile, FAM is an empowering tool for maintaining basic gynecological health by giving her the knowledge to identify everything from true vaginal infections and abnormal bleeding to normal cyclical pains and potential menstrual disorders.

Can anybody use FAM?

Virtually all women of reproductive age will benefit from learning the basic principles of Fertility Awareness, if for no other reason then to discover how much they can learn about their own bodies. Of course, it takes a certain amount of motivation and discipline to chart cycles on a daily basis. Yet, when informed of the choice, countless women have concluded that FAM is both easy to learn and well worth the couple of minutes a day it actually takes.

⅋ə PRACTICAL TIPS WHEN BEGINNING TO TREAT A PATIENT DESIRING PREGNANCY

- Since infertility affects men and women equally, treat the couple together, ordering a semen analysis on him at the same time that you pursue diagnostic tests on her.
- Given that ovulation can vary from cycle to cycle, use her past temperature charts as a general guideline, but don't rely on them to predict future fertility. Instead, encourage your patient to chart her cervical fluid in addition to BBTs, since this will enable her to identify her most fertile time, and you to diagnose and advise her based on each unique cycle as it unfolds.
- Advise patients to focus on *cervical fluid* rather than *temperature* in order to properly time intercourse for conception. The woman is only fertile when her cervical fluid or vaginal sensation is wet and slippery, which usually occurs before the temperature shift. Her Peak Day of fertility is the last day of wet and slippery cervical fluid or vaginal sensation, whichever comes last.
- Encourage your patients to time intercourse *before* the day of the temperature shift, since by the time the temperatures rise, the egg will most likely be dead and gone.
- Don't advise your patients to time intercourse for the preovulatory drop in temperature, since that fortuitous sign only occurs in about 10% of cycles.

- Time various diagnostic tests based on when your patient actually ovulates, and not on a standard Day 14 ovulation. (Commonly mistimed procedures include postcoitals, endometrial biopsies, and progesterone blood tests.)

- Determine if your patient is ovulating on her own before routinely prescribing Clomid. If you decide that Clomid is necessary to either induce ovulation or correct a potential luteal phase problem, be sure that you address the possibility of the drug drying up her cervical fluid.

- If you perform vaginal insemination, make sure it is timed when your patient is about to ovulate that particular cycle rather than automatically around Day 14, which occurs in less than 15% of cycles. Ideally, she should be observing her cervical fluid so that she knows when to most efficiently start testing with an ovulation predictor kit. If she doesn't produce fertile-quality cervical fluid, intrauterine insemination would be more likely to succeed.

SCIENTIFIC PRINCIPLES UPON WHICH THE FERTILITY AWARENESS METHOD IS BASED

A. A woman's menstrual cycle is directly influenced by estrogen and progesterone. Estrogen dominates the first (or follicular) phase of the cycle, progesterone the latter (or secretory) phase. Luteinizing hormone is the catalyst that actually causes ovulation.

B. A woman produces three primary fertility signs that signal impending and completed ovulation: basal body temperature, cervical fluid, and cervical changes.

C. The woman's egg can only live a short time, from about 12 to 24 hours. If a second egg is released within one cycle (as in the case of fraternal twins), it will be released within 24 hours of the first.

D. Sperm can live in women's fertile-quality cervical fluid for up to 5 days.

E. The corpus luteum, the remnant of the egg's follicle, releases progesterone, which acts to inhibit further eggs from being released until the following cycle.

If you would like to learn about FAM software or download master charts for your patients, please visit www.TCOYF.com. Or you can copy the charts in this tear-out for your patients, enlarging by 130%.

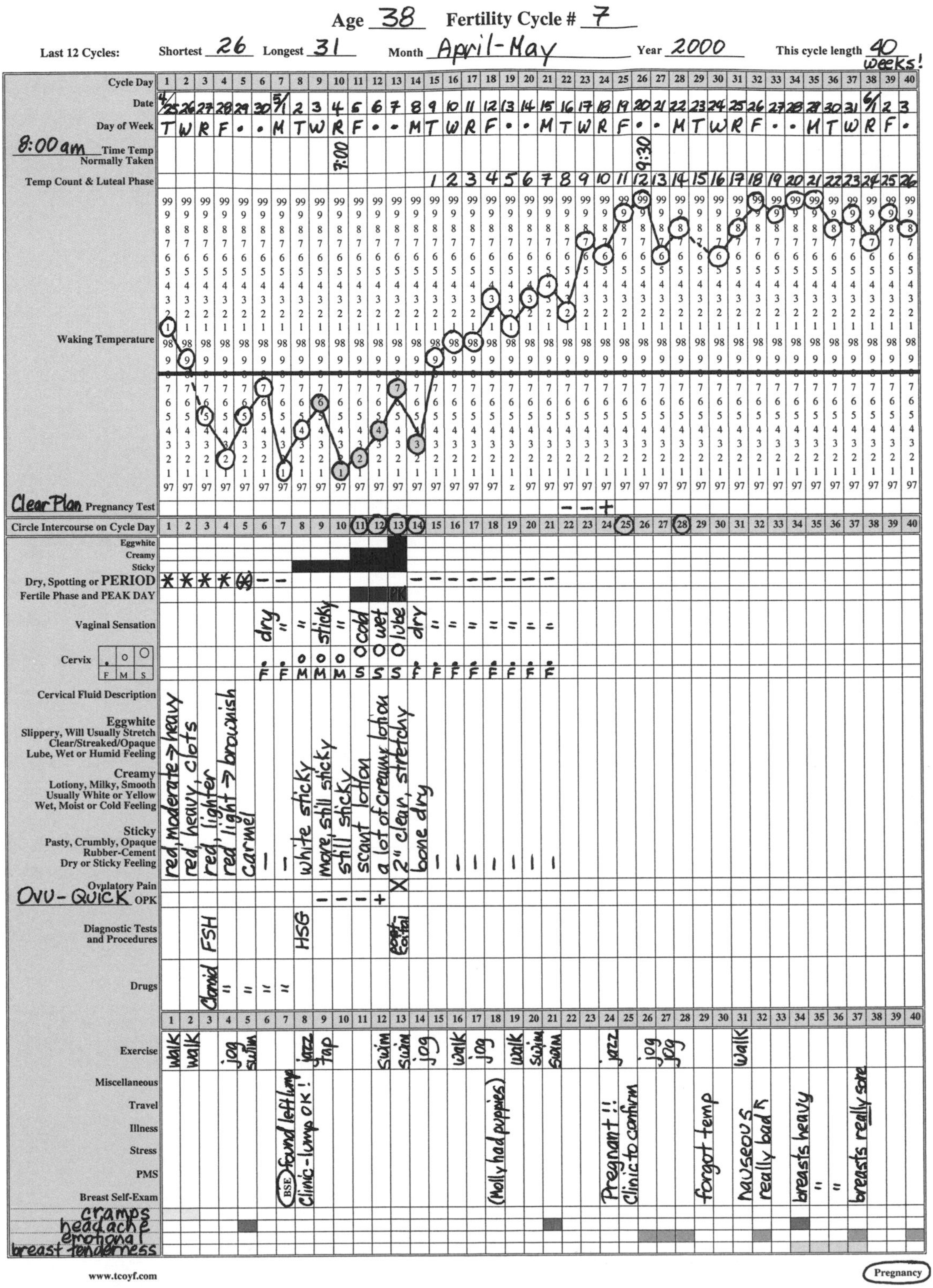

Chart O.1. Pregnancy Achievement.

Age **38**   Fertility Cycle # **7**

Last 12 Cycles: Shortest **26**   Longest **31**   Month **April-May**   Year **2000**   This cycle length **40 weeks!**

Cycle Day	1	2	3	4	5	6	7	8	9	10	11	12	13	14	15	16	17	18	19	20	21	22	23	24	25	26	27	28	29	30	31	32	33	34	35	36	37	38	39	40
Date	4/25	26	27	28	29	30	5/1	2	3	4	5	6	7	8	9	10	11	12	13	14	15	16	17	18	19	20	21	22	23	24	25	26	27	28	29	30	31	6/1	2	3
Day of Week	T	W	R	F	•	•	M	T	W	R	F	•	•	M	T	W	R	F	•	•	M	T	W	R	F	•	•	M	T	W	R	F	•	•	M	T	W	R	F	•

Time Temp Normally Taken: **8:00 am**

Temp Count & Luteal Phase: 1 2 3 4 5 6 7 8 9 10 11 12 13 14 15 16 17 18 19 20 21 22 23 24 25 26

OvU-QUICK OPK

Clear Plan Pregnancy Test: — — +

| Circle Intercourse on Cycle Day | 1 | 2 | 3 | 4 | 5 | 6 | 7 | 8 | 9 | 10 | (11) | 12 | 13 | 14 | 15 | 16 | 17 | 18 | 19 | 20 | 21 | 22 | 23 | 24 | (25) | 26 | 27 | (28) | 29 | 30 | 31 | 32 | 33 | 34 | 35 | 36 | 37 | 38 | 39 | 40 |

Eggwhite / Creamy / Sticky

Dry, Spotting or **PERIOD**: ✗ ✗ ✗ ✗ ⊙⊙ — — — — — — — — — —

Fertile Phase and PEAK DAY

Vaginal Sensation: dry " " sticky occd wet lube dry

Cervix: F F M M M S S S f f F F F F F F

Cervical Fluid Description

Eggwhite: Slippery, Will Usually Stretch / Clear/Streaked/Opaque / Lube, Wet or Humid Feeling

Creamy: Lotiony, Milky, Smooth / Usually White or Yellow / Wet, Moist or Cold Feeling

Sticky: Pasty, Crumbly, Opaque / Rubber-Cement / Dry or Sticky Feeling

Handwritten cervical fluid notes: red, moderate→heavy; red, heavy, clots; red, lighter; red, light→brownish; carmel; white sticky; more still sticky; still sticky; scant lotion; a lot of creamy lotion; X 2" clean, stretchy; bone dry

Ovulatory Pain OPK: — — — +

Diagnostic Tests and Procedures: Clomid; FSH; HSG; post coital

Drugs: Clomid " " "

| | 1 | 2 | 3 | 4 | 5 | 6 | 7 | 8 | 9 | 10 | 11 | 12 | 13 | 14 | 15 | 16 | 17 | 18 | 19 | 20 | 21 | 22 | 23 | 24 | 25 | 26 | 27 | 28 | 29 | 30 | 31 | 32 | 33 | 34 | 35 | 36 | 37 | 38 | 39 | 40 |

Exercise: walk, walk, jog, swim, jazz, tap, swim, swim, jog, walk, jog, walk, swim, sauna, jazz, jog, jog, walk

Miscellaneous / Travel / Illness / Stress / PMS / Breast Self-Exam:
- BSE found left lump
- Clinic - lump OK!
- (Molly had puppies)
- Pregnant!! Clinic to confirm
- forgot temp
- nauseous; really bad R
- breasts heavy "
- breasts really sore

cramps / headache / emotional / breast-tenderness

www.tcoyf.com

Fertile Phase

Pregnancy

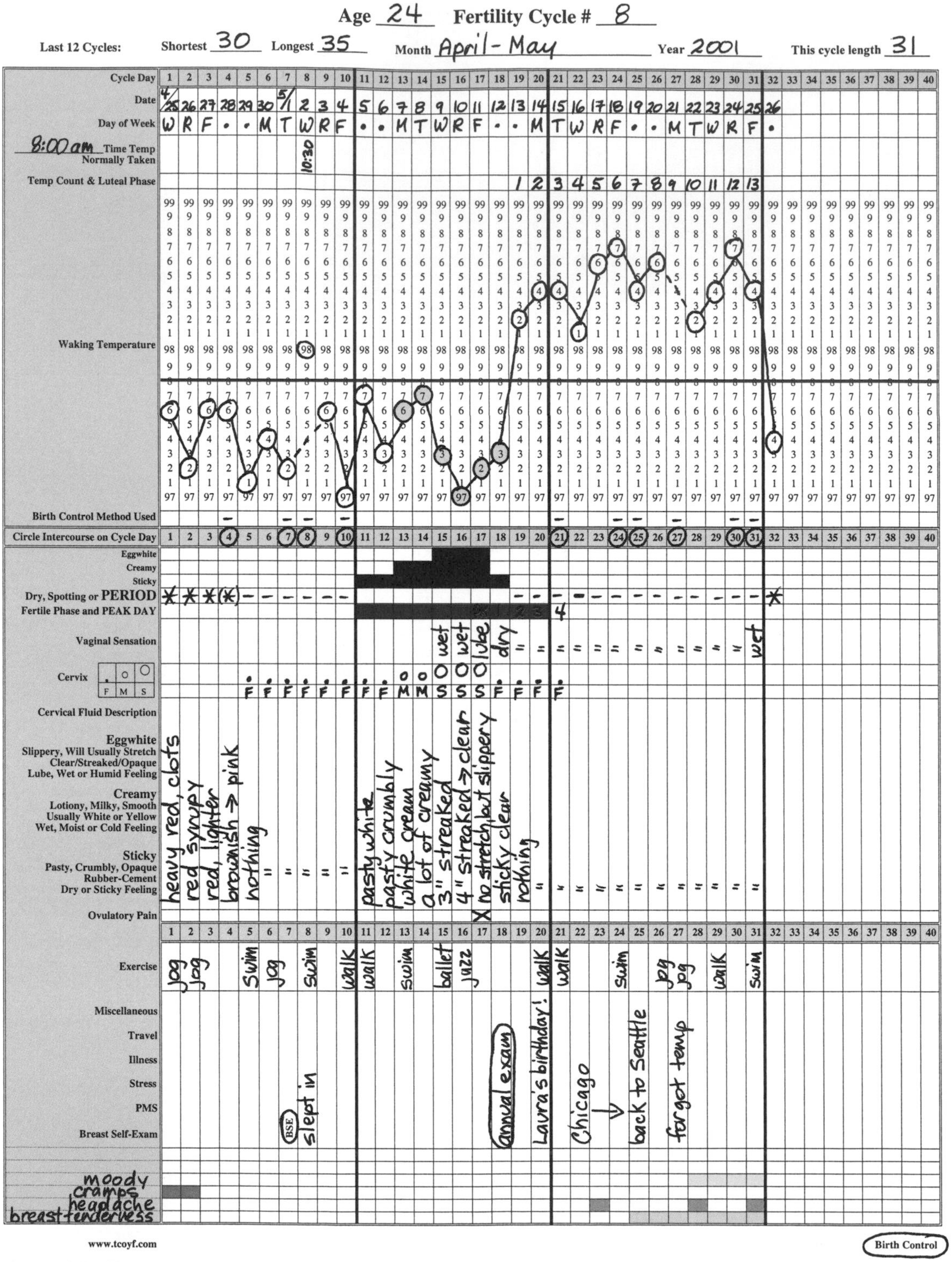

Age **24** Fertility Cycle # **8**

Last 12 Cycles: Shortest **30** Longest **35** Month **April - May** Year **2001** This cycle length **31**

Cycle Day	1	2	3	4	5	6	7	8	9	10	11	12	13	14	15	16	17	18	19	20	21	22	23	24	25	26	27	28	29	30	31	32	33	34	35	36	37	38	39	40
Date	4/25	26	27	28	29	30	5/1	2	3	4	5	6	7	8	9	10	11	12	13	14	15	16	17	18	19	20	21	22	23	24	25	26								
Day of Week	W	R	F	•	•	M	T	W	R	F	•	•	M	T	W	R	F	•	•	M	T	W	R	F	•	•	M	T	W	R	F	•								

Time Temp Normally Taken **8:00 am**

Temp Count & Luteal Phase: (starting cycle day 21) 1 2 3 4 5 6 7 8 9 10 11 12 13

Waking Temperature

Birth Control Method Used

| Circle Intercourse on Cycle Day | 1 | 2 | (3) | 4 | 5 | 6 | (7) | 8 | 9 | (10) | 11 | 12 | 13 | 14 | 15 | 16 | 17 | 18 | 19 | 20 | (21) | 22 | 23 | (24) | (25) | 26 | (27) | 28 | 29 | (30) | (31) | 32 | 33 | 34 | 35 | 36 | 37 | 38 | 39 | 40 |

Eggwhite / Creamy / Sticky

Dry, Spotting or PERIOD: X X X (X) — — — — — ... — — — — — — — — — — X

Fertile Phase and PEAK DAY

Vaginal Sensation: wet wet lube dry

Cervix

Cervical Fluid Description

Eggwhite — Slippery, Will Usually Stretch, Clear/Streaked/Opaque, Lube, Wet or Humid Feeling

Creamy — Lotiony, Milky, Smooth, Usually White or Yellow, Wet, Moist or Cold Feeling

Sticky — Pasty, Crumbly, Opaque, Rubber-Cement, Dry or Sticky Feeling

heavy red, clots / red syrupy / red, lighter / brownish → pink / nothing / pasty white / pasty crumbly white cream / a lot of creamy / 3" streaked / 4" streaked → clear / no stretch, but slippery / sticky clear / nothing

Ovulatory Pain

Exercise: jog / jog / swim / jog / swim / walk / walk / swim / ballet / jazz / walk / walk / swim / jog / jog / walk / swim

Miscellaneous / Travel / Illness / Stress / PMS / Breast Self-Exam

BSE / slept in / annual exam / Laura's birthday! / Chicago / back to Seattle / forgot temp

moody / cramps / headache / breast tenderness

www.tcoyf.com

Birth Control

Chart O.2. Natural Birth Control. ■ **Fertile Phase**

Age _____ **Fertility Cycle #** _____

Cycle Day	1	2	3	4	5	6	7	8	9	10	11	12	13	14	15	16	17	18	19	20	21	22	23	24	25	26	27	28	29	30	31	32	33	34	35	36	37	38	39	40
Date																																								
Day of Week																																								

_____ Time Temp
Normally Taken

Temp Count & Luteal Phase

Waking Temperature

(Temperature grid: each cycle day column 1–40 shows the scale 99, 9, 8, 7, 6, 5, 4, 3, 2, 1, 98, 9, 8, 7, 6, 5, 4, 3, 2, 1, 97)

_____ Pregnancy Test

Circle Intercourse on Cycle Day	1	2	3	4	5	6	7	8	9	10	11	12	13	14	15	16	17	18	19	20	21	22	23	24	25	26	27	28	29	30	31	32	33	34	35	36	37	38	39	40
Eggwhite																																								
Creamy																																								
Sticky																																								
Dry, Spotting or PERIOD																																								
Fertile Phase and PEAK DAY																																								
Vaginal Sensation																																								
Cervix																																								

Cervix: [.] [o] [O]
F   M   S

Cervical Fluid Description

Eggwhite
Slippery, Will Usually Stretch
Clear/Streaked/Opaque
Lube, Wet or Humid Feeling

Creamy
Lotiony, Milky, Smooth
Usually White or Yellow
Wet, Moist or Cold Feeling

Sticky
Pasty, Crumbly, Opaque
Rubber-Cement
Dry or Sticky Feeling

Ovulatory Pain
_____ OPK

Diagnostic Tests
and Procedures

Drugs

	1	2	3	4	5	6	7	8	9	10	11	12	13	14	15	16	17	18	19	20	21	22	23	24	25	26	27	28	29	30	31	32	33	34	35	36	37	38	39	40
Exercise																																								
Miscellaneous																																								
Travel																																								
Illness																																								
Stress																																								
PMS																																								
Breast Self-Exam							BSE																																	

Age _____ **Fertility Cycle #** _____

Cycle Day	1	2	3	4	5	6	7	8	9	10	11	12	13	14	15	16	17	18	19	20	21	22	23	24	25	26	27	28	29	30	31	32	33	34	35	36	37	38	39	40
Date																																								
Day of Week																																								

_____ Time Temp Normally Taken

Temp Count & Luteal Phase

Waking Temperature

Values repeated for each column (Cycle Day 1–40):
99 9 8 7 6 5 4 3 2 1 98 9 8 7 6 5 4 3 2 1 97 ... 98 9 8 7 6 5 4 3 2 1 97

Birth Control Method Used

Circle Intercourse on Cycle Day	1	2	3	4	5	6	7	8	9	10	11	12	13	14	15	16	17	18	19	20	21	22	23	24	25	26	27	28	29	30	31	32	33	34	35	36	37	38	39	40
Eggwhite																																								
Creamy																																								
Sticky																																								
Dry, Spotting or **PERIOD**																																								
Fertile Phase and PEAK DAY																																								
Vaginal Sensation																																								

Cervix: (· o O / F M S)

| Cervical Fluid Description | | | | | | | | | | | | | | | | | | | | | | | | | | | | | | | | | | | | | | | | |

Eggwhite
Slippery, Will Usually Stretch
Clear/Streaked/Opaque
Lube, Wet or Humid Feeling

Creamy
Lotiony, Milky, Smooth
Usually White or Yellow
Wet, Moist or Cold Feeling

Sticky
Pasty, Crumbly, Opaque
Rubber-Cement
Dry or Sticky Feeling

Ovulatory Pain

	1	2	3	4	5	6	7	8	9	10	11	12	13	14	15	16	17	18	19	20	21	22	23	24	25	26	27	28	29	30	31	32	33	34	35	36	37	38	39	40
Exercise																																								
Miscellaneous																																								
Travel																																								
Illness																																								
Stress																																								
PMS																																								
Breast Self-Exam							BSE																																	

Glossary

Abortion: The spontaneous or induced termination of pregnancy before the embryo or fetus is viable.

Abstinence: Avoidance of intercourse. To avoid pregnancy using Natural Family Planning (NFP), abstinence from intercourse includes avoiding all genital contact during the fertile phase of the cycle.

Acquired immune deficiency syndrome: See **AIDS**.

Adhesion: Fibrous tissue that abnormally binds organs or other body parts. It is usually the result of inflammation or abnormal healing of a surgical wound.

AI: See **Artificial insemination**.

AIDS: Acquired immune deficiency syndrome. A fatal disease that is most often transmitted sexually. It is caused by a virus that damages the body's immune system, resulting in infections and cancers.

Amenorrhea: Prolonged absence of menstruation. Causes include stress, fatigue, psychological disturbance, obesity, weight loss, anorexia nervosa, hormonal contraceptives, and medical disorders.

Amniocentesis: Puncture of the fluid sac surrounding the fetus through the abdominal wall and uterus to obtain a sample of the amniotic fluid for testing. The procedure, performed around the 16th week of pregnancy, can be used to identify various birth defects.

Androgens: Male sex hormones, responsible for the development of male secondary sex characteristics including facial hair and a deep voice. Most androgens, including the principal one, testosterone, are produced in the testes. Small amounts of androgens are also produced in a woman's ovaries and adrenal glands.

Anovulation: The absence of ovulation.

Anovulatory (Anovular) cycles: A cycle in which ovulation does not occur.

A.P.L.: A natural HCG fertility drug used to stimulate the ovaries. Administered by injection.

Arousal fluid: The colorless, lubricative fluid secreted around the vaginal opening in response to sexual stimulation, in preparation for intercourse. Arousal fluid should not be confused with fertile cervical fluid, which is secreted in a cyclical pattern around ovulation.

ART: Assisted Reproductive Technologies, such as IVF and GIFT.

Artificial insemination: A procedure in which a syringe is used to insert the man's sperm just outside or inside the cervix. The sperm may be from the husband (AIH) or a donor (AID). See **IUI**.

Bacteria: Microscopic single-celled organisms. Some types of bacteria live in or on the body without doing any harm and are beneficial to health. Pathogenic bacteria cause disease on entering the body, such as gonococcus, which causes gonorrhea.

Barrier methods of contraception: Any method of contraception that uses a physical barrier to prevent sperm from reaching the ovum, such as the condom or diaphragm.

Bartholin's glands: Two tiny glands on each side of the vaginal opening that produce a thin lubricant when a woman becomes sexually aroused.

Basal body temperature (BBT): See **Waking temperature.**

Basal body temperature method: See **BBT method.**

Basic Infertile Pattern (BIP): An extended, unchanging pattern of sticky cervical fluid or dryness that women occasionally experience instead of the normal pattern of progressively wetter (and more fertile) cervical fluid. Such a pattern generally indicates relative inactivity of the ovaries and low oestrogen levels.

BBT: Basal body temperature. See **Waking temperature.**

BBT Method: Basal body temperature method. A type of natural birth control in which the postovulatory infertile phase of the menstrual cycle is identified exclusively by a sustained rise in basal body temperature. Because those who use this method do not chart cervical fluid, they must either abstain or use barriers during the entire preovulatory phase of the cycle.

Billings Method: A natural method of fertility control in which days of fertility are identified exclusively by observations of cervical fluid at the vaginal opening. Developed by Drs. John and Evelyn Billings.

Billings Ovulation Method: See **Billings Method.**

Biopsy: Removal of tissue from the body for microscopic examination and diagnosis, for example, a cone-shaped biopsy of the cervix is for diagnosis and treatment of cervical cancer.

BIP: See **Basic Infertile Pattern.**

Biphasic temperature pattern: A temperature chart that shows a pattern of relatively low temperatures in the preovulatory phase of the cycle, followed by a higher postovulatory level for about 12 to 16 days, until the next menstruation.

Blastocyst: The newly created fertilized ovum, before implantation occurs.

Blighted ovum: A pregnancy in which no fetus ever developed in the pregnancy sac.

Breakthrough bleeding: Bleeding due to excessive oestrogen production, which causes the endometrium to grow beyond the point that it can sustain itself. It usually occurs during anovulatory cycles.

Breastfeeding: The act of suckling, on the part of the infant, and the act of giving milk from the breast, directly to the infant, on the part of the mother. *Full* breastfeeding means that you are not giving your baby *any* supplements or pacifiers; *nearly* full breastfeeding means that you supplement no more than 15% of all feedings. Both mean that intervals between feedings should not exceed 4 hours during the day or 6 hours at night. *Partial* breastfeeding means that supplements such as juices and solids are regularly given. It also means that you are nursing less frequently than every 4 hours during the day, and less than every 6 hours at night.

Calendar Rhythm Method: See **Rhythm Method.**

Centrifuge: An apparatus consisting of a component spun around a central axis to separate contained materials of different density. Used in the process of sperm washing.

Cervical crypts: Pockets in the lining of the cervix where cervical fluid is produced and that function as a temporary shelter for sperm during the woman's fertile phase.

Cervical erosion: The condition of the cervix when the cells lining the cervical canal grow over the lip of the cervix.

Cervical fluid: The secretion produced within the cervix that acts as a medium in which sperm can travel. Its presence and quality is directly related to the production of oestrogen and progesterone. Analogous to a man's seminal fluid. It is one of the three primary fertility signs, along with cervical position and waking temperature. Cervical fluid typically gets progressively wetter as ovulation approaches. See **Creamy, Eggwhite-quality, Fertile-quality,** and **Sticky cervical fluid.**

Cervical fluid ferning test: See **Ferning test.**

Cervical mucus: See **Cervical fluid.**

Cervical os: The opening of the cervix, which itself is the lower portion of the uterus.

Cervical palpation: Feeling the cervix with your middle finger to determine its height, softness, and opening.

Cervical polyp: An overgrowth of normal tissue that lines the cervical canal, often protruding out of the cervical os. May be asymptomatic or cause spotting or even cramping if they push down on the cervix.

Cervical position: The term used to describe one of the three primary fertility signs. In this book, cervical position refers to three facets of the cervix: its height, softness, and opening.

Cervical tip: See **Cervical os.**

Cervix: The lower portion of the uterus that projects into the vagina.

Change of life: The menopausal years during which reproductive functions cease.

Chlamydia: A highly prevalent sexually transmitted disease. It can lead to infertility through scarring of the fallopian tubes.

Chromosome: One of the 46 microscopic units within each cell that carries the genetic material responsible for inherited characteristics.

Climacteric: See **Menopause.**

Clitoris: A small knob of very sensitive erectile tissue. The female counterpart of the male penis, it is situated outside of the vagina under a hood of skin where the labia unite.

Clomid: A commonly prescribed drug used primarily to induce ovulation.

Clomiphene Citrate: See **Clomid.**

Coitus: Sexual intercourse.

Coitus interruptus: See **Withdrawal.**

Colposcopy: A procedure used to examine the vagina and cervix under magnification through an instrument known as a colposcope. It is of particular value in the early detection of cancer of the cervix.

Conceive: To become pregnant.

Conception: Fusion of the sperm and egg.

Condom: A sheath of thin rubber worn over the penis to prevent conception.

Contraception: The prevention of conception by artificial means.

Contraceptive pill: See **Pill**.

Corpus luteum: The yellow gland formed by the ruptured follicle after ovulation. If the egg is fertilized, the corpus luteum continues to produce progesterone to support the early pregnancy until the placenta is formed. If fertilization does not occur, the corpus luteum degenerates within 12 to 16 days.

Corpus luteum cyst: A rare and temporary condition in which the corpus luteum doesn't disintegrate after its typical 12- to 16-day life span. It may lead women to mistakenly believe they are pregnant by delaying their periods and maintaining their high postovulatory temperatures beyond 16 days.

Coverline: A line used to help delineate pre- and postovulatory temperatures on a fertility chart.

Cowper's gland: One of a pair of small glands that secretes the lubricative pre-ejaculatory fluid in the male.

Creamy cervical fluid: The cervical-fluid quality that is generally wet and often similar to the consistency of hand lotion. It is considered fertile, although not as fertile as the eggwhite cervical fluid that usually follows it.

Creighton model/ovulation method: A cervical fluid method developed by Dr. Thomas Hilgers.

Curettage: See **Dilation and curettage**.

Cyst: An abnormal saclike structure containing fluid or semisolid material that may be present as a lump in various parts of the body. Most cysts are benign (nonmalignant) and cause no discomfort, but some may become cancerous.

D and C: See **Dilation and curettage**.

Danazol: A synthetic hormone used to treat endometriosis.

Danocrine: See **Danazol**.

Depo-Provera: An injectable hormonal contraceptive that lasts for 3 months.

Diaphragm: A soft rubber device that is inserted in the vagina to cover the cervix and prevent conception. Must be used with a spermicide.

Dilation and curettage (D and C): A surgical procedure used to scrape the surface of the endometrium with an instrument called a curette. Prior to curettage, the cervix is gradually opened with instruments called dilators.

Discharge: An emission from the vagina. In this book, it refers to an unhealthy symptom of an infection.

Double ovulation: The release of two separate eggs in one menstrual cycle. Both eggs are released within a 24-hour period.

Douche: A cleansing fluid flushed through the vagina. The practice is unnecessary and should be strongly discouraged since the normal vaginal environment is altered and the physiological self-cleansing mechanism is destroyed.

Dry Day Rule: One of the four natural birth control rules. It states that before ovulation, you are safe for unprotected intercourse the evening of every dry day (after 6 P.M.).

Dry days: Days when you observe no cervical fluid or bleeding and have a dry vaginal sensation.

Dysmenorrhea: Painful menstruation. Painful spasmodic contractions of the uterus usually arise just prior to or for the first few hours of menstruation and then gradually subside.

Dyspareunia: Painful or difficult intercourse.

Early ovulation: Release of the egg earlier in the cycle than usual or anticipated.

Ectopic pregnancy: The implantation and development of a fertilized ovum outside the uterus, usually in the fallopian tube.

Egg (cell): See **Ovum.**

Eggwhite-quality cervical fluid: The most fertile type of cervical fluid a woman produces. It typically resembles raw eggwhite and tends to be clear, slippery, and stretchy. It usually appears in the 2 or 3 days preceding ovulation.

Ejaculation: The release of seminal fluid from the penis during orgasm.

Embryo: The initial stages of development from the fertilized egg to around 6 weeks after conception.

Endocrinologist: A physician who specializes in the function of hormones.

Endometrial biopsy: The removal of a small part of the uterine lining (endometrium) for examination under the microscope. Used to determine whether the woman's lining is developing appropriately.

Endometrial polyp: An overgrowth of normal endometrial tissue that may grow into the cervical canal. As with cervical polyps, may be asymptomatic or cause spotting or cramping if they push down on the cervix.

Endometriosis: The growth of endometrial tissue in areas other than the uterus; for example, the fallopian tubes or the ovaries. A woman may be asymptomatic, or she may have lower abdominal pain that worsens during menstruation, pain during intercourse, and unusually long menstrual periods. Hormone therapy, surgery, and pregnancy may improve the condition. Endometriosis may cause infertility.

Endometritis: An inflammation of the endometrium, or lining of the uterus, usually causing pelvic pain and a thick, unpleasant-smelling yellowish discharge.

Endometrium: The lining of the uterus, which is shed during menstruation. If conception occurs, the fertilized egg implants within it.

Epididymis: The beginning of the sperm duct where sperm are stored, matured, and transported. It is attatched to the testicles.

Episiotomy: A cut made through the perineum to facilitate childbirth if the vaginal opening doesn't stretch enough to allow the baby to pass through.

Estriol (E3): The oestrogen produced by the placenta during pregnancy.

Estrone (E1): The dominant oestrogen found in post-menopausal women.

Fall-back temperature shift pattern: A type of thermal shift in which the temperature drops on or below the coverline on the second day after having already risen above it.

Fallopian tube: One of a pair of tubes connected to either side of the uterus. Sperm travel up to potentially unite with an egg in the outer third of the tube, after which the fertilized egg is transported toward the uterus through the tube.

False temperature rise: A temperature rise due to causes other than ovulation, such as fever, restless sleep, or drinking alcohol the night before. It is also caused by taking your temperature substantially later than usual.

Ferning test: The characteristic pattern produced by fertile cervical fluid when dried on a glass slide. So named because it resembles a fern.

Fertile phase: The days of the menstrual cycle during which sexual intercourse or insemination may result in pregnancy. It includes several days leading up to and immediately following ovulation.

Fertile-quality cervical fluid: Cervical fluid that is wet, slippery, stretchy, or resembles raw eggwhite. This type of cervical fluid appears around the time of ovulation, allowing sperm to live and travel in it for about 3 to 5 days.

Fertility: The ability to produce offspring.

Fertility Awareness Method (FAM): A means of determining your fertility through observing the three primary fertility signs: waking temperature, cervical fluid, and cervical position. Unlike Natural Family Planning, users of FAM choose whether they would like to use a barrier method or abstain during the fertile phase.

Fertility drugs: Drugs used to stimulate ovulation. The two most common are Clomid (clomiphene citrate) and Pergonal.

Fertilization: The fusion of a sperm with an egg (ovum), normally in the outer third of the fallopian tube.

Fetal age: The most accurate way of dating the age of a fetus, based on determining the date of conception.

Fetus: A name for a developing embryo from 6 weeks after fertilization until the time of birth.

Fibrocystic breast disease: A misleading term for nothing more than a common benign condition characterized by the formation of fluid-filled sacs in one or both breasts.

Fibroid: A fibrous and muscular growth of tissue in or on the wall of the uterus.

Fimbria: The end of the fallopian tube near the ovary. The fimbriae pick up the egg immediately after ovulation.

First 5 Days Rule: One of the four natural birth control rules. It states that you are safe the first 5 days of the menstrual cycle *if* you had an obvious temperature shift 12 to 16 days before. This rule is not considered as effective if you have had cycles of less than 24 days or have premenopausal symptoms.

Follicle: A small fluid-filled structure in the ovary that contains the egg (ovum). The follicle ruptures the surface of the ovary, releasing the ovum at ovulation.

Follicle-stimulating hormone (FSH): The hormone produced by the pituitary gland that stimulates the ovaries to produce mature ova and the hormone oestrogen.

Follicular phase: See **Preovulatory phase.**

FSH: See **Follicle-stimulating hormone.**

Gamete: The mature reproductive cells of the sperm and ovum.

Gamete Intra-Fallopian Transfer: See **GIFT.**

Genetic: Relating to hereditary characteristics.

Genital: Pertaining to the reproductive organs.

Genital contact: Contact between the penis and the vulva without penetration.

Genitalia (Genitals): The organs of reproduction, especially external.

Gestation: The period of development from conception to the end of pregnancy and birth.

Gestational age: The age of the fetus, based on dating the pregnancy from the first day of the last menstrual period (LMP) rather than the date of conception. The gestational age, by definition, is usually at least two weeks older than the fetus really is.

GIFT: Gamete Intra-Fallopian Transfer. A procedure in which the woman's eggs are removed from her ovaries and then placed in her fallopian tube with her partner's sperm. Unlike IVF, fertilization takes place in the fallopian tube, and not a petri dish.

Gland: Organ that produces chemical substances, including hormones.

GnRH: See **Gonadotropin-Releasing Hormone.**

Gonadotropin-Releasing Hormone (GnRH): A chemical substance produced by the hypothalamus in the brain. It stimulates the pituitary gland to produce and release both FSH and LH, hormones which in turn lead to follicular development and ovulation.

Gonadotropins: The hormones produced by the pituitary gland of males and females that regulates maturation of the sperm and egg. The most important gonadotropins are FSH and LH.

Gonads: The primary sex glands of the ovaries and testes.

Gonorrhea: A highly contagious sexually transmitted disease.

Guaifenesin: An expectorant often taken to increase the fluidity of cervical fluid.

Gynecologist: A doctor who specializes in women's reproductive health.

HCG: Human chorionic gonadotropin, typically referred to as the "pregnancy hormone." It is produced by the developing embryo when it implants in the uterine lining. Its main action is to maintain the corpus luteum and hence the secretion of oestrogen and progesterone until the placenta has developed sufficiently to take over hormonal production. See **Pregnancy test.**

Hemorrhage: Excessively heavy bleeding.

Herpes: A sexually transmitted viral infection that can cause painful, recurring blisters.

HIV: Human immuno-deficiency virus. The virus that causes AIDS.

Hormone: A chemical substance produced in one organ and carried by the blood to another organ where it exerts its effect. An example is FSH, which is produced in the pituitary gland and travels via the blood to the ovary where it stimulates the growth and maturation of follicles.

Hormone replacement therapy: The use of manufactured hormones, particularly oestrogen, to replace the perimenopausal woman's diminished natural supply of hormones. Prescribed to alleviate menopausal symptoms such as vaginal dryness and hot flashes, as well as prevent osteoporosis and possibly heart disease.

Hot flash: A feeling of heat that usually affects the face and neck and lasts a few seconds to a few minutes. It may spread over the upper part of the body and be accompanied by sweating. Most menopausal women will experience them.

HRT: See **Hormone replacement therapy.**

HSG: Hysterosalpingogram. An X ray taken after a special dye is injected through the cervix to produce an image of the inside of the uterus and fallopian tubes. Used to determine whether the tubes are blocked or have scarring.

Huhner's test: See **Postcoital test.**

Human chorionic gonadotrophin: See **HCG.**

Human immuno-deficiency virus: See **HIV.**

Hymen: The typically thin membrane that protects and partially blocks the entrance of the vagina from birth. May or may not be present in girls, depending on factors such as physical trauma.

Hypermenorrhea: Heavy bleeding.

Hypomenorrhea: Unusually light menstrual flow or spotting.

Hypothalamus: A part of the brain located just above the pituitary gland that controls several functions of the body. It produces hormones that influence the pituitary gland and regulate the development and activity of the ovaries and testes.

Hysterectomy: The surgical removal of the uterus.

Hysterosalpingogram: See **HSG.**

Hysteroscopy: Exploratory surgery to view the uterus.

Idiopathic infertility: Infertility of unknown cause.

Implantation: The process by which the fertilized egg embeds in the uterine lining, or endometrium.

In Vitro Fertilization: See **IVF.**

Infertile phases: The phases of the cycle when pregnancy cannot occur. Women have a preovulatory and postovulatory infertile phase.

Infertile-quality cervical fluid: A thick, sticky, or opaque-quality cervical fluid that produces a vaginal sensation of dryness or stickiness. It is very difficult for sperm to survive within it.

Infertility: Inability to conceive or maintain a pregnancy, or to provide viable sperm.

Intermenstrual pain: See **Ovulatory pain.**

Intra-uterine device (IUD): A device placed in the cavity of the uterus to prevent pregnancy. Certain types release hormones while in place.

Intra-Uterine Insemination: See **IUI.**

IUD: See **Intra-uterine device.**

IUI: Intra-Uterine Insemination. A procedure in which a catheter is used to insert the man's sperm through the cervix directly into the uterus.

IVF: In Vitro Fertilization. A procedure in which several eggs from the woman's ovaries are fertilized with her partner's sperm in a petri dish outside her body, then placed in the uterus 2 days later.

Kegel exercise: An exercise to contract and relax the vaginal muscles in order to strengthen them. It is also used to help push cervical fluid and semen out of the vaginal opening.

Labia: The two sets of lips surrounding the vaginal opening, forming part of the female external genitalia.

Lactation: The production of milk by the breasts.

Lactational Amenorrhea Method (LAM): A natural method of family planning used by breastfeeding women whose periods have not yet returned. It is considered highly effective if she is fully or nearly fully breastfeeding and is less than 6 months postpartum.

LAM: See **Lactational Amenorrhea Method.**

Laparoscopy: A procedure in which a laparoscope, a thin telescopic instrument, is inserted through a small incision in the navel to examine the inside of the abdomen, particularly the ovaries. Often used to diagnose endometriosis.

Laparotomy: A surgical operation involving opening the abdomen.

LH: See **Luteinizing hormone.**

Libido: Sexual desire.

LMP: Abbreviation for *last menstrual period,* the first day of the last menstrual period before a pregnancy is suspected or confirmed. The most commonly used means of dating a pregnancy, even though the date of conception is more accurate.

Lochia: Bloody secretions from the uterus and vagina the first few weeks after childbirth.

Lube: Abbreviation for "lubricative," the slippery vaginal sensation you feel when extremely fertile.

Lubricative sensation: The slippery and wet vaginal sensation you feel, usually when fertile-quality cervical fluid is present. If you feel it when no cervical fluid is present, you are still fertile.

LUFS: Luteinized Unruptured Follicle Syndrome. A condition in which the ovum remains stuck within the luteinized follicle, unable to pass through the ovarian wall to a possible conception. It is now believed to be a major cause of unexplained infertility.

Lupron: A drug used to induce a "pseudo-menopause" to provide a clean slate for high-tech procedures, as well as to treat endometriosis and fibroids.

Luteal phase: The phase of the menstrual cycle from ovulation to the onset of the next menstruation. It typically lasts from 12 to 16 days, but rarely varies by more than a day or two within individual women.

Luteal phase defect: See **short luteal phase.**

Luteinized Unruptured Follicle Syndrome: See **LUFS.**

Luteinizing hormone (LH): A hormone from the pituitary gland that is released in a surge, causing ovulation and development of the corpus luteum.

Menarche: The age at which menstruation begins.

Menopausal signs: Those signs that perimenopausal women generally experience, including hot flashes, vaginal dryness, and irregular cycles.

Menopause: The permanent cessation of ovulation, and hence menstruation. A woman is said to have gone through menopause after not having had a period for a full year.

Menorrhagia: Exceptionally heavy or prolonged bleeding during regular menstrual periods. "Gushing" or "open-faucet" bleeding is considered abnormal. Clots may be considered normal.

Menses: See **Menstruation.**

Menstrual cycle: The cyclical changes in the ovaries, cervix, and endometrium under the influence of the sex hormones. The length of the menstrual cycle is calculated from the first day of menstruation to the day before the following menstruation.

Menstrual cycle, phases of: There are 3 specific phases in the menstrual cycle:

1. The preovulatory infertile phase, which starts at the onset of menstruation and ends at the onset of the fertile phase.
2. The fertile phase, which includes the days before and after ovulation when intercourse may result in pregnancy.
3. The postovulatory infertile phase, which starts at the completion of the fertile phase and ends at the onset of the next menstruation.

Menstruation: The cyclical bleeding from the uterus as the endometrium is shed. True menstruation is usually preceded by ovulation 12 to 16 days earlier. Day 1 of menstruation is the first day of true red bleeding.

Method failure rate: This refers to the effectiveness of a contraceptive method under ideal conditions, when always used correctly.

Metrorrhagia: Bleeding between periods.

Micromanipulation: A procedure in which a single sperm is inserted directly into the ovum through the assistance of high-tech instruments. The newly created embryo is then transferred from the petri dish to the woman's uterus.

Midcycle pain: See **Ovulatory pain.**

Midcycle spotting: Light bleeding between two menstrual periods. Usually occurs around the time of ovulation and is often considered a secondary fertility sign.

Mini-pill: A type of contraceptive pill that contains progesterone but no oestrogen.

Miscarriage: The spontaneous loss of the embryo or fetus from the uterus.

Missed abortion: A fetus that has miscarried, or died, but has not emerged naturally.

Mittelschmerz: See **Ovulatory pain.**

Molar pregnancy: A rare condition in which a normal pregnancy goes awry, becoming a benign tumor at about 10 weeks.

Monophasic temperature pattern: A chart that does not show the biphasic pattern of low and high temperatures, indicating a probable absence of ovulation that cycle.

Mons pubis: The soft fleshy tissue beneath the pubic hair that protects the internal reproductive organs.

Mucus: See **Cervical fluid.**

Mucus Method: See **Billings Method.**

Mucus plug: The accumulation of sticky, infertile-quality cervical fluid in the cervical opening. It generally impedes the passage of sperm through the cervix.

Multiple ovulation: The release of at least two separate eggs in one menstrual cycle. Each of the eggs is released within a 24-hour period of time.

Nabothian cyst: A harmless cyst on the surface of the cervix.

Natural Family Planning (NFP): Method for planning or preventing pregnancy by observation of the naturally occurring signs and symptoms of the fertile and infertile phases of the menstrual cycle. Unlike the Fertility Awareness Method, users of NFP abstain rather than consider using contraceptive barriers during the fertile phase.

Norplant: A hormonal contraceptive in which six matchstick-sized capsules are inserted just beneath the skin of the upper arm. Lasts for 5 years.

Obstetrician: A physician who specializes in pregnancy, labor, and delivery.

Oestradiol (E2): The principal type of oestrogen produced by the ovaries, which stimulates follicle growth and ovulation and, along with progesterone, helps prepare the uterine lining for the implantation of a fertilized egg. It is also the form of oestrogen that is responsible for the development of secondary female sex characteristics. (Often referred to as 17-beta estradiol.)

Oestrogen: The hormone produced mainly in the ovaries responsible for the development of female secondary sex characteristics, as well as one of the primary hormones that control the menstrual cycle. Increasing oestrogen levels in the first part of the menstrual cycle produce significant changes in the cervical fluid and cervix, indicating fertility.

Oestrogenic phase: The oestrogen-dominated first phase of the menstrual cycle before ovulation. Also referred to as the Follicular Phase or Preovulatory Phase.

Oligomenorrhea: Menstrual periods that occur more than 35 days apart.

OPK: See **Ovulation predictor kits.**

Orgasm: The culmination of sexual excitement in the male or female. Ejaculation accompanies male orgasm.

Osteoporosis: A condition older women may get in which the loss of calcium and other substances leads to their bones becoming more brittle and fragile.

Ova: Two or more ovum.

Ovarian cyst: A follicle on the ovary that stops developing before ovulation, forming a fluid-filled cyst on the ovarian wall.

Ovary: One of a pair of female sex organs that produces mature ova, and in turn produces oestrogen.

Ovulation: The release of a mature egg (ovum) from the ovarian follicle.

Ovulation method: See **Billings Method.**

Ovulation predictor kits (OPK): Kits that detect the impending release of an egg, usually by testing urine for the presence of LH.

Ovulatory cycle: A cycle in which ovulation occurs.

Ovulation pain: Lower abdominal pain occurring around the time of ovulation. It is most likely caused by the irritation of the pelvic lining due to a slight amount of blood loss or from the actual breakthrough of the egg through the ovarian wall.

Ovum: The mature female sex cell, or egg. Analogous to the male sperm.

Ovum transfer: A procedure in which a man's sperm is used to fertilize the egg of a donor woman. The resulting embryo is then placed in the uterus of his partner, who may even be a postmenopausal woman.

Parlodel (Bromocriptine): A drug used to decrease the over-production of the hormone prolactin.

Patch Rule: One of the two natural birth control rules used during phases of anovulation. It states that you are safe the evening of every day that your 2-week Basic Infertile Pattern remains the same. But as soon as you see a change in your BIP, you must consider yourself fertile until the evening of the fourth consecutive nonwet day after the Peak Day.

PC muscles: Popular term for the pubococcygeous muscles of the pelvic floor. Their function is to support the bladder, rectum, and uterus.

PCOS: See **Polycystic Ovarian Syndrome.**

Peak Day: The last day that you produce fertile cervical fluid or have a wet vaginal sensation for any given cycle. It usually occurs either a day before you ovulate or on the day of ovulation itself.

Peak Day Rule: One of the four natural birth control rules. It states that you are safe the evening of the fourth consecutive day after your Peak Day.

Pelvic cavity: The lower portion of the body surrounded by the hips, containing reproductive and other organs.

Pelvic inflammatory disease (PID): Infection involving inflammation of the internal female reproductive organs, particularly the fallopian tubes and ovaries.

Penis: The external male organ that is inserted into the vagina during intercourse.

Pergonal: A powerful drug used to stimulate ovulation. It often triggers the release of more than one egg.

Perimenopause: The period of months or years preceding menopause during which time there may be emotional and physical changes, including irregularities in the menstrual cycle due to fluctuating hormone levels.

Perineum: The membrane between the vulva and the anus that remarkably stretches during childbirth to allow a baby's head to emerge through the vaginal opening.

Period: See **Menstruation.**

Periodic abstinence: Various methods of family planning based on voluntarily abstaining from intercourse during the fertile phase of the cycle in order to avoid pregnancy.

PID: See **Pelvic inflammatory disease.**

Pill: Synthetic hormone(s) taken orally to prevent pregnancy. It works by preventing ovulation, changing the cervical fluid to an infertile quality, and altering the uterine lining.

Pituitary gland: The master gland at the base of the brain that produces many important hormones, some of which trigger other glands into making their own hormones. The pituitary functions include hormonal control of the ovaries and testes.

PMS: A collection of physical and emotional signs and symptoms that appear during the postovulatory (luteal) phase and disappear at the onset of menstruation. Premenstrual symptoms are experienced by most women in varying degrees.

Polycystic Ovarian Syndrome (PCOS): A common endocrine disorder that usually leads to irregular cycles and other hormonal problems, in which developing follicles often remain trapped inside the ovary, later becoming cysts on the internal ovarian wall. Thought to be caused by high blood insulin levels.

Polymenorrhea: Frequent bleeding, usually due to anovulation.

Polyp: A soft, fleshy, non-cancerous tumor, usually teardrop-shaped, attached to normal tissue by a stem. Often found in the cervix or endometrium.

Postcoital contraception: Emergency contraceptive measure in the form of high-dose pills or insertion of an IUD within a specified time following unprotected intercourse.

Postcoital test: The examination of cervical fluid shortly after intercourse to determine whether sperm survive in it.

Postovulatory phase: See **Luteal phase.**

Pre-ejaculatory fluid: A small amount of lubricating fluid that is emitted from the penis before ejaculation during sexual excitement. May contain sperm.

Pregnancy: The condition of nurturing the embryo or fetus within the woman's body, lasting from conception to birth. Its normal duration is approximately 265 days, though most doctors calculate it from the first day of the last normal period, or approximately 280 days.

Pregnancy test: An early-morning urine sample or blood test to determine the presence of human chorionic gonadotrophin (HCG), the pregnancy hormone. Blood tests tend to be more sensitive and can therefore be done earlier than a urine test.

Pregnancy wheel: A calculating device used by doctors to determine a pregnant woman's due date. It is based on the assumption that ovulation occurs on Day 14, and is therefore often inaccurate.

Pregnanediol: A metabolite (breakdown product) of progesterone, excreted in the urine.

Premarin: A commonly prescribed oestrogen used in Hormone Replacement Therapy.

Premenopause: See **Perimenopause.**

Premenstrual syndrome: See **PMS.**

Preovulatory phase: The variable-length phase of the cycle from the onset of menstruation to ovulation. See **Menstrual cycle.**

Progesterone: A hormone produced mainly by the corpus luteum in the ovary following ovulation. It prepares the endometrium for a possible pregnancy. It is also responsible for the rise in basal body (waking) temperature, and for the change in cervical fluid in the postovulatory infertile state.

Progesterone phase: See **postovulatory phase.**

Prolactin: A pituitary hormone that stimulates the production of breast milk and inhibits the ovarian production of oestrogen.

Proliferative phase: See **preovulatory phase.**

Prostaglandins: A group of fatty acids that is believed to be responsible for severe menstrual cramps.

Prostate gland: A gland situated at the base of the male bladder. Its nutritive secretions help make up the seminal fluid.

Puberty: The time of life in boys and girls when the reproductive organs become functional and the secondary sexual characteristics appear.

Pubococcygeous: See **PC muscles.**

RC: Rubber cement-type cervical fluid that feels dry but has a springy or possibly stretchy quality.

Reproductive endocrinologist: A doctor who specializes in reproductive hormones.

Rhythm Method: An unreliable method of family planning in which the fertile phase of the cycle is calculated according to the lengths of previous menstrual cycles. Because of its reliance on regular menstrual cycles and long periods of abstinence, it is neither effective nor widely accepted as a modern method of natural family planning.

Rule of Thumb: A guideline in which aberrant waking temperatures are ignored, particularly when calculating the coverline.

Scrotum: Pouch of skin containing the testes.

Secondary fertility signs: Physical and emotional changes that may provide supplementary evidence of the fertile phase. Secondary signs include *mittelschmerz* (ovulatory pain), spotting, breast tenderness, and mood changes.

Secondary infertility: When a couple is unable to get pregnant or carry a pregnancy to term after already having a child.

Secondary sex characteristics: Features of masculinity or femininity that develop at puberty under hormonal control. In the male, this includes deepening voice in addition to the growth of beard and underarm and pubic hair. They are influenced by androgens. In the female, such characteristics include rounding of breasts, waist, and hips, as well as the growth of underarm and pubic hair. They are influenced by oestrogens.

Secretory phase: See **postovulatory phase.**

Semen: The fluid ejaculated from the penis at orgasm. The viscous fluid contains sperm and secretions from the seminal vesicles and prostate gland.

Semen Emitting Technique (SET): The use of Kegel exercises (and tissue) in order to eliminate semen from the vagina.

Seminal fluid: See **Semen.**

Seminal vesicle: One of a pair of sacs that open into the top of the male urethra. Its secretions form part of the seminal fluid.

Seminiferous tubules: Microscopic tubes in the testes in which sperm are produced.

Serophene: See **Clomid.**

SET: See **Semen Emitting Technique.**

Sexually transmitted diseases (STDs): Any infection that is transmitted by sexual contact or intercourse.

Short luteal phase: The second phase of the cycle that in some women is deficient in progesterone, typically leading to a phase that is not long enough to allow for successful implantation. A woman usually needs a luteal phase of at least 10 days.

Slow-rise temperature shift pattern: A type of thermal shift in which temperatures rise by merely one-tenth of a degree per day over several days.

Speculum: A two-bladed stainless steel or plastic instrument used to examine the inside of the vagina and the cervix.

Sperm: The mature male sex cell analogous to the female ovum.

Sperm count: A measure of a man's fertility that calculates the total number of sperm per ejaculate as well as the percent of sperm that are both forwardly moving (motility) and of normal shape and size (morphology).

Sperm washing: The process by which the motility of the sperm is dramatically increased through mixing them in a culture media and then placing them in a centrifuge.

Spermicidal: Having sperm-destroying properties.

Spermicides: Vaginal creams, jellies, films, or sponges that can immobilize or destroy sperm.

Spinnbarkeit: Fertility-quality cervical fluid that is generally stretchy, slippery, and clear.

Spotting: Small amounts of red, pink, or brownish blood occurring during the menstrual cycle at times other than the true menstrual period.

Stair-step temperature shift pattern: A type of thermal shift in which an initial rising spurt of temperatures occurs over several days, followed by a higher pattern of temperatures usually resembling a bell curve.

STDs: See **Sexually transmitted diseases.**

Sterility: The inability of a woman to conceive, or of a man to produce functional sperm.

Sterilization: A procedure that renders an individual permanently unable to reproduce.

Sticky cervical fluid: The type of cervical fluid that often has the texture of library paste or rubber cement. It is usually the first type of cervical fluid that appears in a woman's cycle following menstruation. It is very difficult for sperm to survive in it.

Subfertility: A state of less than normal fertility.

Sympto-thermal method (STM): A natural method of family planning combining observation of the basal body (waking) temperature, cervical fluid, and cervical position, along with any other secondary fertility signs. The most comprehensive and effective natural method, and the one taught in this book under the name Fertility Awareness Method (see **FAM**).

Syphilis: A highly contagious sexually transmitted disease.

Temperature chart: A graph showing variation in daily waking temperature. See **Biphasic and Monophasic temperature pattern.**

Temperature method: See **BBT method.**

Temperature shift: The rise in waking temperature that divides the preovulatory low temperatures from the later, postovulatory high temperatures on a biphasic chart. It usually results in temperatures that are at least two-tenths of a degree higher than the previous 6 days.

Temperature Shift Rule: One of the four natural birth control rules. It states that you are safe the evening of the third consecutive day your temperature is above the coverline.

Testes: Plural of testicle.

Testicle: One of a pair of male sex organs that produces sperm and the male sex hormones (androgens), including testosterone.

Testosterone: A hormone produced by the testes, responsible for the development of male secondary sex characteristics and functioning of the male reproductive organs.

Thermal shift: See **Temperature shift.**

Thyroid gland: A butterfly-shaped endocrine gland in the lower part of the neck that produces thyroid hormones (including thyroxin) and regulates hormone use and balance in the body. Hyperthyroidism (an overactive thyroid) and hypothyroidism (an underactive thyroid) are thyroid disorders that can affect a woman's fertility.

Triphasic temperature shift: A temperature shift pattern that usually reflects a pregnancy. About 7 to 10 days after the first thermal shift, a second, more subtle shift often occurs due to the effect of the pregnancy hormone, HCG.

Tubal ligation: The surgical sterilization procedure that ties a woman's fallopian tubes to prevent the sperm and egg from uniting.

Tubal pregnancy: An ectopic pregnancy in which the fertilized egg starts to implant in the fallopian tube rather than the uterus.

Ultrasound: A diagnostic technique that uses sound waves, rather than X rays, to visualize internal body structures.

Unchanging Day Rule: One of the two natural birth control rules used during phases of anovulation. It states that if your 2-week Basic Infertile Pattern (BIP) is dry or the same-quality sticky cervical fluid day after day, you are safe for unprotected intercourse the evening of every dry or unchanging sticky day.

Urethra: The tube that carries urine from the bladder to the outside. The female urethra is very short, extending from the bladder to the urinary opening at the vulva. The male urethra is longer, extending along the length of the penis. It also carries the seminal fluid.

User failure rate: A measure of the effectiveness of a contraceptive method under real-life conditions.

Uterus (womb): The pear-shaped muscular organ in which the fertilized ovum implants and grows for the duration of pregnancy. Muscular contractions of the uterus push the infant out through the birth canal at the time of birth. If implantation does not occur, the uterine lining (endometrium) is shed at menstruation.

Vagina: The muscular canal extending from the cervix to the opening at the vulva. Sperm are deposited in the vagina during intercourse. It is also through this canal that the baby is delivered (birth canal).

Vaginal discharge: See **Discharge.**

Vaginal infection: An abnormal bacterial or viral growth in the vagina.

Vaginismus: A painful spasm of the vagina that prevents comfortable penetration of the penis.

Vaginitis: An inflammation of the vagina caused by an infection or other irritation.

Vanishing Twin Syndrome: A surprisingly common phenomenon in which one of two fraternal twin embryos is spontaneously miscarried or reabsorbed early in a pregnancy, resulting in a single-baby birth.

Varicocele: A varicose-type vein in a man's scrotum that can impede his fertility by increasing the testicular temperature.

Vas deferens: One of a pair of tubes that carries the seminal fluid from the testes to the urethra.

Vasectomy: A male sterilization procedure in which each vas deferens is cut to prevent the passage of sperm.

VD: Venereal disease. See **Sexually transmitted diseases.**

Venereal disease (VD): See **Sexually transmitted diseases.**

Vulva: The external female genitalia comprising the clitoris and two sets of labia.

Vulvodynia: Pain in the vulva, characterized by itching, burning, stinging, or stabbing at the opening of the vagina.

Waking temperature: The temperature of the body at rest, taken immediately upon awakening, before any activity. Often referred to as basal body temperature (BBT).

Withdrawal: Act of removing the penis from the vagina before ejaculation occurs. Often used as a form of contraception.

Withdrawal bleeding: Vaginal bleeding resulting from an insufficient level of oestrogen to maintain the uterine lining. It usually occurs during anovulatory cycles.

Womb: See **Uterus.**

ZIFT: Zygote Intra-Fallopian Transfer. A procedure in which a woman's egg is fertilized by her partner's sperm in a petri dish. The resulting zygote is then placed back in her fallopian tube.

Zygote: The fertilized ovum. A single fertilized cell resulting from fusion of the sperm and the egg. After further cell division the zygote is known as a blastocyst, then as an embryo.

Zygote Intra-Fallopian Transfer: See **ZIFT.**

Bibliography

Many of the recommended books found in Appendix N are also used as source material.

AIDS/STDS

Articles

Bylund, David J., M.D., Ulrike H. M. Ziegner, M.D., Ph.D., and Dennis G. Hooper, M.D., Ph.D. "Review of Testing for Human Immunodeficiency Virus," *Clinics in Laboratory Medicine* 12 (June 1992): 305–333.

Kassler, W. J. "Advances in HIV Testing Technology and Their Potential Impact on Prevention," *AIDS Education and Prevention* 9 (June 1997) (3 Suppl): 27–40.

Sloand, Elaine M., M.D., et al. "HIV Testing: State of the Art," *Journal of the American Medical Association* 266 (November 27, 1991): 2861–2866.

Books

Berer, Marge. *Women and HIV/AIDS: An International Resource Book.* San Francisco: Harper-Collins, 1993.

Marr, Lisa, M.D. *Sexually Transmitted Diseases: A Physician Tells You What You Need to Know.* Baltimore: Johns Hopkins University Press, 1999.

Vargo, Marc E., M.S. *The HIV Test: What You Need to Know to Make an Informed Decision.* New York: Pocket Books, 1992.

BREASTFEEDING

Articles

Family Health International. Consensus Statement. "Breastfeeding as a Family Planning Method," *The Lancet* (November 19, 1988): 1204–1205.

Gray, Ronald H., Oona M. Campbell, Ruben Apelo, Susan S. Eslami, Howard Zacur, Rebecca M. Ramos, Judith C. Gehret, and Miriam H. Labbok. "Risk of Ovulation During Lactation," *The Lancet* 335 (January 6, 1990): 25–29.

Howie, P. W., A. S. McNeilly, M. J. Houston, A. Cook, and H. Boyle. "Fertility After Childbirth: Post-Partum Ovulation and Menstruation in Bottle and Breast-Feeding Mothers," *Clinical Endocrinology* 17 (October 1982): 323–332.

Kennedy, Kathy I., et al. "Breastfeeding and the Symptothermal Method." *Studies in Family Planning* 26 (1995): 107–115.

Kennedy, Kathy J., and Cynthia M. Visness. "Contraceptive Efficacy of Lactational Amenorrhoea," *The Lancet* 339 (January 25, 1992): 227–229.

Labbok, Miriam, Kristin Cooney, and Shirley Coly. *Guidelines: Breastfeeding, Family Planning, and the Lactational Amenorrhea Method-LAM.* Washington, DC: Institute for Reproductive Health, 1994.

Lewis, Patricia R., Ph.D., et al. "The Resumption of Ovulation and Menstruation in a Well-Nourished Population of Women Breastfeeding for an Extended Period of Time," *Fertility and Sterility* 55 (March 1991): 520–535.

Paranteau-Carreau, Suzanne, M.D., IFFLP, and Kristin A. Cooney, M.A., IRH. *Breastfeeding, Lactational Amenorrhea Method, and Natural Family Planning Interface: Teaching Guide,* 1–35. Washington, DC: Institute for Reproductive Health, 1994.

Perez, Alfredo, Miriam H. Labbok, and John T. Queenan. "Clinical Study of the Lactational Amenorrhoea Method for Family Planning," *The Lancet* 339 (April 18, 1992): 968–970.

Tay, Clement C. K. "Mechanisms Controlling Lactational Infertility," *Journal of Human Lactation* 7 (March 1991): 15–18.

Books

Riordan, Jan, Ed.D., R.N., and Kathleen G. Auerbach, Ph.D., *Breastfeeding and Human Lactation.* Boston and London: Jones and Bartlett Publishers, 1993.

CONTRACEPTIVE EFFECTIVENESS

Articles

Barbato, Michele, M.D., and Giancarlo Bertolotti, M.D. "Natural Methods for Fertility Control: A Prospective Study—First Part," *International Fertility Supplement* (1988): 48–51.

The European Natural Family Planning Study Groups. "European Multicenter Study of Natural Family Planning (1989–1995): Efficacy and Dropout." *Advances in Contraception* 15 (1999): 69–83.

Flynn, Anna M., and John Bonnar. "Natural Family Planning." In *Contraception: Science and Practice,* edited by Marcus Filshie and John Guillebaud, 203–205. London: Butterworth's Press, 1989.

Frank-Hermann, Petra, M.D., et al. "Effectiveness and Acceptability of the Symptothermal Method of Natural Family Planning in Germany," *American Journal of Obstetrics & Gynecology* 165 (December 1991): 2052–2054.

———. "Natural Family Planning With and Without Barrier Method Use in the Fertile Phase: Efficacy in Relation to Sexual Behavior: A German Prospective Long-term Study." *Advances in Contraception* 13 (June–Sept. 1997): 179–189.

Ghosh, A. K., S. Saha, and G. Chattergee. "Symptothermia Vis-à-Vis Fertility Control," *Journal of Obstetrics and Gynecology of India* 32 (1982): 443–447.

Guida, M. "An Overview of the Effectiveness of Natural Family Planning," *Gynecological Endocrinology* (June 1997): 203–219.

Hume, K. "Fertility Awareness in the 1990s—The Billings Ovulation Method of Natural Family Planning, Its Scientific Basis, Practical Application and Effectiveness," *Advances in Contraception* 7 (June-September 1991): 301–311.

Lamprecht, V., and J. Trussel. "Natural Family Planning Effectiveness: Evaluating Published Reports," *Advances in Contraception* 13 (1997): 155–165.

Lethbridge, Dona J., R.N., Ph.D. "Coitus Interruptus: Considerations as a Method of Birth Control," *Journal of Obstetrics, Gynecologic and Neonatal Nursing* 20 (1991): 80–85.

Petotti, Diana B. "Statistical Aspects of the Evaluation of the Safety and Effectiveness of Fertility Control Methods." In *Fertility Control,* edited by Stephen L. Corson, Richard J. Dennan, and Louise B. Tyrer, pp. 13–25. Boston: Little, Brown, 1985.

Rice, Frank J., Ph.D., Claude A. Lanctôt, M.D., and Consuelo Farcia-DeVesa, Ph.D. "Effectiveness of the Sympto-Thermal Method of Natural Family Planning: An International Study," *International Journal of Fertility* 26 (1981): 222–230.

Royston, J. P. "Basal Body Temperature, Ovulation and the Risk of Conception, with Special Reference to the Lifetimes of Sperm and Egg," *Biometrics* 38 (June 1982): 397–406.

Ryder, R. E. J. " 'Natural Family Planning': Effective Birth Control Supported by the Catholic Church," *British Medical Journal* 307 (September 18, 1993): 723–726.

Trussell, James, and Laurence Grummer-Strawn. "Contraceptive Failure of the Ovulation Method of Periodic Abstinence," *Family Planning Perspectives* 22 (March/April 1990): 65–75.

Trussell, James, and Kathryn Kost. "Contraceptive Failure in the United States: A Critical Review of the Literature," *Studies in Family Planning* 18 (September-October 1987): 237–283.

Trussell, James, Ph.D., et al. "Contraceptive Failure in the United States: An Update," *Studies in Family Planning* 21 (January-February 1990): 51–54.

———. "A Guide to Interpreting Contraceptive Efficacy Studies," *Obstetrics & Gynecology* 76 (September 1990): 558–567.

Wade, Maclyn E., M.D., et al. "A Randomized Prospective Study of the Use-Effectiveness of Two Methods of Natural Family Planning," *American Journal of Obstetrics & Gynecology* 141 (October 1981): 368–376.

Woolley, Robert J., M.D. "Contraception—A Look Forward, Part I: New Spermicides and Natural Family Planning," *Journal of the American Board of Family Practice* (January 1991): 33–44.

World Health Organization, Task Force. "A Prospective Multicentre Trial of the Ovulation Method of Natural Family Planning. II. The Effectiveness Phase," *Fertility and Sterility* 36 (November 1981): 591–598.

———. "A Prospective Multicentre Trial of the Ovulation Method of Natural Family Planning. III. Characteristics of the Menstrual Cycle and of the Fertile Phase," *Fertility and Sterility* 40 (December 1983): 773–778.

Books

Hatcher, Robert A., M.D., M.P.H., et al. *Contraceptive Technology,* 17th rev. ed., New York: Irvington Publishers, Inc., 1998.

FERTILITY AND THE MENSTRUAL CYCLE

Articles

Badwe, R. A., et al. "Timing of Surgery During Menstrual Cycle and Survival of Premenopausal Women with Operable Breast Cancer," *The Lancet* 337 (May 25, 1991): 1261–1264

Banks, A. Lawrence, M.D. "Does Adoption Affect Infertility?" *International Journal of Fertility* (1962): 23–28.

Barnes, Ann B., M.D. "Menstrual History and Fecundity of Women Exposed and Unexposed in Utero to Diethylstilbestrol," *Journal of Reproductive Medicine* 29 (September 1984): 651–655.

———. "Menstrual History of Young Women Exposed in Utero to Diethylstilbestrol," *Fertility and Sterility* 32 (August 1979): 148–153.

Bartuska, Doris G., M.D. "Thyroid and Parathyroid Disease." In *Textbook of Woman's Health,* edited by Lila A. Wallis, M.D., pp. 525–532. New York: Lippincott-Raven Publishers, 1998.

Brown, James B., D.Sc., Joanne Holmes, B.A., and Gillian Barker. "Use of the Home Ovarian Monitor in Pregnancy Avoidance," *American Journal of Obstetrics and Gynecology* 165 (December 1991): 2008–2011.

Burger, Henry G., M.D. "Neuroendocrine Control of Human Ovulation," *International Journal of Fertility* 26 (1981): 153–160.

Campbell, Doris M. "Aetiology of Twinning." In *Twinning and Twins,* edited by I. MacGillivray, D. M. Campbell, and B. Thompson, pp. 27–36. London: John Wiley & Sons, Ltd., 1988.

Canfield, R. E., et al. "Development of an Assay for a Biomarker of Pregnancy and Early Fetal Loss," *Environmental Health Perspectives* 74 (October 1987): 57–66.

Chard, T. "Pregnancy Tests: A Review," *Human Reproduction* 7 (May 1992): 701–710.

Check, Jerome H., M.D., et al. "Comparison of Various Therapies for the Leutinized Unruptured Follicle Syndrome," *International Journal of Fertility* 37 (January/February 1992): 33–40.

Croxatto, H. B., et al. "Studies in the Duration of Egg Transport by the Human Oviduct. II. Ovum Location at Various Intervals Following Luteinizing Hormone Peak," *American Journal of Obstetrics & Gynecology* 132 (November 15, 1978): 629–634.

Cunha, G. R., Ph.D., et al. "Teratogenic Effects of Clomiphene, Tamoxifen, and Diethylstilbestrol on the Developing Human Female Genetic Tract," *Human Pathology* 18 (November 1987): 1132–1143.

Daly, Douglas C., M.D., et al. "Ultrasonographic Assessment of Luteinized Unruptured Follicle Syndrome in Unexplained Infertility," *Fertility and Sterility* 43 (January 1985): 62–65.

Darland, Nancy Wilson, R.N.C., M.S.N. "Infertility Associated with Luteal Phase Defect," *Journal of Obstetric, Gynecologic and Neonatal Nursing* (May/June 1985): 212–217.

Daviaud, Joëlle, et al. "Reliability and Feasibility of Pregnancy Home-Use Tests: Laboratory Validation and Diagnostic Evaluation by 638 Volunteers," *Clinical Chemistry* 39 (January 1993): 53–59.

De Mouzon, Jacques, M.D., et al. "Time Relationships Between Basal Body Temperature and Ovulation or Plasma Progestins," *Fertility and Sterility* 41 (February 1984): 254–259.

DeVane, Gary W., M.D. "Prolactin Measurement: What Is Normal?" *Contemporary Ob/Gyn* (September 1989): 99–117.

Djerassi, Carl, Ph.D., "Fertility Awareness: Jet-Age Rhythm Method?" *Science* (June 1990): 1061–1062.

Domar, Alice D., Ph.D., et al. "Impact of Group Psychological Interventions on Pregnancy Rates in Infertile Women." *Fertility and Sterility* 73 (April 2000), 805–811.

———. "The Prevalence and Predictability of Depression in Infertile Women." *Fertility and Sterility* (December 1992): 1158–1163.

Eggert-Kruse, W., I. Gerhard, W. Tilgen, and B. Runnebaum. "The Use of Hens' Egg White as a Substitute for Human Cervical Mucus in Assessing Human Infertility," *International Journal of Andrology* 13 (August 1990): 258–266.

Eisenberg, Esther, M.D. "Infertility." In *Textbook of Woman's Health,* edited by Lila A. Wallis, M.D., pp. 679–685. New York: Lippincott-Raven Publishers, 1998.

Fehring, Richard J., R.N., DNSc. "Methods Used to Self-Predict Ovulation: A Comparative Study," *Journal of Obstetric, Gynecologic, and Neonatal Nursing* 19 (May/June 1990): 233–237.

Field, Charles S., M.D. "Dysfunctional Uterine Bleeding," *Primary Care* 15 (September 1988): 561–573.

Filer, Robert B., M.D., and Chung H. Wu, M.D. "Coitus During Menses: Its Effect on Endometriosis and Pelvic Inflammatory Disease," *Journal of Reproductive Medicine* 34 (November 1989): 887–890.

Filicori, Marco, et al. "Evidence for a Specific Role of GnRH Pulse Frequency in the Control of the Human Menstrual Cycle," *American Journal of Physiology* 257 (December 1989): 930–936.

Fish, Lisa H., M.D., and Cary N. Mariash, M.D. "Hyperprolactinemia, Infertility, and Hypothyroidism," *Archives of Internal Medicine* 148 (March 1988): 709–711.

Flynn, Anna M., and John Bonnar. "Natural Family Planning." In *Contraception: Science and Practice,* edited by Marcus Filshie and John Guillebaud, pp. 203–205. London: Butterworth's Press, 1989.

Ford, Judith Helen, and Lesley MacCormac. "Pregnancy and Lifestyle Study. The Long-term use of the Contraceptive Pill and the Risk of Age-Related Miscarriage," *Human Reproduction* 10 (1995): 1397–1402.

Fordney-Settlage, Diane, M.D., M.S. "A Review of Cervical Mucus and Sperm Interactions in Humans," *International Journal of Fertility* 26 (1981): 161–169.

France, John T., Ph.D. "Overview of the Biological Aspects of the Fertile Period," *International Journal of Fertility* 26 (1981): 143–152.

Freidson, Eliot, Ph.D. "The Professional Mind." In *The Sociology of Medicine, a Structural Approach,* pp. 130–131. New York: Dodd, Mead and Company, 1968.

Glatstein, Isaac Z., M.D., et al. "The Reproducibility of the Postcoital Test: A Prospective Study," *Obstetrics and Gynecology* 85 (1995): 396–400.

Gnant, Michael F. X., et al. "Breast Cancer and Timing of Surgery During Menstrual Cycle: A 5-Year Analysis of 385 Pre-Menopausal Women," *International Journal of Cancer* 52 (November 11, 1992): 707–712.

Goldenberg, Robert L., M.D., and Roberta White, R.N. "The Effect of Vaginal Lubricants on Sperm Motility in Vitro," *Fertility and Sterility* 26 (September, 1975): 872–873.

Goldhirsch, A. "Menstrual Cycle and Timing of Breast Surgery in Premenopausal Node-Positive Breast Cancer: Results of the International Breast Cancer Study Group Trial VI," *Annals of Oncology* 8 (1997): 751–756.

Gondos, Bernard, M.D., and Daniel H. Riddick, M.D., Ph.D., eds. "Cervical Mucus and Sperm Motility." In *Pathology of Infertility: Clinical Correlations in the Male and Female,* pp. 337–351. New York: Thieme Medical Publishers, Inc., 1987.

Grodstein, Francine, et al. "Relation of Female Infertility to Consumption of Caffeinated Beverages," *American Journal of Epidemiology* 137 (June 15, 1993): 1353–1359.

Guerrero, R., O. Rojas, and A. Cifuentes. "Natural Family Planning Methods." In *Human Ovulation,* edited by E. S. E. Hafez, pp. 477–479. Amsterdam and New York: Elsevier North-Holland Biomedical Press, 1979.

Guyton, Arthur C., M.D. "Endocrinology and Reproduction." In *Textbook of Medical Physiology,* 8th ed, p. 912. Philadelphia: W. B. Saunders Company, 1991.

Hardy, M. L. "Herbs of Special Interest to Women." *Journal of the American Pharmaceutical Association* 40 (2000): 232–234.

Hamilton, Mark P. R., M.D., et al. "Luteal Cysts and Unexplained Infertility: Biochemical and Ultrasonic Evaluation," *Fertility and Sterility* 54 (July 1990): 32–37.

Hibbard, Lester T., M.D. "Corpus Luteum Surgery," *American Journal of Obstetrics & Gynecology* 135 (November 1, 1979): 666–667.

Hilgers, Thomas W., M.D., Guy E. Abraham, M.D., and Denis Cavanagh, M.D. "Natural Family Planning. I. The Peak Symptom and Estimated Time of Ovulation," *The American College of Obstetricians and Gynecologists* 52 (November 1978): 575–582.

Hilgers, Thomas W., M.D., Guy E. Abraham, M.D., and Ann M. Prebil. "The Length of the Luteal Phase," *International Review* (Spring/Summer 1989): 99–106.

Hilgers, Thomas W., M.D., and Alan J. Baile MSW, ACSW. "Natural Family Planning. II. Basal Body Temperature and Estimated Time of Ovulation," *Obstetrics & Gynecology* 55 (March 1980): 333–339.

Howles, Colin M. "Follicle Growth and Luteinization." In *Encyclopedia of Human Biology,* vol. 3, pp. 627–635. London: Academic Press, 1991.

Huggins, George R., M.D., and Vanessa E. Cullins, M.D. "Fertility After Contraception or Abortion," *Fertility and Sterility* 54 (October 1990): 559–570.

Hull, M. G. R., et al. "Expectations of Assisted Conception for Fertility," *British Medical Journal* 304 (June 6, 1992): 1465–1469.

Joesoef, M. Riduan, et al. "Are Caffeinated Beverages Risk Factors for Delayed Conception?" *The Lancet* (January 20, 1990): 136–137.

Jones, Howard W., Jr., M.D., and James P. Toner, M.D., Ph.D. "The Infertile Couple," *New England Journal of Medicine* 7 (December 2, 1993): 1710–1715.

Kerin, John F., M.D., et al. "Incidence of the Luteinized Unruptured Follicle Phenomenon in Cycling Women," *Fertility and Sterility* 40 (November 1983): 620–626.

Knee, Gerald R., M.S., et al. "Detection of the Ovulatory Luteinizing Hormone (LH) Surge with a Semiquantitative Urinary LH Assay," *Fertility and Sterility* 44 (November 1985): 707–709.

Koninckx, P. R., and I. A. Brosens. "The Luteinized Unruptured Follicle Syndrome." In *The Inadequate Luteal Phase: Pathophysiology, Diagnostics, Therapy,* edited by H. D. Taubert and H. Kuhl, pp. 145–151. Lancaster: MTP Press Ltd., 1983.

Koukolis, G. N. "Hormone Replacement Therapy and Breast Cancer Risk," *Annals of the New York Academy of Sciences* 900 (2000): 422–428.

Lamb, Emmet J., M.D., and Sue Luergans, Ph.D. "Does Adoption Affect Subsequent Fertility?" *American Journal of Obstetrics and Gynecology* 134 (May 15, 1979): 138–144.

Lambert, Hovey, Ph.D., et al. "Sperm Capacitation in the Human Female Reproductive Tract," *Fertility and Sterility* 43 (February 1985): 325–327.

Landy, Helain J., M.D., et al. "The 'Vanishing-Twin': Ultrasonographic Assessment of Fetal Disappearance in the First Trimester," *American Journal of Obstetrics and Gynecology* (July 1986): 14–19.

LeMaire, Gail Schoen, R.N., M.S.N. "The Luteinized Unruptured Follicle Syndrome: Anovulation in Disguise," *Journal of Obstetric, Gynecologic and Neonatal Nursing* (March/April 1987): 116–120.

Lenton, Elizabeth A., Britt-Marie Landgren, and Lynne Sexton. "Normal Variation in the Length of the Luteal Phase of the Menstrual Cycle: Identification of the Short Luteal Phase," *British Journal of Obstetrics and Gynecology* 91 (July 1984): 685–689.

Luciano, Anthony A., M.D., et al. "Temporal Relationship and Reliability of the Clinical, Hormonal, and Ultrasonographic Indices of Ovulation in Infertile Women," *Obstetrics & Gynecology* 75 (March 1990): 412–416.

MacGillivray, Ian, Mike Samphier, and Julian Little. "Factors Affecting Twinning." In *Twinning and Twins,* edited by I. MacGillivray, D. M. Campbell, and B. Thompson, pp. 67–92. London: John Wiley & Sons, Ltd., 1988.

March, C. M. "Ovulation Induction," *Journal of Reproductive Medicine* 38 (May 1993): 335–346.

Marik, Jaroslav, M.D., and Jaroslav Hulka, M.D. "Luteinized Unruptured Follicle Syndrome: A Subtle Cause of Infertility," *Fertility and Sterility* (March 1978): 270–274.

Masha, Mahadevan, M., et al. "Yeast Infection of Sperm, Oocytes, and Embryos After Intravaginal Culture for Embryo Transfer." *Fertility and Sterility* 65 (1996): 481–483.

McCarthy, John J., Jr., M.D., and Howard E. Rockette, Ph.D. "A Comparison of Methods to Interpret the Basal Body Temperature Graph," *Fertility and Sterility* 39 (May 1983): 640–646.

Messinis, I. E., et al. "Changes in Pituitary Response to GnRH During the Luteal-Follicular Transition of the Human Menstrual Cycle," *Clinical Endocrinology* 38 (February 1993): 159–163.

Miller, Karen K., et al. "Decreased Leptin Levels in Normal Weight Women with Hypothalmic Amenorrhea: The Effects of Body Composition and Nutritional Intake." *Journal of Clinical Endocrinology and Metabolism* 83 (1998): 2309–2312.

Nesse, Robert E., M.D. "Abnormal Vaginal Bleeding in Perimenopausal Women," *American Family Physician* (July 1989): 185–189.

Nicholson, Roberto, M.D. "Vitality of Spermatozoa in the Endocervical Canal," *Fertility and Sterility* 16 (November-December 1965): 758–764.

O'Herlihy, C., MRCOG, MRCPI, and H.P. Robinson, M.D., MRCOG. "Mittelschmerz Is a Preovulatory Symptom," *British Medical Journal* (April 1980): 986.

Olsen, Jorn. "Cigarette Smoking, Tea and Coffee Drinking, and Subfecundity," *American Journal of Epidemiology* (April 1, 1991): 734–739.

Overstreet, James W., David F. Katz, and Ashley I. Yudin. "Cervical Mucus and Sperm Transport in Reproduction," *Seminars in Perinatology* 15 (April 1991): 149–155.

Padilla, Santiago L., M.D., and Kathryn S. Craft, RNC. "Anovulation: Etiology, Evaluation and Management," *Nurse Practitioner* (December 1985): 28–44.

Pillet, M. Christine, M.D., et al. "Improved Prediction of Postovulatory Day Using Temperature Recording, Endometrial Biopsy, and Serum Progesterone," *Fertility and Sterility* 53 (April 1990): 614–619.

Pritchard, Jack P., Paul C. MacDonald, and Norman F. Gant, "Multifetal Pregnancy." In *Williams Obstetrics*, 17th ed., pp. 503–524. Norwalk, CT: Appleton-Century-Crofts, 1985.

Profet, Margie. "Menstruation as a Defense Against Pathogens Transported by Sperm," *Quarterly Review of Biology* 68 (September 1993): 335–381.

Rebar, Robert W. "Premature Ovarian Failure." In *Treatment of the Post-Menopausal Woman: Basic and Clinical Aspects*, edited by Rogerio A. Lobo, pp. 25–33. New York: Raven Press, Ltd., 1994.

Ross, G. T. "HCG in Early Human Pregnancy." In *Maternal Recognition of Pregnancy,* edited by Julie Whelan, pp. 198–199. New York: Ciba Foundation Press, 1979.

Rossing, Mary Anne, D.V.M., Ph.D., et al. "Ovarian Tumors in a Cohort of Infertile Women," *New England Journal of Medicine* (September 22, 1994), 771–776.

Rousseau, Serge, M.D., et al. "The Expectancy of Pregnancy for 'Normal' Infertile Couples," *Fertility and Sterility* 40 (December 1983): 768–772.

Salle, B. "Another Two Cases of Ovarian Tumours in Women Who Had Undergone Multiple Ovulation Induction Cycles," *Human Reproduction* 12 (1997): 1732–1735.

Sanders, Katherine A., and Bruce, Neville W. "Psychosocial Stress and the Menstrual Cycle," *Journal of Biosocial Sciences* 31 (1999): 393–402.

Scholes, D., et al. "Vaginal Douching as a Risk Factor for Acute Pelvic Inflammatory Disease," *Obstetrics & Gynecology* 81 (April 1993): 601–606.

Simmer, Hans H. "Placental Hormones." In *Biology of Gestation,* edited by N. S. Assali, pp. 296–299. New York: Academic Press, 1968.

Smith, S. K., Elizabeth A. Lenton, and I. D. Cooke. "Plasma Gonadotrophin and Ovarian Steroid Concentrations in Women with Menstrual Cycles with a Short Luteal Phase," *Journal of Reproduction and Fertility* 75 (November 1985): 363–368.

Smith, Stephen K., et al. "The Short Luteal Phase and Infertility," *British Journal of Obstetrics and Gynecology* 91 (November 1984): 1120–1122.

Souka, Abdel Razek, et al. "Effect of Aspirin on the Luteal Phase of Human Menstrual Cycle," *Contraception* 29 (February 1984): 181–188.

Thomas, R., M.D., and R. L. Reid, M.D. "Thyroid Disease and Reproductive Dysfunction: A Review," *Obstetrics & Gynecology* 70 (November 1987): 789–792.

Thrush, Parke, M.D., and Deborah Willard, M.D. "Pseudo-Ectopic Pregnancy: An Ovarian Cyst Mimicking Ectopic Pregnancy," *West Virginia Medical Journal* 85 (November 1989): 488–489.

Tulandi, Togas, M.D., and Robert A. McInnes, M.D. "Vaginal Lubricants: Effect of Glycerin and Egg White on Sperm Motility and Progression in Vitro," *Fertility and Sterility* 41 (January 1984): 151–153.

Tulandi, Togas, M.D., Leo Plouffe, Jr., M.D., and Robert A. McInnes, M.D. "Effect of Saliva on Sperm Motility and Activity," *Fertility and Sterility* 38 (December 1982): 721–723.

Vermesh, Michael, M.D., et al. "Monitoring Techniques to Predict and Detect Ovulation," *Fertility and Sterility* 47 (February 1987): 259–264.

Veronesi, Umberto, et al. "Effect of Menstrual Phase on Surgical Treatment of Breast Cancer," *The Lancet* 343 (June 18, 1994): 1545–1547.

Weir, William C., M.D., and David R. Weir, M.D. "Adoption and Subsequent Conceptions," *Fertility and Sterility* (March/April 1966): 283–288.

Wilcox, Allen, David Dunson, and Donna Baird. "The Timing of the 'Fertile Window' in the Menstrual Cycle: Day-Specific Estimates from a Prospective Study. *British Medical Journal* 321 (November 18, 2000): 1259–1262.

Wilcox, Allen, Clarine Weinberg, and Donna Baird. "Caffeinated Beverages and Decreased Fertility," *The Lancet* (December 24–31, 1988): 1453–1455.

Wood, James W. "Fecundity and Natural Fertility in Humans," *Oxford Review of Natural Fertility in Humans* (1989): 61–109.

Worley, Richard J., M.D. "Dysfunctional Uterine Bleeding," *Postgraduate Medicine* 9 (February 15, 1986): 101–106.

Yong, Eu Leong, MRCOG, et al. "Simple Office Methods to Predict Ovulation: The Clinical Usefulness of a New Urine Luteinizing Hormone Kit Compared to Basal Body Temperature, Cervical Mucus and Ultrasound," *Aust NZ Journal of Obstetrics & Gynecology* 29 (May 1989): 155–159.

Zacur, Howard A., M.D., Ph.D., and Machelle M. Seibel, M.D. "Steps in Diagnosing Prolactin-Related Disorders," *Contemporary Ob/Gyn* (September 1989): 84–96.

Zuspan, Kathryn J., and F. P. Zuspan, "Basal Body Temperature." In *Human Ovulation,* edited by E. S. E. Hafez, pp. 291–298. Amsterdam and New York: Elsevier North-Holland Biomedical Press, 1979.

Books

Biale, Rachel. *Women and Jewish Law: An Exploration of Women's Issues in Halakhic Sources.* New York: Schocken Books, 1984.

Bryan, Elizabeth M., M.D., MRCP, DCH. *The Nature and Nurture of Twins.* London: Baillière Tindall, 1983.

Clubb, Elizabeth, M.D., and Jane Knight, *Fertility: Fertility Awareness and Natural Family Planning.* United Kingdom: David and Charles, 1996.

Danforth's Obstetrics and Gynecology, 8th ed. Philadelphia: J. B. Lippincott Company, 1999.

Edwards, Robert G. *Conception in the Human Female.* London: Academic Press/Harcourt Brace Jovanovich, 1980.

Gondos, Bernard, M.D., and Daniel H. Riddick, M.D., Ph.D., eds. *Pathology of Infertility: Clinical Correlations in the Male and Female.* New York: Thieme Medical Publishers, Inc., 1987.

Hafez, E. S. E., ed. *Human Reproduction: Conception and Contraception,* 2nd ed. New York: Harper & Row, 1980.

Herbst, Arthur L., M.D., and Howard A. Bern, Ph.D., eds. *Developmental Effects of Diethylstilbestrol (DES) in Pregnancy.* New York: Thieme-Stratton, Inc., 1981.

Jones, Richard E. *Human Reproductive Biology.* New York: Academic Press, 1997.

Kaplan, Abraham. *The Conduct of Inquiry: Methodology for Behavioral Science.* San Francisco: Chandler Publishing Company, 1964.

Lauersen, Niels H., M.D., and Colette Bouchez. *Getting Pregnant: What You Need to Know Right Now.* New York: Simon and Schuster, 2000.

Marrs, Richard, M.D. *Dr. Richard Marrs' Fertility Book.* New York: Dell Books, 1998.

Mishell, Daniel R., Jr., M.D., and Val Davajan, M.D., eds. *Infertility, Contraception & Reproductive Endocrinology,* 2nd ed. Oradell, NJ: Medical Economics Books, 1986.

Older, Julia. *Endometriosis.* New York: Charles Scribner's Sons, 1984.

Sachs, Judith. *What Women Can Do About Chronic Endometriosis.* New York: Dell Medical Library, 1991.

Taymor, Melvin L., M.D. *Infertility: A Clinician's Guide to Diagnosis and Treatment.* New York and London: Plenum Medical Book Company, 1990.

Wallis, Lila A., M.D., ed. *Textbook of Woman's Health.* New York: Lippincott-Raven Publishers, 1998.

GENDER PRESELECTION

Articles

France, John T., Ph.D., D.Sc., et al. "Characteristics of Natural Conceptual Cycles Occurring in a Prospective Study of Sex Preselection: Fertility Awareness Symptoms, Hormone Levels, Sperm Survival, and Pregnancy Outcome," *International Journal of Fertility* 37 (July/August 1992): 244–255.

Levin, R. J. "Human Sex Preselection," *Oxford Review of Reproductive Biology* 9 (1987): 161–191.

McSweeney, L. "A Prospective Study of Sex Preselection in Ondo, Nigeria, Using the Billings Ovulation Method of Natural Family Planning," *Victoria Bulletin* 20 (December 1993): 9–16.

Reubinoff, Benjamin E., M.D., Ph.D., and Joseph G. Schenker. "New Advances in Sex Preselection," *Fertility and Sterility* 66 (September 1996) 343–350.

Books

Shettles, Landrum, M.D., Ph.D., and David Rorvik. *How to Choose the Sex of Your Baby.* New York: Doubleday, 1997.

MALE FERTILITY

Articles

Ahlgren, M., Kerstin Boström, and R. Malmqvist. "Sperm Transport and Survival in Women with Special Reference to the Fallopian Tube," *The Biology of Spermatozoa,* INSERM Int. Symp., Nouzilly, France (1973): 63–73.

Amelar, Richard D., M.D., Lawrence Dubin, M.D., and Cy Schoenfeld, Ph.D. "Sperm Motility," *Fertility and Sterility* 34 (September 1980): 197–215.

Anderson, L., et al. "The Effects of Coital Lubricants on Sperm Motility in Vitro," *Human Reproduction* (December 13, 2000): 3351–3356.

Austin, G. R. "Sperm Fertility, Viability and Persistence in the Female Tract," *Journal of Reproduction and Fertility,* Suppl. 22 (1975): 75–89.

Dawson, Earl B., William A. Harris, and Leslie C. Powell. "Relationship Between Ascorbic Acid and Male Fertility," *World Review of Nutrition and Diet* 62 (1990): 2–26.

Giblin, Paul T., Ph.D., et al. "Effects of Stress and Characteristic Adaptability on Semen Quality in Healthy Men," *Fertility and Sterility* 49 (January 1988): 127–132.

Harris, William A., Thaddeus E. Harden, B.S., and Earl B. Dawson, Ph.D. "Apparent Effect of Ascorbic Acid Medication on Semen Metal Levels," *Fertility and Sterility* 32 (October 1979): 455–459.

Jaszczak, S., and E. S. E. Hafez. "Physiopathology of Sperm Transport in the Human Female," *The Biology of Spermatozoa,* INSERM Int. Symp., Nouzilly, France (1973): 250–256.

Kutteh, William H., M.D., et al. "Vaginal Lubricants for the Infertile Couple: Effect on Sperm Activity," *International Journal of Fertility* 41 (1996): 400–404.

Levin, Robert M., Ph.D., et al. "Correlation of Sperm Count with Frequency of Ejaculation," *Fertility and Sterility* 45 (March 1986): 732–734.

Makler, Amnon, M.D., et al. "Factors Affecting Sperm Motility. IX. Survival of Spermatozoa in Various Biological Media and Under Different Gaseous Compositions," *Fertility and Sterility* 41 (March 1984): 428–432.

Medical News. "Sperm Swim Singly After Vitamin C. Therapy," *Journal of the American Medical Association* 249 (May 27, 1983): 2747–2751.

Megory, E., H. Zuckerman, Z. Shoham (Schwartz), and B. Lunenfeld. "Infections and Male Fertility," *Obstetrical and Gynecological Survey* 42 (1987): 283–290.

Schlegel, Peter N., M.D., Thomas S. K. Chang, Ph.D., and Gray F. Marshall, M.D. "Antibiotics: Potential Hazards to Male Fertility," *Fertility and Sterility* 55 (February 1991): 235–242.

Tulandi, Togas, M.D., Leo Plouffe, Jr., M.D., and Robert A. MacInnes, M.D. "Effect of Saliva on Sperm Motility and Activity," *Fertility and Sterility* 38 (December 1982): 721–723.

Zinaman, Michael, et al. "The Physiology of Sperm Recovered from the Human Cervix: Acrosomal Status and Response to Inducers of the Acrosome Reaction," *Biology of Reproduction* 41 (November 1989): 790–797.

Books

Glover, T. D., C. L. R. Barratt, J. P. P. Tyler, and J. F. Hennessey. *Human Male Fertility and Semen Analysis.* London: Academic Press/Harcourt Brace Jovanovich, 1990.

Tanagho, Emil, and Jack W. McAninch. *Smith's General Urology,* 13th ed., Norwalk, CT: Appleton and Lange, 1992.

Thomas, Anthony, M.D., and Leslie R. Schover. *Overcoming Male Infertility: Understanding Its Causes and Treatments.* New York: John Wiley and Sons, 2000.

MENOPAUSE

Articles

Cummings, D. C., "Menarche, Menses, and Menopause: A Brief Review," *Cleveland Clinical Journal of Medicine* 57 (March-April 1990): 169–175.

Flynn, Anna M., M.D., et al., "Sympto-Thermal and Hormonal Markers of Potential Fertility in Climacteric Women," *American Journal of Obstetrics and Gynecology* 165 (December 1991): 1987–1989.

Fox, Susan C., M.D., and Lila A. Wallis, M.D. "Transition at Menopause." In *Textbook of Woman's Health,* edited by Lila A. Wallis, M.D., pp. 117–123. New York: Lippincott-Raven Publishers, 1998.

Rosenberg, Leon E. "Endocrinology and Metabolism." In *Harrison's Principles of Internal Medicine,* edited by Jean D. Wilson, et al., pp. 1780–1781. New York: McGraw Hill, 1991.

Shideler, S. E., et al. "Ovarian-Pituitary Hormone Interactions During the Peri-Menopause," *Maturitas* 11 (December 1989): 331–339.

Wallis, Lila A., M.D., and Dorothy M. Barbo, M.D. "Hormone Replacement Therapy." In *Textbook of Woman's Health,* edited by Lila A. Wallis, M.D., pp. 731–746. New York: Lippincott-Raven Publishers, 1998.

Books

Love, Susan, M.D. *Dr. Susan Love's Hormone Book: Making Informed Choices About Menopause.* London: Little, Brown & Company, 1999.

Utian, Wulf H. *Menopause in Modern Perspective: A Guide to Clinical Practice.* New York: Appleton-Century Crofts, 1980.

PMS

Articles

Chakmakjian, Z. H., M.D., C. E. Higgins, B.S., and G. E. Abraham, M.D. "The Effect of a Nutritional Supplement, Optivite for Women, on Premenstrual Tension Syndromes," *Journal of Applied Nutrition* 37 (1985): 12–17.

Endicott, Jean, "The Menstrual Cycle and Mood Disorders," *Journal of Affective Disorders* 29 (October-November 1993): 193–200.

Faccinetti, Fabio, M.D., et al. "Premenstrual Fall of Plasma β-Endorphin in Patients with Premenstrual Syndrome," *Fertility and Sterility* 47 (April 1987): 570–573.

Johnson, Susan, M.D. "Premenstrual Syndrome." In *Textbook of Woman's Health,* edited by Lila A. Wallis, M.D., pp. 691–697. New York: Lippincott-Raven Publishers, 1998.

Books

Lark, Susan M., M.D. *Premenstrual Syndrome Self-Help Book.* Berkeley, CA: Celestial Arts, 1989.

Severino, Sally K., M.D., and Margaret L. Moline, Ph.D. *Premenstrual Syndrome: A Clinician's Guide.* New York: The Guilford Press, 1989.

Index

Master Charts

These final pages are master charts that I designed for various stages in your life. For the most part, I think one of the classic charts on either side of the last page of the book will meet your needs perfectly, depending on whether you want to avoid or achieve pregnancy. But I would still encourage you to skim through the differences among them to see if one is more appropriate for your particular situation. If you would like to chart your cycles simply to keep track of your general health, and not specifically for contraception, you will still probably want to use the classic birth control chart on the second to last page, since it is the most basic.

Whichever one you choose as your master chart, you should enlarge it by about 130%. Then before you copy from that, list the various signs you would like to color code in the narrow rows at the bottom, such as breast tenderness, headaches, or cramps, to name a few.

The map on the next page lets you scan the 9 charts to choose the one most appropriate for your needs. The purpose of each chart is listed in tiny print in the bottom right-hand corner of each one. If you would prefer to access them online, they are available at TCOYF.com

I recommend keeping your fertility charts organized in a three-ring binder with your most recent on top. Ideally, you may want to use a plastic sheet cover after each is complete. You will probably want to keep 3 sheets in the inside cover of the notebook: your master fertility chart, annual exam form, and color-coding key of the signs you plan to record in the narrow columns at the bottom of the master. Keeping all your charts in chronological order is a great way to get an overview of your reproductive health over time, and is an invaluable resource for your doctor, if and when problems or changes arise.

Master Charts Map
Guide to the last ten pages of the book.
Most frequently used charts appear at the end for ease in copying.

<table>
<tr>
<td>

(Master Charts Map)

</td>
<td>

Annual Physical Exam Form
Copy the blank form onto the back of the chart during the cycle in which you have your annual exam.

</td>
</tr>
<tr>
<td>

Pregnancy—Celsius
Exactly the same as the classic pregnancy chart, but temperatures are in Celsius rather than Fahrenheit.

</td>
<td>

Birth Control—Celsius
Exactly the same as the classic birth control chart, but temperatures are in Celsius rather than Fahrenheit.

</td>
</tr>
<tr>
<td>

Pregnancy—Premenopause
Exactly the same as the classic pregnancy chart, with 3 color-coded menopausal symptoms: vaginal dryness, night sweats, and hot flashes.

</td>
<td>

Birth Control—Premenopause
Exactly the same as the classic birth control chart, with 3 color-coded menopausal symptoms: vaginal dryness, night sweats, and hot flashes.

</td>
</tr>
<tr>
<td>

Pregnancy—Optional Symbols
Exactly the same as the classic pregnancy chart, but uses the cervical fluid symbols from the first edition of this book.

</td>
<td>

Birth Control—Optional Symbols
Exactly the same as the classic birth control chart, but uses the cervical fluid symbols from the first edition of this book.

</td>
</tr>
<tr>
<td>

Birth Control—Internal and External Cervical Fluid Checking
Similiar to the classic birth control chart, but with a separate row for checking cervical fluid at the cervical os.

</td>
<td>

Birth Control (Classic)
The classic birth control chart, which can also be used as a basic reproductive health chart, with a special row for recording method of birth control used.

</td>
</tr>
<tr>
<td>

Pregnancy (Classic)
The classic pregnancy chart, with special rows for pregnancy tests, ovulation predictor kits, diagnostic tests and procedures, and drugs taken.

</td>
<td>

(blank)

</td>
</tr>
</table>

Annual Physical Examination
Health Practitioner
_____

Cholesterol _____ Ratio _____ HDL _____ LDL _____   Day of cycle ____ Date _____

Blood (CBC) _____   Age at time of examination ___

Urine test _____   Height _____ Weight _____

Cervical smear _____   Pulse _____

Chlamydia test (optional) _____   Blood pressure _____/_____

Other Tests _____   Shots/Boosters/Vaccines

_____   _____

_____   _____

_____   _____

	Status	Comments
Breast examination		
Mammogram		
Cervix		
Uterus		
Ovaries		
Heart		
Lungs		

Prescriptions _____

Recommendations _____

_____

Referrals _____

Age **33**   Fertility Cycle # _____

Last 12 Cycles: Shortest _____   Longest _____   Month **JUNE → JULY**   Year **2012**   This cycle length _____

Cycle Day	1	2	3	4	5	6	7	8	9	10	11	12	13	14	15	16	17	18	19	20	21	22	23	24	25	26	27	28	29	30	31	32	33	34	35	36	37	38	39	40
Date	24	25	26	27	28	29	30	1	2	3	4	5	6	7	8	9	10	11	12	13	14	15	16	17	18	19	20													
Day of Week	S	M	T	W	T	F	S	S	M	T	W	T	F	S	S	M	T	W	T	F	S	S	M	T	W	T	F													

Time Temp Normally Taken: 6:30 am

Temp Count & Luteal Phase

Waking Temperature (scale 36.05 through 37.10 °C, no temperatures recorded)

Pregnancy Test

Circle Intercourse on Cycle Day	1	2	3	4	5	6	7	8	9	10	11	12	(13)	14	(15)	16	17	18	19	20	21	22	23	24	25	26	27	28	29	30	31	32	33	34	35	36	37	38	39	40
Eggwhite																																								
Creamy													✓	✓																										
Sticky																																								
Dry, Spotting or **PERIOD**	✕	✕	✕																																					
Fertile Phase and PEAK DAY																																								
Vaginal Sensation													∿	∿																										

Cervix F · M o S O

Cervical Fluid Description

Eggwhite — Slippery, Will Usually Stretch, Clear/Streaked/Opaque, Lube, Wet or Humid Feeling

Creamy — Lotiony, Milky, Smooth, Usually White or Yellow, Wet, Moist or Cold Feeling

Sticky — Pasty, Crumbly, Opaque, Rubber-Cement, Dry or Sticky Feeling

Ovulatory Pain

OPK

Diagnostic Tests and Procedures

Drugs

	1	2	3	4	5	6	7	8	9	10	11	12	13	14	15	16	17	18	19	20	21	22	23	24	25	26	27	28	29	30	31	32	33	34	35	36	37	38	39	40
Exercise																																								
Miscellaneous																																								
Travel																																								
Illness																																								
Stress																																								
PMS																																								
Breast Self-Exam						BSE																																		

Pregnancy (celsius)

Age _____   Fertility Cycle # _____

Last 12 Cycles: Shortest _____   Longest _____   Month _____   Year _____   This cycle length _____

Cycle Day	1	2	3	4	5	6	7	8	9	10	11	12	13	14	15	16	17	18	19	20	21	22	23	24	25	26	27	28	29	30	31	32	33	34	35	36	37	38	39	40
Date																																								
Day of Week																																								
_____Time Temp Normally Taken																																								
Temp Count & Luteal Phase																																								

Waking Temperature (rows of values: 10, 05, 37, 95, 90, 85, 80, 75, 70, 65, 60, 55, 50, 45, 40, 35, 30, 25, 20, 15, 10, 36 — repeated across all 40 columns)

| Birth Control Method Used | | | | | | | | | | | | | | | | | | | | | | | | | | | | | | | | | | | | | | | | |

Circle Intercourse on Cycle Day	1	2	3	4	5	6	7	8	9	10	11	12	13	14	15	16	17	18	19	20	21	22	23	24	25	26	27	28	29	30	31	32	33	34	35	36	37	38	39	40

Eggwhite
Creamy
Sticky
Dry, Spotting or **PERIOD**
Infertile Phase and PEAK DAY

Vaginal Sensation

Cervix [· ○ ○] F M S

Cervical Fluid Description

Eggwhite
Slippery, Will Usually Stretch
Clear/Streaked/Opaque
Lube, Wet or Humid Feeling

Creamy
Lotiony, Milky, Smooth
Usually White or Yellow
Wet, Moist or Cold Feeling

Sticky
Pasty, Crumbly, Opaque
Rubber-Cement
Dry or Sticky Feeling

Ovulatory Pain

	1	2	3	4	5	6	7	8	9	10	11	12	13	14	15	16	17	18	19	20	21	22	23	24	25	26	27	28	29	30	31	32	33	34	35	36	37	38	39	40

Exercise

Miscellaneous

Travel

Illness

Stress

PMS

Breast Self-Exam — BSE (cycle day 7)

Age __33__ Fertility Cycle # _____

Age _____ Last 12 Cycles: Shortest _____ Longest _____ Month JUNE → JULY Year 2012 This cycle length _____

Cycle Day	1	2	3	4	5	6	7	8	9	10	11	12	13	14	15	16	17	18	19	20	21	22	23	24	25	26	27	28	29	30	31	32	33	34	35	36	37	38	39	40
Date	24	25	26	27	28	29	30	1	2	3	4	5	6	7	8	9	10	11	12	13	14	15	16	17	18	19	20	21	22											
Day of Week	S	M	T	W	T	F	S	S	M	T	W	T	F	S	S	M	T	W	T	F	S	S	M	T	W	T	F	S	S											

Time Temp Normally Taken: 6:30AM

Temp Count & Luteal Phase

Waking Temperature (99 down to 97 scale per day)

Pregnancy Test

| Circle Intercourse on Cycle Day | 1 | 2 | 3 | 4 | 5 | 6 | 7 | 8 | 9 | 10 | 11 | 12 | (13) | 14 | (15) | 16 | 17 | (18) | 19 | 20 | 21 | 22 | 23 | 24 | 25 | 26 | 27 | 28 | 29 | 30 | 31 | 32 | 33 | 34 | 35 | 36 | 37 | 38 | 39 | 40 |

Eggwhite

Creamy

Sticky

Dry, Spotting or **PERIOD**: X X X (Days 1–3)

Fertile Phase and PEAK DAY

Vaginal Sensation: WET (Day 13), WET (Day 14), WET (Day 15)

Cervix: F M S (o o O)

Cervical Fluid Description

Eggwhite — Slippery, Will Usually Stretch Clear/Streaked/Opaque Lube, Wet or Humid Feeling: "Arthur home!" (Day 13)

Creamy — Lotiony, Milky, Smooth Usually White or Yellow Wet, Moist or Cold Feeling

Sticky — Pasty, Crumbly, Opaque Rubber-Cement Dry or Sticky Feeling: "3 GLASSES WINE" (Day 15)

Ovulatory Pain

OPK

Diagnostic Tests and Procedures

Drugs

| | 1 | 2 | 3 | 4 | 5 | 6 | 7 | 8 | 9 | 10 | 11 | 12 | 13 | 14 | 15 | 16 | 17 | 18 | 19 | 20 | 21 | 22 | 23 | 24 | 25 | 26 | 27 | 28 | 29 | 30 | 31 | 32 | 33 | 34 | 35 | 36 | 37 | 38 | 39 | 40 |

Exercise

Miscellaneous

Travel

Illness

Stress

PMS

Breast Self-Exam: BSE (Day 7)

Vaginal Dryness

Night Sweats

Hot Flashes

Age _____   Fertility Cycle # _____

Last 12 Cycles: Shortest _____   Longest _____   Month _____   Year _____   This cycle length _____

Cycle Day	1	2	3	4	5	6	7	8	9	10	11	12	13	14	15	16	17	18	19	20	21	22	23	24	25	26	27	28	29	30	31	32	33	34	35	36	37	38	39	40
Date																																								
Day of Week																																								
_____ Time Temp Normally Taken																																								
Temp Count & Luteal Phase																																								

Waking Temperature

Each column shows the scale: 99, 9, 8, 7, 6, 5, 4, 3, 2, 1, 98, 9, 8, 7, 6, 5, 4, 3, 2, 1, 97 (repeated across all 40 cycle days)

Birth Control Method Used																																								

Circle Intercourse on Cycle Day	1	2	3	4	5	6	7	8	9	10	11	12	13	14	15	16	17	18	19	20	21	22	23	24	25	26	27	28	29	30	31	32	33	34	35	36	37	38	39	40
Eggwhite																																								
Creamy																																								
Sticky																																								
Dry, Spotting or **PERIOD**																																								
Fertile Phase and PEAK DAY																																								
Vaginal Sensation																																								

Cervix · o ◯
          F M S

Cervical Fluid Description																																								

Eggwhite
Slippery, Will Usually Stretch
Clear/Streaked/Opaque
Lube, Wet or Humid Feeling

Creamy
Lotiony, Milky, Smooth
Usually White or Yellow   Wet,
Moist or Cold Feeling

Sticky   Pasty,
Crumbly, Opaque Rubber-
Cement   Dry or
Sticky Feeling

Ovulatory Pain

	1	2	3	4	5	6	7	8	9	10	11	12	13	14	15	16	17	18	19	20	21	22	23	24	25	26	27	28	29	30	31	32	33	34	35	36	37	38	39	40
Exercise																																								
Miscellaneous																																								
Travel																																								
Illness																																								
Stress																																								
PMS																																								
Breast Self-Exam						BSE																																		
Vaginal Dryness																																								
Night Sweats																																								
Hot Flashes																																								

Birth Control   (premenopause)

Age _____ Fertility Cycle # _____

Last 12 Cycles: Shortest _____   Longest _____   Month _____   Year _____   This cycle length _____

Cycle Day	1	2	3	4	5	6	7	8	9	10	11	12	13	14	15	16	17	18	19	20	21	22	23	24	25	26	27	28	29	30	31	32	33	34	35	36	37	38	39	40
Date																																								
Day of Week																																								
_____ Time Temp Normally Taken																																								
Temp Count & Luteal Phase																																								

Waking Temperature

Each cell column shows the temperature scale:
99 9 8 7 6 5 4 3 2 1
98 9 8 7 6 5 4 3 2 1
97

| _____ Pregnancy Test | | | | | | | | | | | | | | | | | | | | | | | | | | | | | | | | | | | | | | | | |

Circle Intercourse on Cycle Day	1	2	3	4	5	6	7	8	9	10	11	12	13	14	15	16	17	18	19	20	21	22	23	24	25	26	27	28	29	30	31	32	33	34	35	36	37	38	39	40

Cervical Fluid
Dry, Spotting or **PERIOD**
Infertile Phase and PEAK DAY

Vaginal Sensation

Cervix . o O / F M S

Cervical Fluid Description

Ovulatory Pain
_____ OPK
Diagnostic Tests and Procedures

Drugs

	1	2	3	4	5	6	7	8	9	10	11	12	13	14	15	16	17	18	19	20	21	22	23	24	25	26	27	28	29	30	31	32	33	34	35	36	37	38	39	40

Exercise

Miscellaneous
Travel
Illness
Stress
PMS
Breast Self-Exam — BSE

Cervical Fluid Symbols	✳	(✳)	—	S	Ⓒ	Ⓔ
Cervical Fluid Description	Menses	Spotting	No Cervical Fluid	Sticky	Creamy	Eggwhite
	Bright Red	Pink or Brown	Nothing	Sticky, Crumbly, Gummy, or Rubbery Yellow or White	Creamy, Lotiony, Milky, or Smooth Yellow or White	Slippery and Usually Stretchy Clear, Streaked or Opaque
Vaginal Sensation	Wet	Moist or Dry	Dry	Dry or Sticky	Wet and/or Cold	Lubricative and Very Wet, May Feel Humid

www.tcoyf.com

Pregnancy (optional symbols)

Age _____   Fertility Cycle # _____

Last 12 Cycles: Shortest _____   Longest _____   Month _____   Year _____   This cycle length _____

Cycle Day	1	2	3	4	5	6	7	8	9	10	11	12	13	14	15	16	17	18	19	20	21	22	23	24	25	26	27	28	29	30	31	32	33	34	35	36	37	38	39	40
Date																																								
Day of Week																																								
Time Temp Normally Taken																																								
Temp Count & Luteal Phase																																								

Waking Temperature (scale 99–97 repeated per column)

| Birth Control Method Used | | | | | | | | | | | | | | | | | | | | | | | | | | | | | | | | | | | | | | | | |

Circle Intercourse on Cycle Day	1	2	3	4	5	6	7	8	9	10	11	12	13	14	15	16	17	18	19	20	21	22	23	24	25	26	27	28	29	30	31	32	33	34	35	36	37	38	39	40

Cervical Fluid
Dry, Spotting or **PERIOD**
Fertile Phase and PEAK DAY

Vaginal Sensation

Cervix . o O
        F M S

Cervical Fluid Description

Ovulatory Pain

	1	2	3	4	5	6	7	8	9	10	11	12	13	14	15	16	17	18	19	20	21	22	23	24	25	26	27	28	29	30	31	32	33	34	35	36	37	38	39	40
Exercise																																								
Miscellaneous																																								
Travel																																								
Illness																																								
Stress																																								
PMS																																								
Breast Self-Exam				BSE																																				

	Menses	Spotting	No Cervical Fluid	Sticky	Creamy	Eggwhite
Cervical Fluid Symbols	✱	(✱)	—	S	C	E
Cervical Fluid Description	Bright Red	Pink or Brown	Nothing	Sticky, Crumbly, Gummy, or Rubbery / Yellow or White	Creamy, Lotiony, Milky, or Smooth / Yellow or White	Slippery and Usually Stretchy / Clear, Streaked or Opaque
Vaginal Sensation	Wet	Moist or Dry	Dry	Dry or Sticky	Wet and/or Cold	Lubricative and Very Wet, May Feel Humid

Birth Control   (optional symbols)

Age _____   **Fertility Cycle #** _____

Cycle Day	1	2	3	4	5	6	7	8	9	10	11	12	13	14	15	16	17	18	19	20	21	22	23	24	25	26	27	28	29	30	31	32	33	34	35	36	37	38	39	40
Date																																								
Day of Week																																								
_____Time Temp Normally Taken																																								
Temp Count & Luteal Phase																																								

Waking Temperature grid (each column repeats, showing 99, 9, 8, 7, 6, 5, 4, 3, 2, 1, 98, 9, 8, 7, 6, 5, 4, 3, 2, 1, 97) for cycle days 1–40.

Birth Control Method Used																																								

Circle Intercourse on Cycle Day	1	2	3	4	5	6	7	8	9	10	11	12	13	14	15	16	17	18	19	20	21	22	23	24	25	26	27	28	29	30	31	32	33	34	35	36	37	38	39	40
Eggwhite																																								
Creamy																																								
Sticky																																								
Dry, Spotting or **PERIOD**																																								
Fertile Phase and PEAK DAY																																								
Vaginal Sensation																																								
Cervix (F M S)																																								
Cervical Fluid at the Vulva																																								
Cervical Fluid at the Cervix																																								
Ovulatory Pain																																								

	1	2	3	4	5	6	7	8	9	10	11	12	13	14	15	16	17	18	19	20	21	22	23	24	25	26	27	28	29	30	31	32	33	34	35	36	37	38	39	40
Exercise																																								
Miscellaneous																																								
Breast Self-Exam						BSE																																		

Temperature Conversion Chart

Celsius	Fahrenheit	Celsius	Fahrenheit
0	32.0	26	78.8
1	33.8	27	80.6
2	35.6	28	82.4
3	37.4	29	84.2
4	39.2	30	86.0
5	41.0	31	87.8
6	42.8	32	89.6
7	44.6	33	91.4
8	46.4	34	93.2
9	48.2	35	95.0
10	50.0	36	96.8
11	51.8	37	98.6
12	53.6	38	100.4
13	55.4	39	102.2
14	57.2	40	104.0
15	59.0	41	105.8
16	60.8	42	107.6
17	62.6	43	109.4
18	64.4	44	111.2
19	66.2	45	113.0
20	68.0	46	114.8
21	69.8	47	116.6
22	71.6	48	118.4
23	73.4	49	120.2
24	75.2	50	122.0
25	77.0		

For greater accuracy, the following formulae can be used:

To convert from Celsius to Fahrenheit: $(°C \times 1.8) + 32 = °F$

To convert from Fahrenheit to Celsius: $(°F - 32) / 1.8 = °C$